TRANSITIONING FROM LPN/VN TO RN

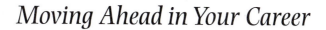

Moving Ahead in Your Career

Second Edition

Gena Duncan, MSEd, MSN, RN

Former Associate Professor of Nursing
Ivy Tech Community College
Fort Wayne, Indiana

René DePew, MSN, FNP-BC

Assistant Professor of Nursing
University of Saint Francis
Fort Wayne, Indiana
Family Nurse Practitioner
Huntington-Inverness Foot Clinic
Huntington & Fort Wayne, Indiana

D0781613

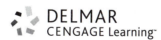

DELMAR
CENGAGE Learning™

Australia • Brazil • Japan • Korea • Mexico • Singapore • Spain • United Kingdom • United States

College of the Ouachitas

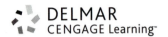
DELMAR
CENGAGE Learning™

**Transitioning from LPN/VN to RN:
Moving Ahead in Your Career,
Second Edition**
Gena Duncan and René DePew

Vice President, Career and Professional
Editorial: Dave Garza

Director of Learning Solutions:
Matthew Kane

Executive Editor: Stephen Helba

Managing Editor: Marah Bellegarde

Editorial Assistant: Meghan Orvis

Vice President, Career and Professional
Marketing: Jennifer Baker

Marketing Director: Wendy Mapstone

Marketing Manager: Michéle McTighe

Marketing Coordinator: Scott Chrysler

Production Director: Carolyn Miller

Production Manager: Andrew Crouth

Content Project Manager: Allyson Bozeth

Art Director: Jack Pendleton

Library of Congress Control Number: 2009943012

ISBN-13: 978-14354-4821-6

ISBN-10: 1-4354-4821-9

Delmar
5 Maxwell Drive
Clifton Park, NY 12065-2919
USA

Cengage Learning is a leading provider of customized learning solutions with office locations around the globe, including Singapore, the United Kingdom, Australia, Mexico, Brazil, and Japan. Locate your local office at:
international.cengage.com/region

Cengage Learning products are represented in Canada by
Nelson Education, Ltd.

To learn more about Delmar, visit **www.cengage.com/delmar**

Purchase any of our products at your local college store or at our preferred online store **www.ichapters.com**

Printed in the United States of America
1 2 3 4 5 6 7 13 12 11 10

Contents

▼ ▼ ▼ ▼ ▼ ▼ ▼

PART I: THE NURSE IN ROLE TRANSITION

PART IV: THE NURSE AS PROFESSIONAL

PART V: THE LPN TO RN STUDENT TRANSITIONING SKILLS

Preface

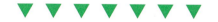

As a LPN/VN, celebrate the accomplishments and goals that you have met thus far. Your decision to commit to life-long learning and to seek new educational goals is to be praised and applauded. Nursing is an awesome career option with a great deal of opportunity for growth, and a chance to serve others at very critical times in their lives. Pursuing further education benefits both the care giver and care receiver. Seize this moment to make the most of every opportunity that arises.

As the authors of this book, we drew from many different resources to develop the transitions course that we taught for LPNs to RNs. Therefore, this concise, applicable book was written to address issues that LPNs face as they transition into the educational process. The content in these pages was written with respect for each individual student continuing her own personal and professional journey. Since there is much diversity in LPN education, a variety of conceptual and clinical areas are addressed, including math review, intravenous (IV) therapy, care plan development, concept mapping, and assessment skills, so the LPN can smoothly transition into the RN role. The content thoroughly delves into changes that the LPN can expect to encounter in the transition from the LPN to RN role. We continually survey faculty teaching LPN-RN courses and former LPN-RN students. We do this to ensure that current topics are addressed and to assess the needs of LPNs as they transition into RN programs.

The content leads to stimulating class discussions and encourages self-reflection through critical thinking and journaling activities.

ORGANIZATION

This book is rich with features. The five sections are thoughtfully organized and follow the professional requirements needed for the RN role: The Nurse in Role Transition, The Nurse as Caregiver, The Nurse as Manager, The Nurse as Professional, and—new in this edition—The LPN to RN Student Transitioning Skills.

Part I: The Nurse in Role Transition prepares the LPN transition students to advance in their education.

Chapter 1 Returning to School reviews basic study skills and strategies, identifies individual learning styles, suggests time-management skills in balancing the responsibilities of home, work, and school. This content is presented to enhance the student's learning and study skills.

Chapter 2 Role Transition addresses the student's socialization needs in transitioning from the LPN role to the RN role. A re-socialization assessment tool assists the student in the socialization process as she explores (for agreement) the change process in transitioning and socializing into the new RN role. Personal and career conflicts encountered while pursuing an RN degree are candidly discussed.

Chapter 3 Enhancing Assessment Skills reviews assessment skills learned as an LPN and are expanded by presenting two methods of assessing clients: systems approach and Gordon's Functional Health Pattern. Critical thinking and Theory to Practice activities guide the LPN to enhance assessment skills.

In Chapter 4 LPN and RN Knowledge and Roles, the student is skillfully guided to take a candid look at the LPN role and the RN role in an objective, non-confrontational manner. The most current NCLEX RN and LPN test plans are used to develop the discussion of the RN and LPN roles. The NCLEX-PN and NCLEX-RN test plans and the NLN roles and responsibilities differentiate the two nursing roles. The student is asked to define the differences between the LPN and RN roles through critical thinking activities.

Part II: The Nurse as Caregiver prepares the LPN for expanded roles and responsibilities in clinical judgment: problem solving; decision making; client teaching; and communication skills with colleagues, clients, and their significant support persons and in crisis situations.

Chapter 5 Communication shares the SBAR communication technique to improve communication with physicians, colleagues, close friends, and significant others. The traditional communication techniques are reviewed and then expanded with the newest communication tool (SBAR).

Chapter 6 Caring: The Heart and Soul of Nursing starts with a self-study to determine personal caring skills and then delves deeper into providing genuine caring in nursing interventions.

Chapter 7 Clinical Decision Making and the Nursing Process integrate and apply the nursing process and Gordon's functional health patterns into the discussion of client care within the clinical setting.

Chapter 8 Client Teaching compares the teaching process to the nursing process in preparing the student to teach clients, a vital component of nursing responsibilities.

Part III: The Nurse as Manager explores the roles of the nurse as a leader and manager, with emphasis on delegation, accountability, time management, conflict management, decision making, and resource management. The roles of leader and manager are defined and explored.

Chapter 9 The Nurse as Leader explores generational attitudes toward leadership styles and behaviors. It defines the leadership role and compares leadership styles and encourages the student to compare and contrast the difference between leadership and management. It explains the RN leadership role and challenges the student to explore their desired leadership style and role.

Chapter 10 Managing Client Care defines conflict resolution and presents effective strategies for resolving conflict. It presents time management tips for the clinical unit and discusses resource management. The student explores conflict management style through a conflict management tool.

Part IV: The Nurse as Professional discusses nursing theory and ethical and legal considerations in real life situations. The RN's role in research is explored.

In Chapter 11 Nursing Theory as a Basis to Practice Nursing the theoretical components of nursing theory are explained and then presented in a practical manner by showing the interrelatedness of theory to practice and research. The chapter content shows how nursing theory defines nursing, delineates nursing theorists' contribution to nursing, relates nursing theory to all levels of nursing, and applies nursing theory to clinical nursing. Critical Thinking questions and the Theory to Practice feature guides students to integrate theory into nursing education and clinical practice.

Chapter 12 Ethical and Legal Considerations examines the theories for Piaget, Erickson, and Kohlberg, so the student comprehends how personal values and beliefs guide personal decision making. The ethical decision process is delineated, and then the student is given the opportunity to use the process to make practical ethical decisions. The student examines the professional standards and expectations of professional nursing organizations that guide their socialization into the nursing profession. Legal terms are defined and explained. Critical Thinking activities and the Theory to Practice feature prepares the LPN transition student to face ethical and legal situations and to function professionally as a leader and a sound decision maker.

Part V: The LPN to RN Student Transitioning Skills

Chapter 13 IV Therapy Skills discusses the purpose of IV therapy, assessment of the IV site, preparation for IV administration, maintenance of the IV site, and termination of IV therapy. A quick-glance table for prompt review of the use and precautions of IV solutions is provided. Geriatric and pediatric special IV administration considerations are presented. The chapter includes step-by-step procedures for administering medication via secondary administration set and adding medication to hanging IV solutions. The introductory Scenario, Chapter Reflection, practical Critical Thinking activities, and the Theory to Practice provide practical clinical scenarios.

Appendix A Déjà Vu: Nursing Exams Today and Licensure Exam Tomorrow presents effective test taking strategy tips along with a preparatory explanation of the NCLEX-RN exam.

Appendix B Medication Preparation and Administration Competency for Registered Nurse provides an opportunity for the student to compute basic math equations. Medication errors often occur because of erroneous dosage calculations.

Appendices C: American Nurses Association Codes of Ethics, D: The International Council of Nurses Codes of Ethics, E: National Student Nurses' Association, Inc. Code of Professional Conduct, and F: National Student Nurses' Association, Inc. Code of Academic and Clinical Conduct provide the student an opportunity to examine the professional standards and expectations of professional nursing organizations and adapt the principles to their nursing values through the discussion in Chapter 12.

FEATURES

- **Learning Objectives** A numbered list of learning objectives opens each chapter and shows what the level of knowledge should be by the end of the chapter.
- **Key Terms** Listed at the beginning of each chapter and bolded within the book, key terms highlight important terminology and concepts for the transitioning nurse.
- **Scenario/Think About It** Each chapter begins with a scenario created from real-life stories and experiences of a typical LPN student pursuing an RN degree and is followed by a series of critical thinking questions. The chapter then presents content that challenges the student to rethink the scenario. At the end of the chapter, the *Chapter Reflections* draws the student back into the scenario to reconsider present thinking.
- **Tables and Figures** Tables and figures are quick references that provide a visual learning tool to enhance concepts and summarize the content.
- **Critical Thinking Activities** The student is guided through activities to critically think about content presented in the book, and how it applies in real-life nursing situations. Students are challenged to think outside the box and encouraged to learn new ideas, change, and grow.
- **Theory to Practice** This *new* feature takes the student through theory content into the real-world issues of nursing. By developing one's critical thinking skills and applying this knowledge to real life situations, student nurses can further their professional development and the image of nursing as a profession.
- **Summary** Each chapter has a brief summary of the chapter content the student has just learned.
- **Chapter Reflections** At the end of the chapter, students are drawn back into the chapter-opening scenario with questions that guide them to internalize the RN role both personally and professionally.
- **Journaling Your Journey** Journaling is a reflective activity to help one grow professionally and can be continued throughout the nursing career. The *new* Journaling Your Journey feature encourages students to tell their unique story by prompting them to answer three questions: Where have you been? Where are you now? and Where are you going or what are you going to do about the new opportunity? This feature offers students an opportunity to reconsider what past experiences they have had, how they thought and responded at that time, and what they think and plan to do about the situation after reading the chapter. Since each person has a different learning style,

this feature is a great tool for those who are able to express themselves better in writing than verbally in class or in group discussions.

- **My Story** My Story is a *new* feature in the second edition. Students will read about real world RNs who share their personal life stories as they began their journey transitioning from LPNs to RNs. Students are encouraged to compare what they read and discuss in class to real-world practice scenarios.
- **References/Suggested Resources** A list of chapter references and suggested resources are provided for the student.

NEW TO THIS EDITION

New pedagogical tools encourage students to think critically and draw from their own experiences as LPNs in order to prepare them for their new role as RNs. These new learning tools are:

- Theory to Practice
- Journaling Your Journey
- My Story

New figures, tables, and key terms have been added to enhance the nurse's understanding and critical thinking skills.

Theory to practice is added to each chapter to enhance the student's current knowledge base and to encourage theory application in clinical practice.

New chapter content adds depth and provides valuable assessment tools that further prepare LPNs for their transition into the RN role.

Chapter 3 *Enhancing Assessment Skills*

- System-by-system symptoms or problems to report to an RN are detailed for the practicing LPN in order to prepare the student in assuming the new RN role.

Chapter 5 *Communication*

- The SBAR communication tool is added to the second edition in order to provide an excellent and concise way to communicate with physicians, coworkers, and clients.
- The Critical Thinking Activities further guide the student in this new, innovative communication technique.

Chapter 7 *Clinical Decision Making and the Nursing Process*

- Concept mapping is added to the second edition as another option to nursing care plans. Concept maps provide a different approach to learning disease processes, client assessment, diagnosis, nursing interventions, and evaluation of client goals; they also assist students in understanding connections and rationale in client care.

- The nursing process section is expanded and includes critical thinking questions for each process step for effectiveness in clinical application. The case scenario at the end of the chapter guides the student in developing a nursing care plan.

Chapter 13 *IV Therapy Skills*

- This new chapter reviews or enhances IV skills for LPNs depending on their past experience with IV therapy.
- A new IV table explains the indications, incompatibilities, precautions, and contraindications for hypotonic, isotonic, and hypertonic IV solutions. This table is a valuable source for the clinical setting as the student pursues the RN degree and in practice.
- Step-by-step procedures are given for preparing the IV bag and tubing, administering medications via secondary administration sets (piggyback), and adding medication to hanging IV fluids.

FOR THE INSTRUCTOR

With Delmar Cengage Learning's Instructor Resources preparing for class and evaluating students has never been easier! As an instructor, you will find this Online Tool offers invaluable assistance by giving you access to all of your resources—anywhere and at any time.

ONLINE COMPANION FEATURES

- The **Chapter Outlines** provide you with at-a-glance information for each chapter.
- The **Computerized Testbank** in **ExamView®** makes generating tests and quizzes a snap. With many questions and different styles to choose from, you can create customized assessments for your students with the click of a button. Add your own unique questions and print rationales for easy class preparation.
- Customizable instructor support slide presentations in **PowerPoint®** format focus on key points for each chapter.

  Visit www.delmarlearning.com/companions/to access the Instructor Resource content. Please contact your sales representative for password information.

ABOUT THE AUTHORS

Gena Duncan has two master's degrees, one in secondary education and the other in community health nursing. She taught LPNs for 15 years at Ivy Tech Community College and then took a teaching position at Lutheran College that had an ASN and BSN completion nursing program. After Lutheran College was acquired by the University of Saint Francis, she was director of the ASN program. During this time, she guided the curriculum development of an

LPN to ASN transition program. She returned to Ivy Tech Community College and, as an associate professor in nursing, taught in the ASN program. In the fall of 2005, Ivy Tech started an LPN to ASN program and she taught in that program, also. Throughout her career, she has taught LPN, ASN, BSN, and master's level students. She has authored five textbooks for LPN nursing programs and the transition book.

René DePew began her nursing career as an LPN in 1987 and moved on to obtain her BSN in 1998 and then her master's, as a family nurse practitioner, in 2000. She is currently a tenured Assistant Professor of nursing at the University of Saint Francis (Fort Wayne, Indiana) in the ASN program. She teaches a medical surgical course to ASN and LPN-RN students and the transitions course to the new LPN to RN students entering the program. She also serves as faculty advisor to the University of Saint Francis Student Nurses Association which is a total membership program and very active at the local, state and national levels. She has mentored students while serving in top leadership roles at all three levels and also functions as a state consultant to the Indiana Association of Nursing Students. Outside of academia, she practices as a Family Nurse Practitioner in the Huntington-Inverness Foot Clinics. She sees this as an opportunity to stay current in practice and continue providing direct patient care while she role models what she teaches. This also is an opportunity to mentor MSN students.

ACKNOWLEDGMENTS

The authors wish to thank the following reviewers:

Eric Mason, MSN, BSEd, RN
    James A. Rhodes State College, School of Nursing, Lima, Ohio
Dodie Serafini RN, BS, MSN
    National American University—Denver Campus; Denver, CO
Martha Tafoya, MSN, RN
    Angelo State University, San Angelo, TX

The authors wish to thank the following:

Steve Helba, executive editor at Delmar Cengage Learning, for his commitment to the book and support throughout the project.

Monica Ohlinger and Brooke Wilson (Ohlinger Publishing Services) for their attention to book detail and content and continuous encouragement and support as the book was developed. We truly enjoyed working with them both.

Kim Penland for her continued support and input regarding the needs of an LPN transitioning into an RN program. She began her nursing career as an LPN and is now pursuing her doctorate.

John Duncan for his assistance, patience, and encouragement as we worked on the book.

LPN to RN nurses for sharing their stories: Charles Burd, Lori Covey, Cindy Deemer, Kyan DiVita, Patty Emrich, Katrina Evans, Stacy Fladhammer, Jennifer Foley, Heather Konger, Monique Myles, Kim Penland, and Julie Richardson.

Becky Jenson for her excellent contributions to Chapter 13 IV Therapy Skills.

Wendy Baumle for graciously granting permission to use sections of the IV chapter from the nursing book that she is co-authoring with Gena Duncan.

Maria Gomez and Heather Krull for their candid answers to transition issues they personally made in advancing from LPNs to RNs.

Mary Spath for her invaluable input into the needs of LPN-RN students as we developed the first edition of the book. She taught a transition course for LPN-RN students at the University of Saint Francis, Fort Wayne, Indiana.

AVENUE FOR FEEDBACK

We value your feedback of questions, suggestions, or comments about the book. You may contact the authors at:

Gena Duncan: email: genaduncan@aol.com; phone: 260-403-1161 or 260-693-3811.

René DePew: email: rdepew@sf.edu; phone: 260-399-7700 Ext. 8512.

Chapter 1
Returning to School

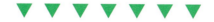

LEARNING OBJECTIVES

By the end of this chapter, you should be able to:

1. Discuss phases students experience throughout the education process.
2. Explain four learning styles.
3. Discover your individual learning style.
4. Identify specific time-management skills.
5. Identify study skills to assist in the education process.
6. Discuss ways to balance home, work, and school responsibilities.

KEY TERMS

Abstract random (AR)
Abstract sequential (AS)
Concrete random (CR)
Concrete sequential (CS)
Conflict phase
Honeymoon phase
Learning style
Resolution phase
Returning to School Syndrome (RTSS)
Time management

SCENARIO

Megan has been an LPN for five years. She is planning to return to college to further her nursing education. Megan works full-time and has two school-age sons, Todd, age 9, and Shane, age 13. Her husband, Jim, travels quite frequently for his job. Megan feels that studying will not be a problem for her because she can study at her children's games, on her work breaks, and in between her other various activities.

THINK ABOUT IT

1. How does your own schedule compare to Megan's schedule?
2. How many hours do you anticipate that you will need for school obligations?
3. Does Megan's schedule seem realistic to accomplish her educational goal?

INTRODUCTION

Welcome back to the world of student nursing! Many will chose to maintain their current working status as Licensed Practical Nurses (LPN) while returning to school to become Registered Nurses (RN). Juggling both nurse and student nurse roles will possibly be challenging from time to time, but what a wonderful time to pursue additional nursing education and obtain an RN degree. Pursuing an RN education is a great opportunity for both professional and personal growth, especially when approached with a positive attitude. Each LPN brings many stories, experiences, skills, and knowledge to these classes. How exciting to build on your own knowledge, enhance current skills, and learn new ones. This is a good time to reflect on where you started in nursing, where you are today, and where you hope to go in the future. Make note: Going back to school requires a great deal of time and energy. This is an opportunity to push beyond your comfort zone and maximize this experience, to make it all it possibly can be. Take the time to establish specific and measurable education goals.

According to a study by Green (1996), licensed practical nurses/licensed vocational nurses (LPNs/LVNs) who chose to pursue a higher degree have frequently received excellent work reviews for nursing competence and critical thinking. These students were successful not only in completing their degrees but in passing state boards and obtaining jobs.

The fact that you are enrolling in school to further your nursing education demonstrates your commitment, desire to learn, and ability to set personal and professional goals. You have given much thought and personal analysis to this decision. Perhaps you experienced some self-doubt and anxiety. Returning to college is a challenge, especially if you have not been in a school environment with classes and lessons in some time. Technological advances may be intimidating. The classroom setting and presentations have changed considerably. However, your nursing instructors want you to succeed, and they are a source of guidance and encouragement (Farley, 2006). A stimulating, enriching experience awaits you in becoming an RN. This will be an adventure of personal and intellectual growth. Many emotions may already have surfaced, and you will experience many more in the next few months as you pursue your educational goal. In an article entitled "Be a Real Survivor," Melissa Ezarik (2001) states, "Take the challenge, and you'll reap the rewards."

In this chapter we will discuss coping skills that will assist you as you pursue your degree. You are introduced to the Gregorc learning styles and given time-management techniques to improve your study habits. Helpful suggestions are given for balancing the demands of school, home, and work. Many of these suggestions may not be new to you, but they serve as reminders to guide you through future successful semesters.

DEVELOPING A POSITIVE ATTITUDE

An important part of success in achieving anything in life is a positive attitude. A nursing student must believe in herself and never give up. For some, self-confidence will come naturally, and for others it will come as knowledge grows and experiences occur. Nursing students must always believe in themselves and their potential to accomplish this goal.

Students pursuing another degree usually are highly motivated and do well academically (Utley-Smith, Phillips, Turner, 2007). By reviewing the experiences of other students who also went through the educational process, students gain insight into ways to cope successfully and avoid some undesirable diversions. In 1983 Donea Shane described the emotional ups and downs students experienced when they returned to school for an associate degree and termed the experience the **Returning to School Syndrome (RTSS)** (see Figure 1–1). During the **honeymoon phase**, the student is fascinated with all the new aspects of academic life. There is an increased awareness of purpose and confidence. This phase lasts until the student encounters a class with in-depth nursing theory or clinical experience. When this occurs, the student experiences anxiety, feels intimidated, and dreads the clinical evaluation.

The second phase is called the **conflict phase**. During this time, new and different nursing concepts are presented and the student experiences conflict with various personal roles, faculty members, and previous knowledge base versus newly acquired knowledge. The student experiences uncertainty and self-doubt and becomes angry, feels overwhelmed, and is fatigued. The college, faculty, home life, or any tangible object is blamed for the lack of perceived success. This phase is divided into two parts: *disintegration* and *reintegration*. During disintegration the student turns anxious feelings inward and becomes depressed and withdrawn. In reintegration, the student shows feelings of frustration by acting hostile toward others, especially the faculty. The student expresses feelings of frustration with the nursing program and the education process in general.

The last phase is the **resolution phase**. Some of the stages in this phase are *chronic conflict*, *false acceptance*, and *biculturalism*. In the chronic conflict stage, the student is constantly angry, failing to see the value of the education process. She spends extensive emotional effort in angry, hostile, aggressive behavior. In false acceptance, the student gives the appearance of accepting and experiencing the educational process yet does not value or embrace the positive aspects of the educational opportunity. In biculturalism, the student meshes more than one culture, such as school and work, or school and personal life. The student begins to understand the demands of the academic experience and adjusts with new coping skills. The student's attention is now focused on maximizing educational opportunities (Utley-Smith, Phillips, Turner, 2007).

A student does not necessarily move through these phases in a linear manner but may move in and out of each phase at different times. Understanding these phases gives insight

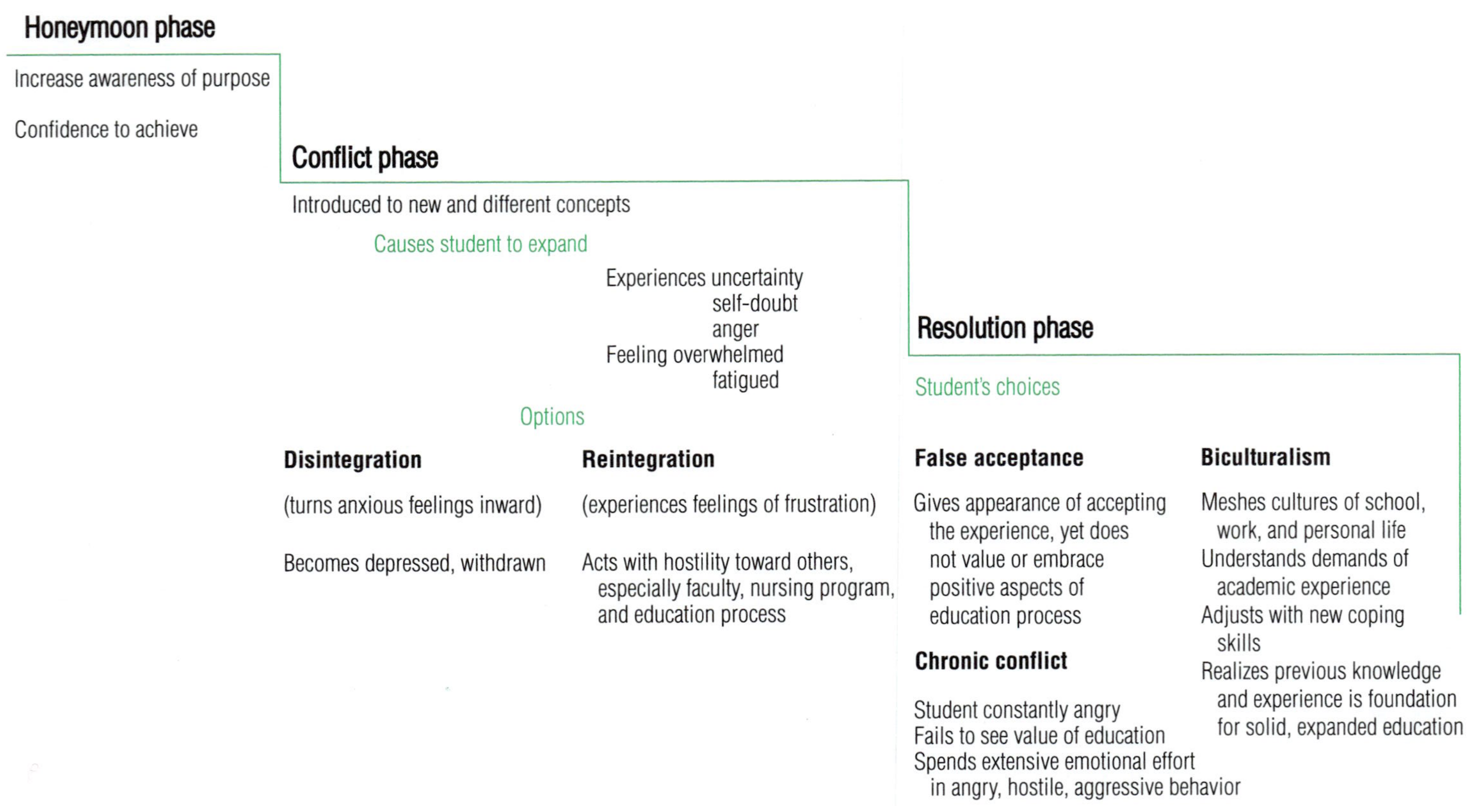

Honeymoon phase

Increase awareness of purpose

Confidence to achieve

Conflict phase

Introduced to new and different concepts

Causes student to expand

Experiences uncertainty
self-doubt
anger

Feeling overwhelmed
fatigued

Options

Disintegration

(turns anxious feelings inward)

Becomes depressed, withdrawn

Reintegration

(experiences feelings of frustration)

Acts with hostility toward others, especially faculty, nursing program, and education process

Resolution phase

Student's choices

False acceptance

Gives appearance of accepting the experience, yet does not value or embrace positive aspects of education process

Chronic conflict

Student constantly angry
Fails to see value of education
Spends extensive emotional effort in angry, hostile, aggressive behavior

Biculturalism

Meshes cultures of school, work, and personal life
Understands demands of academic experience
Adjusts with new coping skills
Realizes previous knowledge and experience is foundation for solid, expanded education

Figure 1–1 Returning to School Syndrome (Shane, 1983).

as various feelings and emotions arise during the educational experience. You can apply this knowledge to your personal life and learn positive coping skills as you feel these emotions surfacing.

COPING SKILLS

From Shane's RTSS study, you become aware of some paths you may want to follow. At first the whole educational experience seems exciting. Then, as new concepts and more difficult material are presented, realize that you have a choice in your response to the educational experience. Recognizing that you have a choice is gaining insight into ways of coping with life situations. A coping skill is choosing a new way to solve a problem. At times you feel overwhelmed and uncertain. Fatigue will set in. These feelings are not new to students in education. Rather than *choosing* to feel overwhelmed and anxious, recall your goals, think positive thoughts, spend time with friends who are upbeat, share your feelings with a friend, and know that using some of the study and coping methods presented in this chapter will sustain you through these times. Rather than striking out at faculty or classmates, realize they may be struggling too, and try to encourage them. Resolve to learn new coping skills to juggle the different responsibilities of home, school, and work. Be open to new nursing concepts and experiences. Compare new concepts with previously learned concepts. By doing this, the educational experience becomes a valuable growth experience.

Develop a sense of humor. Appropriate humor and laughter can relieve stressful times when you are caring for clients. Reading comic strips, humorous books, and good jokes from Internet friends can develop your sense of humor. If you learn not to take life so seriously and to laugh at your own mistakes, you will release a lot of stress. Some doctors say a good belly laugh a day is good medicine. Laughter definitely gives a more positive outlook on any situation.

Taking a few minutes to play a simple game with your family also relieves stress. Playing board games and cards breaks the monotony of the daily routine. Conversing and laughing with your family offer great opportunities for bonding and many future positive memories.

Interaction with a pet also relieves the day's frustration and provides a break in a hectic schedule. Emotionally bonding with a pet provides warmth and security.

THEORY TO PRACTICE

Yesterday: Where You Started

A nurse is blessed with the opportunity to make a difference in the lives of others every single day. The journey of a nurse is generally very individual and personal. This journey is one that will present challenges, celebratory moments, and an opportunity for a lifetime of growth and rewards. Enjoy the moments, both the good and the bad, for it is the combination of all those experiences that shape and mold an individual into a nurse.

Decision to Become an LPN

Reflecting on the decision to become an LPN probably stimulates a wealth of memories. Individuals choose their nursing paths for a wide variety of reasons. Maybe that particular opportunity was the most convenient, affordable, or flexible at the time. Maybe the program seemed easier than another nursing program or met a time-sensitive need at that point in life. Maybe a mentor or life role model encouraged this path. Or, maybe the strong personal desire to care for people was the driving force of the decision. Being a nurse could provide independence, job security, and flexibility. Maybe the real reason was that nursing best suited your needs at that particular time in life.

Experience as an LPN

LPNs are valuable members of the health care team. They are exposed to a vast array of experiences and opportunities. It is these experiences and opportunities for LPNs that build strong assessment skills, physical care skills, therapeutic communication skills, poise and confidence, as well as the ability to multi-task. All of these are very valuable skills for any nurse. It is very important for LPNs to respect this knowledge and build on it for future nursing practice.

Personal and Professional Lessons to Hold On To

While moving forward in nursing, try to remember lessons learned along the way and acknowledge the accomplishments already made at this point in your journey. Not only recognize, but take time to celebrate those accomplishments and know that challenges and hurdles have already been crossed. Think about what lessons as an LPN will be important to maintain and blend with the new skills being obtained as a registered nurse (RN). Use those current skills to help meet your new goals as an RN.

Today: Where You Are Headed

Your life has led you back to nursing school. Choices are made, and action is required to accomplish new goals—life continues to happen one day at a time. Time marches on. Yesterday you were an LPN, today you are a registered nursing student on the way to becoming an RN.

Deciding to Go Back to School

Seize the moment! Opportunity has knocked, and your journey has led you back to nursing school. Why today? Why this degree? Why this university? Those details may not be completely understood and again that is OK, but chances are, it is the option that best meets your needs for today.

Establishing Personal Goals and Expectations

Now that you have made these decisions, it is important to establish some personal goals and expectations. Our goals and expected outcomes should be specific and measurable.

This will provide a nursing student with the opportunity to evaluate the experience. It will give focus, meaning, and purpose to the journey. It is also important to have both short and long-term goals. The accomplishment of the short-term goals is more realistic and more within reach throughout the educational journey. Reaching these short-term goals provides reasons to celebrate and offers a chance to maintain enthusiasm and stamina through the challenges of life as a nursing student. Long-term goals give focus and insight to the future. Write down your personal and professional goals and expectations to help you along the way.

- Goals for the next year
- Goals for the next three years
- Goals for the next five years
- Goals for the next ten years

DEVELOPING BASIC SKILLS

The nursing environment is constantly changing and nurses need a variety of new skills to be successful in the work environment. Computer skills are a must. Many clinics and other health care facilities are going paperless and are using electronic medical records (EMRs). The health care provider may use a computer in the exam room to record the client's concerns and make assessments as the client relates her symptoms to them. On clinical units nurses record nursing notes on the computer; order medications, supplies, and equipment; and obtain medications from computer-accessed supplies. If uncertain about computer skills, a basic computer course makes for a smoother transition back into nursing education.

Basic math and/or algebra are often required in nursing program curricula. Even though many medications are dispensed in unit dose, math skills are still needed to verify the correct medication dose. If your math skills need a boost, take a math refresher course so you are ready for the algebra course (see Appendix C for basic math skill practice). Math and algebra courses also broaden people intellectually and improve critical thinking problem-solving skills.

An English course is often required when pursuing your nursing education. It is important for a nurse to have solid English grammar skills. Misspelling words and using poor grammar taint the nursing profession's image. It also causes legal issues if the wrong subject is referred to in a sentence or if syntax is inaccurate. In administration, nurses write many memos and important documents or apply for grants. Good writing skills are needed for these tasks. Therefore, it is important for a nurse to learn basic rules of English grammar and spell correctly.

CRITICAL THINKING ACTIVITIES

1. What phase of the RTSS describes your present feelings?
2. How can you prevent or cope with the conflict phase of the RTSS?
3. What will help you move into the biculturalism stage of the resolution phase of the RTSS?

DISCOVERING YOUR LEARNING STYLE

Learning styles are "a particular way in which the mind receives and processes information" (Katz, Carter, Bishop, and Kravitis, 2004, p. 73). Your particular learning style is the unique way you perceive information, process it, and then relate the information to others. Determining your learning style maximizes learning, produces more effective study habits and an increased understanding of others' behaviors and learning needs. Refer to the Suggested Resources at the end of the chapter for on-line methods to determine your learning style.

As you discover your particular **learning style**, your scope of learning is broadened. You will understand how learning occurs and the reason learning occurs more easily in some classes than in others, or the reason that taking a class on-line appeals to you. You will also understand the rationale of some professors' teaching methods. Discovering your particular learning style allows you to adapt and learn more effectively.

As an adult learner, take time to identify strategies that work best for your individual learning style. Some class presentations will not "fit" your learning style. Be flexible with the different methods of presentation and learn to adjust to make the most of all opportunities (Farley, 2006). Be an engaged learner by listening in class and never fearing to ask questions or clarifying information.

Anthony Gregorc (1982) describes four learning styles: concrete sequential (CS), concrete random (CR), abstract sequential (AS), and abstract random (AR). He believes one's learning style determines one's preferred study method (Gregorc & Butler, 1984). Therefore, by determining your learning style, you learn effective studying methods. Gregorc also applied learning styles to personality traits and to behaviors in the work environment. By studying learning styles, you gain insight into your own behavior and the behavior of those with whom you work.

Each of Gregorc's four learning styles is described in the next few paragraphs. Try to identify which one is most like your preferred learning style, and see if the characteristics of that style match your personal characteristics and preferences. By using the study methods listed under the learning style, learning becomes much easier. For example, if your style suggests that you learn best in an environment without distractions, try to find a quiet place to make the most of your study time.

People with a **concrete sequential (CS)** learning style are practical, organized, and structured. The person with a dominant CS style is calm, collected, precise, and strives for perfection. A person scoring high in the CS style works step-by-step, following specific instructions until a project is completed (Gregorc, 1982). Concrete sequential learners prefer a structured, orderly presentation; step-by-step directions; and time for a hands-on experience. They do not tolerate environmental distractions (Gregorc & Ward, 1977). To retain information, the CS learner memorizes or drills. Study method preferences of the CS learner are using workbooks and lab manuals, programmed instruction, computer-aided instruction, organized field trips, demonstration teaching, direct application problems, assembly kits, and hands-on opportunities.

Individuals with a dominant **concrete random (CR)** learning style are creative, independent, and curious. They tend to make quick, impulsive, intuitive decisions. In the workplace, they are the ideas people who do not want to be fenced in but want to be free to express themselves. Their curiosity and competitiveness rarely allow them to accept another's word as fact; instead, the fact must be proven by personal trial and error (Gregorc, 1982). Such people work well on an individual basis and do not respond well to assistance from a teacher in their learning pursuits (Gregorc & Ward, 1977). A person with dominant CR prefers independent study, computer games, open-ended problem solving, simulations, supplemental reading assignments, interactive video, and short lectures with the opportunity to try new methods (Gregorc & Butler, 1984).

Abstract sequential (AS) learners prefer abstract ideas and pictures. Individuals with AS styles may appear flighty or absent-minded, but they love to gather facts, find answers, and debate issues extensively. They are often respected for their intellectual ability. This factor, along with their ability to make long-term plans, leads them into higher education (Gregorc, 1982). Abstract sequential learners prefer lectures, textbooks, supplemental readings, audiotapes, guided individual study, and audiovisual aids, such as videotapes and slide tapes (Gregorc & Butler, 1984). They prefer few environmental distractions (Gregorc & Ward, 1977).

Abstract random (AR) learners are sensitive and flexible. Their approach to the world is based on intuition, emotions, and gut feelings. They are often viewed as daydreamers. Abstract random learners experience the entire learning environment through their emotions (Gregorc, 1982). They prefer to receive information in an unstructured manner and then assimilate the material by reflecting on it (Gregorc & Ward, 1977). They want to belong to the group, and they work well with others, especially in a noncompetitive environment. People with dominant AR style prefer group discussion and enjoy studying with background music. Abstract random learners prefer television, movies, short lectures with questions and answers, guided imagery, and contemplative assignments (Gregorc & Butler, 1984).

A person's cognitive style (the way one processes information) is not limited to learning situations but actually is responsible for one's personality. The behavior patterns evidenced by individual cognitive style have much in common with behavior patterns known as learning style, decision-making style, and social style.

Making Learning Style Adjustments

If the classroom style does not match the student's learning style, the student can still adjust to the classroom mode. Because the student knows how she learns best or her preferred learning style, she can attempt to adjust to the presented style and then make personal adjustments by learning the difficult concepts in her preferred style. For example, if an AR learner is in a class that is presented in a CS manner—using workbooks, computer-aided instruction, and demonstrations—the learner can obtain videos from the library to review concepts, meet with other students to discuss concepts presented in class, or ask questions in class to have the needed personal interaction. This helps the student adapt to styles that are not the preferred style and assists in learning the needed information.

If a student knows her preferred learning style, she also has a preferred study method. The student uses that information to obtain the material needed to assist in the learning process.

Communicating Learning Style to Faculty

There are several learning style assessment tools, such as Anthony Gregorc, Gregorc Style Delineator: A Self-Assessment Instrument for Adults; Dave Kolb (1984), Learning Style Inventory; Peter Honey, Learning Style Questionnaire; and Neil Fleming, VARK: A Guide to Learning Styles (www.vark-learn.com). Additional resources are available through an Internet search for learning style tools or learning style assessment. A student can share her personal learning style with the professor and discuss learning style concepts with faculty members. By working together, faculty and student grow and assist each other in providing a mutually effective learning environment whether that environment is a traditional classroom, online, or another distant learning method.

Ideally, faculty members use a variety of methods in presenting information to a class. A student who finds certain concepts difficult can ask the faculty member where those concepts can be found in a different medium. Online courses that have an interactive option built in can assist some learners.

If the faculty member assists in the student's learning and the student takes personal responsibility for learning, a productive, challenging environment is created that hurtles many learning obstacles. Utilizing learning style concepts and providing varied learning methods impact the learning environment in a dramatic way.

CRITICAL THINKING ACTIVITY

1. What is your personal learning style according to the description of each learning style presented in the text? Within that learning style, what are your own best study methods? You may desire to complete a learning style inventory, either online or by obtaining a learning style assessment tool.

2. Knowing your personal learning style and other learning styles, identify ways to adapt to a classroom setting in which your personal learning style is not the dominant presentation.

3. How could a person's learning style affect her personality? How could learning style affect a person's work ethic?

TIME MANAGEMENT

Often we vacillate between the feelings expressed in two phrases: "Where has the time gone?" and "Will this time never end?" We all have the same amount of time, but some people use time more effectively and accomplish more than others. Time can either control us, or we can control time by learning to manage activities within an allotted time frame. Goodman

(2007) states lack of time management is like a hamster running in a wheel without rhyme or reason. In this mode, it is easy to lose sight of why we are doing what we are doing. However, we profit if we view time as a continuous growth opportunity to effectively organize activities. That is **time management**: effectively prioritizing and organizing responsibilities and activities within a set time frame.

As a returning student, time becomes a precious commodity. Often academic tasks take twice as long as expected. The juggling of all your roles and responsibilities may seem overwhelming at times. Therefore, a segment of unexpected time is a gift. That is the reason daily judicious prioritizing and organizing of activities is vital.

The academic semester schedule contains monthly, weekly, and daily time segments. At the beginning of each semester, review each course syllabus and record on a monthly calendar project due dates, exam dates, presentation dates, and any special assignment dates for all classes. Also record personal items such as birthdays, ball games, your work schedule, date nights or times with spouse or children, exercise time, and special personal events. Review this for conflicts and possible overload, and adjust the schedule as needed. It is important to maintain this habit, and as each new commitment arises, record it on the monthly calendar. Committing the plan to a written schedule provides direction and a visual reminder.

Some people prefer to break the monthly calendar into weekly or daily calendars. The monthly calendar gives the long-term view, the weekly calendar gives a short-term view offering an opportunity for needed adjustments in preventing a crisis or scheduling conflicts, and the daily view assists with prioritization of activities. By viewing the monthly calendar, you can get an early start on assignments and complete them before their due dates. This decreases physical and emotional stress. Purchasing a computer program that automatically transfers monthly listings to weekly- or daily-planning pages may be very helpful.

One of the best ways to effectively manage responsibilities and time is to complete a daily time plan (see Table 1–1). To make this time plan effective, combine it with a "to do" list. List all items that need completing. The list may seem overwhelming at first, but when you divide it into segments, it will begin to look manageable. Once you have completed the "to do" list, prioritize the items. One way to do this is to number the tasks—for instance, 1 to 10. Another way is to prioritize the items as A (must be done today), B (good if done today), or C (not necessary to do today). Then place all 1 through 5 or A items in the time frames of your daily planner. The time frames should be small segments of time—15 minutes, 30 minutes, or 60 minutes. Experiment with this to see what time segments are most appropriate for you (see Table 1–2 for an example using 30-minute segments). You can make a personal day planner on a computer or purchase one at an office supplies store or campus bookstore.

At the end of each day, marking off completed items gives a sense of satisfaction. Once you have done that, review the "to do" list again and reorganize the next day. Some items that were not completed may drop off the "to do" list if they have lost their importance. It is best to complete this task at the end of each day, when items that need completing are still fresh in your mind. This way, you can start the next day with purpose, without letting less pressing activities take control of valuable time. Some prefer to prioritize items in the morning when feeling fresh. Experiment with different times of the day for completing this activity and see what works best.

Table 1–1 Sample daily planner

Done	Time	Schedule	"To do" list	Priority
	7:00			
	7:30			
	8:00			
	8:30			
	9:00			
	9:30			
	10:00			
	10:30			
	11:00			
	11:30			
	12:00			
	12:30			
	1:00			
	1:30			
	2:00			
	2:30			
	3:00			
	3:30			
	4:00			
	4:30			
	5:00			
	5:30			
	6:00			
	6:30			
	7:00			
	7:30			
	8:00			
	8:30			
	9:00			
	9:30			
	10:00			
			Phone calls to make	

Table 1–2 Completed sample daily planner

Done	Time	Schedule	"To do" list	Priority
	7:00		Complete care plan for clinical	B
	7:30		Prep for pharmacology class	A
	8:00	Drop car at repair shop	Buy paint for house	C
	8:30	Study for geriatric nursing exam	Physical therapy on arm	A
	9:00		Pay electric bill	C
	9:30		Drop car at repair shop	A
	10:00	Call Brad's teacher	Get money at bank	B
	10:30		Call Linda	B
	11:00	Prep for pharmacology class	Study for geriatric nursing exam	A
	11:30		Schedule parent-teacher conference	A
	12:00		Mow yard	C
	12:30	Lunch		
	1:00	Pharmacology class		
	1:30			
	2:00			
	2:30			
	3:00			
	3:30			
	4:00			
	4:30	Pick up car at repair shop		
	5:00	Physical therapy on arm		
	5:30			
	6:00	Geriatric nursing class		
	6:30			
	7:00			
	7:30			
	8:00			
	8:30			
	9:00			
	9:30			
	10:00			
			Phone calls to make	
			Call Linda	

STUDY STRATEGIES

By now you may already have developed study methods that work well for you. A review of some survival study skills follows.

Time-Saving Tips

One way to plan your time effectively and be organized is to use a daily planner to record all assignments, test dates, paper due dates, and study time. Set aside a specific area in your home, at school, or at the library to study. Keep your study area neat and organized. Have a place to file old papers and assignments. Keep separate folders or filing cartons for each class to assist in quickly finding specific papers without sorting through all of them. Use five-minute time segments to make phone calls, contact a classmate to clarify a question or assignment, or review notes. Because most computer paper and assignment papers are 8 1/2 × 11 inches, purchase a 9 × 12–inch zippered notebook to hold your monthly, weekly, and daily planners, phone numbers, and articles or homework that you can work on while waiting in an office or to meet a family member or friend. Some people prefer storing needed information in a PDA type device for easy access. Accomplish two tasks at once, such as talking on the phone and folding clothes or feeding a pet. Developing effective planning and organizational skills as a student will pay dividends as a nurse.

Class Preparation

Prepare for each week's assignment before class in order to glean more from the class content and increase personal participation. Also, advance preparation allows time to review material for exams, and not study it for the first time just before an exam. It also prevents the last-minute rush to complete assignments at the end of the semester, which leads to stress.

Effective Note Taking

Learn to take good notes. Devise personal abbreviations for frequently used words. Write phrases, not complete sentences. If note taking is difficult, outline reading assignments and then add to or highlight the class members' or instructor's input. The use of a tape recorder in class frees a student from the stress of having to write down all the information. Review the recorded material after class to fill in any gaps in your notes. Taking notes on a laptop computer is another viable option. Some faculty members prefer that students request permission prior to using a laptop or tape recorder in class. Review your notes after class while the material is fresh in your mind to cement the information and complete fragmented notes.

Some classes may not have a lecture, note-taking format. Instead, the professor prefers discussion, presentations, case study review, and other creative educational methods. These offer opportunities for students to adjust to a different type of learning environment. More learning styles are addressed when faculty vary their presentation methods.

Study Time

Set aside study time and inform friends and family of the designated time to prevent interruptions. Let the telephone answering machine record messages during this time so your concentration on study material is not interrupted. Use the designated study time to study; do not allow other activities to fill this scheduled time. The general rule is that a student should spend two to three hours studying for every hour spent in the classroom. The amount of time needed for studying varies depending on your previous knowledge base of class content. Schedule breaks to prevent sluggishness. If you become drowsy, stand up and move; have a healthy snack of carrots, celery, or an apple; or take a short power nap.

Paper Writing

When writing papers, ask your professor for specific information regarding the expectations for the paper, such as general content, format, inclusion of articles or other references, and specific information to be included. Obtain a copy of the required style guidelines for use at home; APA (American Psychological Association) and MLA (Modern Language Association) are the most frequently required. The APA has a formatting supplement in an electronic version. There are electronic supplement tools as well as online resources to assist with assignments.

Start work early on papers and projects so library personnel can obtain articles, computer information, and books as you need them when writing the paper or completing the project. Begin your own computer searches early so the articles will be available when you need them. Complete the paper early and put it aside for a day, then review it for content change or other needed revisions. Working ahead of schedule decreases stress.

Exam Preparation

Ask your professor as much as possible about exams such as type (multiple choice, true–false, matching, essay); length (timed exam, whole class period); and items you need to bring (calculator, number 2 pencil, book for open-book quiz, or one-page notes if allowed). This information makes your study time more effective because preparation is different for each type of exam. Some students find study groups effective to review class material, quiz one another on content, and discuss concepts. Use study groups effectively. Do not substitute personal study time for group study. Study the material first so that you are prepared to contribute to and benefit from the study group. Cramming leads to insecurity when taking exams. Adequate preparation; materials comprehension; and a positive, self-confident attitude decrease test anxiety and lead to test-taking success.

Before beginning the exam "brain dump," jot down on the answer sheet or exam paper rhymes or information that will assist you in recalling information (see Figure 1–2). Ask the professor for clarification if you do not understand the exam material. Pace yourself throughout the exam so that you will have time to complete it. Refer to Appendix A for test-taking skills and NCLEX preparation.

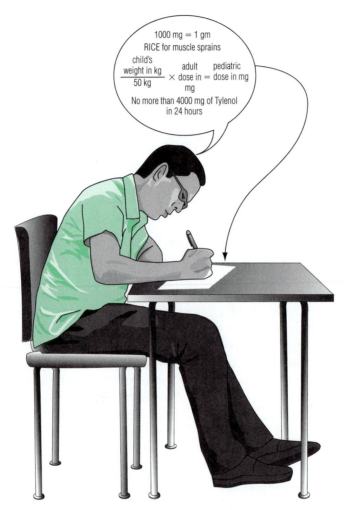

Figure 1–2 "Brain dump" at the start of the exam by jotting down on the answer sheet or exam paper rhymes or information that will assist you in recalling information.

Grade Games

Some students get caught up in an intense concern and competition for grades that leads to a mental battle for self-esteem. This allows the grade to determine their identity and self-worth. The focus of learning becomes the grade rather than acquiring meaningful information for present and future application. But grades do not always represent the time or energy put into the project. And a grade less than A does not diminish one's identity or self-worth.

CRITICAL THINKING ACTIVITY

1. Review the study strategies and choose two or three methods that you have not used in the past but would like to incorporate into your study skills this semester. Write them down and describe how you will integrate the strategies into your current schedule.

BALANCING HOME, WORK, AND SCHOOL

In a study of older adults returning to school, Scala (1996) found that students stopped attending classes because of health problems and lack of time for school. In returning to school, a nurse takes on a new role, that of student. Time and energy for each life role (parent, family member, nurse, friend, student, home care provider, employee) come from a finite source. Some students return to school with the "superman complex," thinking that nurses are invincible and can do all things and be all things to all people. Some students attempt to work forty-plus hours a week and still take a full academic load. In the process, their health fails and/or their grades suffer. Failure to review and revise personal schedules and work commitments often leads to health issues and lack of study time. Adequate planning decreases the number of conflicts encountered in the educational venture.

Family support is essential when returning to school. Significant support persons and family members may not realize the demands or pressures of school. Communicating the demands and expectations of courses and professors can help your family understand the new pressures on you. Role reversals and delegation of household chores may be helpful during this time. Show family members and friends that their assistance is valued. Perfection is not the name of the game. Clothes do not have to be folded with all corners lined up. Simple meals are a luxury. A basic cleaning will do. Pay to have the lawn mowed. If a child or friend is computer literate and can assist with a project, encourage and prize the help. If a friend offers to carpool or baby-sit, accept the assistance. Helping you gives your family and friends a sense of contributing to the project. Therefore, when you finally receive your degree, in essence, your entire family and significant support persons celebrate the accomplishment with you.

Working while going to school can be a stressor or a refreshing outlet. If you are working, discuss a schedule with your supervisor that will accommodate study time, class time, and personal time. Some organizations and companies offer students tuition reimbursement. Working only on weekends may offer more pay along with the freedom to study and spend some leisure time with friends or family during the weekdays.

When students are juggling so many schedules, their physical, emotional, nutritional, and spiritual lives are often neglected. Neglecting social contacts, physical exercise, and spiritual needs can lead to emptiness, isolation, and depression. Have regular contact with a friend over a cup of coffee, in the gym, or at a movie. Exercising three to four times weekly helps maintain a positive attitude and keeps you physically fit. Find an activity you enjoy and participate in it regularly. There are so many good activities to chose, such as walking, biking, racquetball, tennis, and golf. Exercising with friends is an added bonus because it can meet a physical and social need. Maintaining a well-balanced, low-fat diet also aids physical stamina and fitness. Engaging in regular spiritual renewal through worship, prayer, meditation, or study groups meets the spiritual needs that keep us whole.

CRITICAL THINKING ACTIVITY

1. How can you put some of these ideas into daily practice?

SUMMARY

Students who return to school often experience a variety of feelings. It is important to understand the RTSS phases to deflect unneeded emotions and take corrective coping actions. Planning for success in nursing education begins prior to stepping into the classroom. First, an individual evaluates personal abilities and selects the appropriate nursing program for skills and life situation. The "plan for success" continues as the nursing student reevaluates, reprioritizes, and succeeds in the educational journey. Want it, commit to it, and pursue it!

CHAPTER REFLECTIONS

1. Refer back to the scenario at the beginning of this chapter. After reading the chapter, what changes do you think Megan may need to make to achieve her educational goals?
2. Do you have trouble managing your time on a daily basis to meet your responsibilities?
3. Identify your learning style and the study skills that will assist you to be successful.
4. Do you have a support network to turn to for assistance?
5. What strategies suggested in this chapter could you apply to your life?
6. How do you feel your personal attitude can influence your educational experience?

Journaling Your Journey

1. Think about the professional goals you set in the Theory to Practice activity and share your personal story of yesterday, today, and tomorrow.
2. Returning to school: what do you find the most exciting and the most intimidating?
3. Describe your current roles and responsibilities. How will you find balance?

‿ﻭ ‿ﻭ ‿ﻭ

CRITICAL THINKING ACTIVITY

1. Identify your strengths and weaknesses that could potentially make your educational experience more stressful if not addressed in an appropriate manner.

2. Identify your strengths that will enhance your educational experience.

My Story...

Working was probably the biggest challenge in going back to school due to class schedules and study time. As with many students, I had to balance the care of a small child, house, work, and school. I tried to focus on the fact that it was just for a certain length of time and the benefits would pay off. I tried to stay "in the moment." Worrying about the past or the future made the whole picture overwhelming.

I was already comfortable with patient interaction when I entered the RN program. The client comfort level gave me a greater opportunity to focus on applying what I learned in the classroom to the clinical situation. When I graduated from the RN program, I obtained a job in a critical care unit. It was a benefit that I was already comfortable with general patient care since there was so much to learn. If I would not have had the experience of being an LPN, I don't believe I would have had the confidence as a new RN to take on this role.

Julie Richardson, MSN, RN

REFERENCES

Chenevert, M. (1997). *PRO-Nurse handbook* (3rd ed.). St. Louis: Mosby.

Ezarik, M. (2001). Be a real survivor. *Career World, 30*(2), 6–10.

Farley, H. (2006). Essential skills for students who are returning to school. *Art & Science Education, 21*(6), 44–48.

Goodman, B. (2007). Get things in perspective. *Nursing Standard 22*(8), 61.

Green, J. (1996, April 8). LPN-to-RN training: A boon for small hospitals? *AHA News, 32*(14), 5–11.

Gregorc, A. (1982). *An adult's guide to style.* Columbia, CT: Gregorc Associates.

Gregorc, A., & Butler, K. (1984). Learning is a matter of style. *Vocational Education, 4,* 27–29.

Gregorc, A., & Ward, H. B. (1977). Implications for learning and teaching: A new definition for individual. *NASSP Bulletin,* 20–26.

Katz, J., Carter, C., Bishop, J. & Kravits, S. (2004). *Keys to nursing success.* (2nd Ed). Pearson Prentice Hall: New Jersey.

Morgenthaler, M. (2009). Too old for school? Barriers nurses can overcome when returning to school. *AORN Journal, 89*(2), 335–344.

Scala, M. (1996). Going back to school: Participation motives and experience of older adults in an undergraduate program. *Educational Gerontology, 22*(8), 747–774.

Shane, D. (1983). *Returning to school: A guide for nurses.* Englewood Cliffs, NJ: Prentice Hall.

Utley-Smith, Q., Phillips, B., & Turner, K. (2007). Avoiding socializations pitfalls in accelerated second-degree nursing education: The returning-to-school syndrome model. *Journal of Nursing Education, 46*(9), 423–426.

SUGGESTED RESOURCES

Brew, C. (2002). Kolb's learning style instrument: Sensitive to gender. *Educational and Psychological Measurement, 62*(2), 373–390.

Delahoussaye, M. (2002). The perfect learner: An expert debate on learning styles. *Training, 39*(5), 28–36.

Fleming, N. (2001). VARK: A guide to learning styles. www.vark-learning.com

Gregorc, A. (1985). *Gregorc style delineator: A self-assessment instrument for adults.* Columbia, CT: Gregorc Associates.

Honey, P., & Mumford, A. (1992). *The manual of learning styles.* Maidenhead, Berkshire: Peter Honey Publications.

Kearney, R. (2001). *Advancing your career: Concepts of professional nursing.* Philadelphia: F.A. Davis Company.

Kolb, D. (1984). *Experiential learning: Experience as the source of learning and development.* Englewood Cliffs, NJ: Prentice Hall.

Mumford, A. & Honey, P. (2000). The learner styles helper's guide. Maidenhead, Berkshire: Peter Honey Publications.

Reese, S. (2002). Understanding our differences. *Techniques, 77*(1), 20–23.

What's your learning style?, www.ldpride.net

What's your learning style?, agelesslearner.com/

Chapter 2
Role Transition

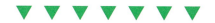

LEARNING OBJECTIVES

By the end of this chapter, you should be able to:

1. Define the term *role*.
2. Define nurse's role.
3. Explain responsibilities of the nurse's role.
4. Discuss the transition process from LPN to RN.
5. Discuss the socialization process in becoming an RN.
6. Explain steps in the change process.
7. Identify ways to use the change process effectively in transitioning from LPN to RN.

KEY TERMS

Advocate
Change agent
Change process
Collaborator
Communicator
Counselor
Educator
Entrepreneur
Leader
Mentor
Researcher
Role
Role conflict
Role model

Role socialization

Role transition

SCENARIO

Jefferson, an LPN, is entering the transitions class in a registered nursing program at a local college. He feels the transitions class is not really necessary because he has been dealing with transitions his entire life. His nursing career began in high school when he worked as a nursing assistant in a nursing home. After high school he became a qualified medical assistant (QMA) and, then, an LPN. Today he is working on his associate degree . . . what is one more step up the nursing ladder? Jefferson feels that making a bed is making a bed . . . passing medication is passing medication . . . nursing is nursing! He says, "What's the big deal? I'm already doing everything the RNs are doing!"

THINK ABOUT IT

1. How did Jefferson's responsibilities change for each of his roles, from QMA to LPN and, finally, RN? Do you think his employer or other members of the health care team had higher expectations as he climbed the nursing ladder?

2. Do changes in roles, such as moving from LPN to RN, affect the attitudes of co-workers toward you and what you are doing?

3. As you move toward your RN role, what are your thoughts about the other nursing positions (QMA, LPN, etc.)? Do people in these positions have value on the health care team, or should they be following in your footsteps in education?

INTRODUCTION

You have just embarked on a new adventure that will require an adjustment in your professional role. In the previous chapter we discussed strategies to assist you as you make the transition to the student role. In this chapter we will focus on the transition and socialization process needed in making the change from LPN to RN, and the role conflicts you may encounter in the transition. We will define the nursing role and look at the components of that role. We will also explore the change process in making the transition from LPN to RN. By the end of the chapter you will have information to assist you in becoming an RN.

TYPES OF ROLE

A **role** is a set of expectations or behaviors society assumes a person in a certain position or occupation will perform (Business Dictionary, 2009; Merriam-Webster online, 2009). Each of us assumes various roles in the course of a day. Some of these roles may be parent, partner, friend, counselor, chauffeur, teacher, chef, and nurse. As a nurse completes his daily personal and professional responsibilities, he assumes many roles to complete the work effectively.

Some LPN students may re-enter nursing education thinking their nursing role will not change once they become an RN. They believe they will still use the clinical skills they have been using as an LPN. Some clinical duties *will* be the same, and the LPN often performs them with expertise. So, what changes are needed to become an RN?

In becoming an RN student, the LPN student will change, or make a role transition, in personal identity and role function (Amos, 2001). Every change or "challenging situation brings the chance to grow wiser and more skillful" (Brunkhorst, 2006). One of the main changes that occurs is performance of the same clinical skills with improved and refined critical thinking. Rather than doing a routine procedure, an LPN-RN student learns to analyze diagnostic test results, analyze the client's overall condition, and evaluate whether the procedure should be done on the client. He will then accept the responsibility of using his own critical thinking skills to determine whether the client's condition may be jeopardized by the procedure. Critical thinking skills are continually refined throughout the education experience. The refinement and application of critical thinking is part of transitioning into the role of RN.

CRITICAL THINKING ACTIVITY

1. What role changes do you anticipate occurring in your life in the next two years?
2. Think of three specific ways your professional role will change by becoming an RN.

ROLE RESPONSIBILITIES

Some of the roles society may place on a nurse are competent worker, organized care provider, knowledgeable caregiver, caring person, and hard worker. In fact, the nurse's roles include advocate, counselor, researcher, mentor, collaborator, change agent, educator, entrepreneur, role model, leader, and communicator (Figure 2–1). We will discuss these role responsibilities to gain a better understanding of the RN's role.

Advocate

An **advocate** speaks for or acts on behalf of another person. At times, this is the role of the nurse. The client may request the nurse to speak to a doctor on his behalf. The nurse's duty is to act on behalf of the client. A nurse asks a physician to repeat an explanation of a scheduled procedure to a nonassertive client. A nurse stands up for a client's right to refuse a procedure. "Because of nursing's presence, patient and family are never alone, never left uncared for or uninformed, and never left without an advocate" (Dickenson-Hazard, 2000, p. 8).

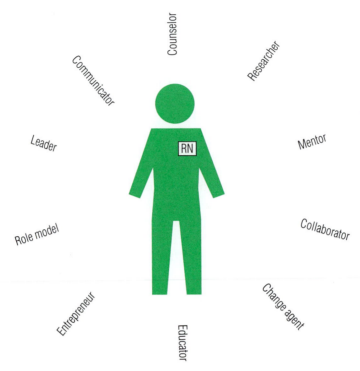

Figure 2–1 Nurses' Roles.

Counselor

The nurse, as a **counselor,** listens to a client and uses therapeutic communication to assist the client in making a choice that determines his health outcome. For example, a nurse lends an ear to a client who is debating two or more choices. It is important for the nurse to explain, define, and review the client's options. The final decision, however, always remains with the client. For example, a client may be deciding whether to proceed with chemotherapy treatment at a local hospital or seek other treatment options at the Mayo Clinic. The nurse answers questions and reviews options with the client, but the treatment decision ultimately lies with the client.

The RN's education prepares him to identify a client's emotional status. The RN identifies the client's anxiety level, assesses the client's coping skills, and determines the client's defense mechanisms. This knowledge assists in counseling the client.

Researcher

Each day nurses are faced with multiple questions to answer and many scientific problems to solve. What is the best way to treat pressure sores? Is a certain type of dressing more absorbent than another, and, if it is, how does that affect the client's healing process? Is medication X more effective for the client than medication Y? What are the benefits and side effects of each? In participating in clinical research on scientific questions such as these, the RN functions as a **researcher**. The goal of nursing research is to improve the quality of client nursing care. An RN develops research questions, collects data for research, values research results, and applies research findings to practice. A master's- or doctorate-prepared RN is usually the nurse who conducts research. However, all RNs can be involved in collecting data for research and in initiating nursing research questions.

Substantiated research can provide quality evidence-based practice. Sigma Theta Tau International (2005) defines evidence-based practice as the "integration of the best evidence available, nursing expertise, and the values and preferences of the individuals, families, and communities who are served." Following the guidelines of the definition, nurses practice according to the best research evidence to meet the uniqueness of each client's need. Sendelbach (2008) gives the example of a client with open-heart surgery who requests not to have a blood transfusion because of religious beliefs. Erythropoietin, a hormone that stimulates red blood cell production, is given instead of the usual blood transfusion. The medical intervention addresses quality evidence-based practice and the client's personal desires. This is quality research-based or evidence-based nursing care.

Mentor

Webster's New World Dictionary and Thesaurus defines **mentor** as "a wise, loyal adviser." As a mentor, the nurse is a wise adviser to a new graduate or new employee and is loyal to that individual by assisting him with unit procedures and policies, explaining unit equipment, and walking alongside the new nurse, easing his adjustment to the unit in every possible way.

Sometimes a mentor is called a *nurse preceptor*. A new nurse or graduate is assigned to another nurse, a preceptor, who assists the new nurse as he transitions onto the unit. The preceptor fulfills the role of a confidant, allowing the new nurse to ask questions in a safe, supportive environment so that the nurse can smoothly adapt to the work environment and the role of nurse. This type of program often enhances recruitment and retention of nurses. An RN fulfills the role of a mentor or preceptor. Even if the mentor/preceptor role is not part of a formal program, it is important that every RN assume the mentor role when a new nurse comes into the work environment.

Collaborator

The nurse **collaborator** interacts with the personnel of several departments to coordinate the client's care. The client may be referred to physical therapy, occupational therapy, radiology, surgery, and social services. The nurse skillfully schedules and communicates the client's needs to each of these departments and fulfills the role of collaborator. An RN assumes the role of collaborator by meeting with multidisciplinary personnel to achieve the client's goal of maximum health and by meeting with family members to plan care with the client. In completing these tasks, the RN may delegate responsibilities to other nurses and then follow up on the delegated tasks.

Change Agent

In our present health care delivery system, changes occur on a daily basis. Often these changes are brought about by nurses or with the nurse's input. The nurse gains an understanding of the change process and becomes a vital **change agent**. The "idea person" is an essential asset to the nursing unit and nursing in general. A creative nurse that possesses personal and communicative skills persuades others that change is needed and is instrumental in facilitating the needed change as smoothly as possible. Some units function more smoothly when nurses work 12-hour shifts or if shift flexibility is provided. The nurse can be a vital change agent to persuade a facility's administration and the nursing staff to try the idea of flexible shift scheduling. The RN is a dynamic change agent by writing proposals, making appointments with administrators and sharing their ideas, actively participating in staff meetings, and becoming an active committee member.

Nurses take an active change agent role in Magnet status hospitals that support nursing involvement in data collection and decision-making in patient care delivery. Nurses' decision-making abilities are valued in providing quality nursing care and attaining excellent patient outcomes. Hospitals open to nurses' input, willing to change to provide evidence-based practice, are cutting-edge hospitals that provide an exciting work environment.

Not only are nurses change agents within the health care system, but they also play a very effective and influential role in the formation of public policy. They can write legislators and influence politicians regarding legislative bills for home health care and health care in general. Issues that still need resolution are prescription coverage for the elderly, large companies' giving kickbacks to physicians for prescribing their branded drugs rather than encouraging physicians to prescribe generic drugs, and staffing issues in nursing homes and hospitals. RNs become aware of and have the opportunity to get involved in current issues by reading newspapers, listening to or watching local and world news programs, reviewing congressional bill proposals on-line, e-mailing politicians, and participating in professional nursing organizations.

Educator

All nurses perform the role of **educator** on a daily basis with clients as they explain procedures, lab tests, disease processes, and care interventions. Through the education process, an RN is taught critical thinking techniques to meet the emotional needs of clients as procedures and diagnostic tests are explained.

The RN often functions as a staff educator. He reads current literature and shares new knowledge with co-workers. As research is published, he shares the findings with co-workers and applies them to client care. It is important that nurses recognize the role of educator and make learning a lifelong process through attending seminars and local presentations and reading current literature.

Entrepreneur

A nurse becomes an **entrepreneur** by venturing into health care businesses. Many are doing so. Nurses willing to take a business challenge and use their professional skills fill gaps in the health care system. These nurses have expanded the scope of nursing and health care. Nurse entrepreneurs are offering health education, ostomy care, aromatherapy, case management, and counseling services. Three LPNs started an adult day care center in a moderate-sized midwestern U.S. city. Nurse practitioners are starting and managing health clinics.

There are several steps to take to embark on this type of venture. First, the nurse sees a need that is not being met in the present health care system. Second, he completes a market analysis (or hires someone to complete one) to see if the product or service is truly needed in the community. Third, he completes a market test with the product or service, followed by a business trial run. Before becoming an entrepreneur, the nurse must have a solid knowledge of the business world and of government policies addressing the desired business (Hood & Leddy, 2005). Health care entrepreneurship is limited only by lack of imagination and initiative.

Role Model

As a **role model** a nurse is a professional example for student nurses and new graduates. Nurses are role models as they interact with clients, health care team members, and co-workers. A nurse who facilitates a positive, encouraging, supportive work environment is one of the best role models on the health care team.

Leader

RNs often assume the role of **leader** as they manage client care, hospital units, and clinics. However, leadership is demonstrated in decisive decision making and in accepting autonomy, responsibility, and accountability in providing competent care. Dickenson-Hazard (2000) states, "Every nurse is a leader . . . [because] every nurse exercises leading-edge authority to influence the health of those in his or her care." It is important for the LPN-RN student to learn leadership skills.

When an RN assumes leadership responsibilities, sometimes co-workers become jealous and make the job more difficult for him. When co-workers become leaders, a professional nurse supports and encourages the RNs to be successful in their new leadership role.

Communicator

The art of therapeutic communication is taught in nursing education because communication skills are essential for nurses. The nurse as **communicator** uses therapeutic communication to relate information and to explore clients' feelings and thoughts. So often, these skills are forgotten in the rush of daily responsibilities. Yet it is important to communicate in a therapeutic manner with a client.

The techniques of therapeutic communication are also effective in interpersonal communication. It is a joy to see nurses communicate effectively with one another as their communication skills become second nature.

CRITICAL THINKING ACTIVITIES

1. List nurse role responsibilities other than those described in the text.
2. How many of the role responsibilities described in the previous section have you fulfilled as an LPN?
3. What entrepreneurial ventures would you like to undertake if money, life responsibilities, or other issues were not a factor?
4. Give an example of effective communication you witnessed at work or on a clinical site.
5. What political nursing issue would you like to address with a legislator?
6. Choose an RN in a role you find interesting in your community. Shadow the RN for one day and then list and describe the responsibilities of his or her role.

ROLE SOCIALIZATION

As you move through the educational process, your clinical nursing skills will expand, you will acquire new critical thinking ability, and you will internalize a new personal identity. Your LPN education is very important and will be utilized in developing this new role. You have chosen to move to a different level in your education and professional status. This involves a process called role socialization. In the role socialization process, personal identity meshes with professional identity. You have professionally identified with the RN nursing role. **Role socialization** is developing an internal attitude toward a profession. When role socialization occurs, you can proudly say, "I am an RN." You had this same feeling when you became an LPN, and now you are in the process of assuming a new identity—that of an RN. The resocialization process began when you decided to enroll in the RN program. During the educational process, you will learn new skills, a new way of thinking, and have a chance to develop new values toward the nursing profession.

As an adult learner, you have some special expectations and goals for the educational process. Lawler (1991) lists nine principles of adult learning. As you read these nine principles, examine their relevance to your present philosophy of education.

1. Adult learning requires an atmosphere of respect.
2. A cooperative, two-way learning environment is essential to adult education.
3. Adult education builds on the education of the participant.
4. Adult education encourages critical contemplative thinking.
5. Adult education presents situational problems and encourages problem solving.

6. Adult education is pertinent and applicable.

7. Adult education is an active, give and take process with the adult learner taking part in the learning process.

8. Adult education gives power and immeasurable opportunity to the learner.

9. Adult education stimulates the learner to be self-directed and independent.

These nine principles are essential for the LPN-RN student. The LPN comes to the learning environment with a foundation of knowledge and experience to be refined and advanced to the next educational level.

It is important for the LPN to have a voice and be involved in the learning process. One way to involve yourself in the learning process is to collaborate with staff nurses and faculty members as you are learning new nursing concepts. In the learning environment, seek to find solutions to clinical and client problems. The staff and nursing faculty serve as role models to demonstrate critical thinking skills. Take the opportunity to interact with staff and faculty members to examine and analyze clinical situations.

Your experience as an LPN provides you with confidence, comfort, and a degree of independence in the clinical environment. As you collaborate with staff and faculty members, seek feedback as to ways you can improve your critical thinking skills and clinical performance. This is an opportunity for the LPN to blossom and reach full potential.

During the process of becoming an RN, it is important for the LPN to value past education and, at the same time, meet the challenge of accepting new ideas, improving critical thinking skills, and learning new nursing techniques. This will be a time of tremendous growth and change.

Hood and Leddy (2003, p. 97) state, "The socialization process involves changes in knowledge, attitudes, values, and skills. These changes can be associated with conflict and strong emotional reactions." The process of acquiring new skills, knowledge, and values may occur several times in your lifetime. Two role socialization transitions that will soon occur in your life are adjusting to the educational process and adapting to the new role of registered nurse. Throwe and Fought (1987) developed a resocialization assessment tool (Table 2–1) that uses Erik Erickson's theory of developmental stages to identify changes that will occur in a nurse's life as he either resists or accepts a new role identity. You can use this tool periodically to evaluate your personal role socialization progress as you advance through your educational experience and move into your role as an RN.

CRITICAL THINKING ACTIVITIES

1. At what point did you truly identify or become socialized in your role as a new LPN? What were the biggest factors in shaping your professional identity?

2. Describe where you are today in the socialization process as an LPN-RN student.

3. Choose three of the nine principles of adult learning that are most important to you. Explain the significance of these three principles to your present educational process.

Table 2–1 Resocialization assessment tool

Developmental Task	Role-Resisting Behaviors Observed	Role-Accepting Behaviors Observed
Trust/mistrust		
Learns to trust the worlds of education and work through consistency and repetitive experiences	Physically isolated from peers both in class, clinical Does not initiate interactions with others Responds only if called on	Involved with classmates Readily and quickly forms/joins groups when directed Initiates discussions with others Asks for clarification
Autonomy/doubt		
Begins to develop independence while under supervision	Delays joining groups for unstructured activities Does not contribute easily Forgets or suppresses assignment dates Does not meet target dates Self-conscious about being evaluated by others	Joins groups for unstructured activities (study groups) Shares information with group, prepares for activities Meets target dates Able to interact in the teaching/learning environment Begins to develop independence with guidance
Initiative/guilt Can independently identify plan, and implement skills/assignments	Perceives objectives and assignments as not worthwhile Stress-related symptoms increase Has difficulty setting priorities Waits for instructor to initiate priority setting Lacks initiative to deal with conflicts Unaware of available resources	Objectives and assignments take on meaning Applies new skills, content to other work settings Effective in time management Renegotiates deadline extensions when appropriate Takes initiative in resolving conflict situations Aware of and uses available resources
Industry/inferiority		
Behavior is dominated by performance of tasks and curiosity—individuals need encouragement to attempt and master skills	Elicits performance rewards and feedback from others Needs direct encouragement especially when performing affective and cognitive skills Last to volunteer to demonstrate new behaviors Seeks rewards by performing old familiar skills rather than those in new dimensions Demonstrates disengaging behaviors (late, uninterested, resistive to learning opportunities)	Able to reward self Confidence thrives Eager to try out new skills; takes risks Volunteers to demonstrate new behaviors Profits from guidance and direction of others Applies self beyond family/work setting Curiosity channeled through education system

Table 2–1 (continued)

Identity/role confusions

The individual searches for continuity and structure, is concerned with how he/she is accepted by others; how he/she is accepted by self; each individual struggles to shape or formulate own identity	Needs a structured clinical setting to further develop ego identity	Searches for continuity and structure but can adapt to unstructured clinical settings
	Sees old job as ideal and denies need for change	Identifies role models in clinical setting
	Serious about learning (content and clinical) practice	Articulates need for change or for modification of job-related roles and procedures
	Frustrated with nursing as a career choice	Appears to enjoy learning and performing in clinical settings
	Too ideological or overly critical of others	Idealistic about own achievements and progress in educational system

Intimacy/isolation

Seeks to combine his/her identity with other self-selected individuals	Participates as a member but resists group leader role	Volunteers to lead work/study groups
	Does not participate in professional meetings	Participates in professional organizations
	Unsupportive of others' educational advancement	Recruits others and represents school
	Feels no increased esteem in performing new role behaviors	Demonstrates pride in new role behaviors and shares with others in work settings
	Meets minimal requirements and sees instructor only in evaluative role	Seeks out instructor for additional learning, information, and professional growth opportunities
	Resists using newly developed skills, more comfortable with previous level of performance	Values symbols of profession (using assessment tools, RN name tags)
	Avoids giving feedback to agency personnel	Evaluates ability of clinical agencies to facilitate meeting learner objectives
		Provides feedback to agency personnel

Table 2–1 (continued)

Generativity/stagnation

Efforts are made to guide and direct incoming students; assists others	Avoids social interaction and information sharing with incoming students Provides minimal care, unconcerned about continuity of patient care Selects patients with common familiar clinical disorders No increased ease of learning or improved test-taking abilities Does not elect to test out of course requirements Stagnates in same job setting	Guides and directs incoming students Provides quality nursing care to patient, family, and community Takes calculated risks (questions level of care, seeks multiple learning opportunities, shares level of expertise, elects to test out required elective courses) Demonstrates critical problem-solving skills Attains mastery of test-taking skills Self-directed learner Demonstrates clinical problem-solving in own work setting Uses holistic approach to delivery of health care

Ego integrity/despair

Acceptance of one's own progress, achievement, and goals through realistic self-appraisal	Frustrated with progress and achievement; stagnated in developing new goals Crisis prone when changing roles Self appraisal unrealistic Does not participate in structured educational opportunities Returns to old job and does not modify role performance Sees no reward in risk-taking High risk for dissatisfaction with profession	Accepts progress, achievement and goal attainment Realistic in self-appraisal Resets professional goals (graduate school, participation in continuing education, certification) Joins new perspectives on old job by use of critical thinking Takes risks (new jobs, different clinical setting, and leadership roles)

(From "Landmarks in the Socialization Process," by A. Throwe and S. Fought, 1987, *Nurse Educator,* 12, pp. 16–17. Reprinted by permission of Lippincott-Raven Publishers.)

ROLE TRANSITION

Role transition implies a change in one's role requirements, expectations, and work responsibilities. It also requires an internal change in the way one thinks about or views the new role. As you move through the process of becoming a registered nurse, your job requirements, expectations, and work responsibilities will change. At first you may think that you are performing the same responsibilities. To a degree you are. You still change dressings, administer medications, and assess clients. However, as you progress in the education process, you will perform these duties with more knowledge, critical thinking skills, and nursing judgment. A role transition is occurring. This is a process, not an overnight change. Abrams (2003) states, "If you see yourself as being in a process of transformation you're more likely to feel—and be—successful than if you see change as black and white. According to Abrams, it takes at least a year for a change or new behaviors to become a habit or routine.

Nicholson and West (1988) describe four stages in work transitions when a company downsizes. These four stages (preparation, encounter, adjustment, and stabilization) also relate to other life transitions (see Figure 2–2).

The preparation stage is mostly concerned with psychological preparedness for the transition that is occurring. When changing roles from LPN to RN, one must psychologically desire the change. The LPN examines personal qualities and decides if he possesses the personal mental and emotional abilities needed to become an RN. During this time, the LPN closely watches RNs to see how they function and what they do. Then, the LPN measures the observed skills against his own abilities.

The encounter phase is the first few days and weeks after the initial psychological decision to change has been made. During the encounter phase, the LPN makes the necessary contacts to enroll in college, makes financial arrangements, and revises personal schedules to accommodate class and clinical schedules. In this stage, the LPN may experience a feeling of loss or disconnectedness.

In the adjustment stage, one focuses on and establishes a new set of priorities. The LPN may find that previous relationships with co-workers change as he makes the appropriate

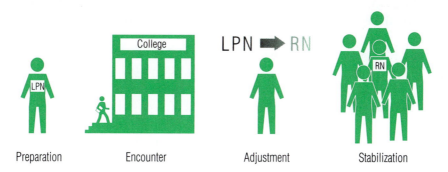

Preparation   Encounter   Adjustment   Stabilization

Figure 2–2 Stages in Work Transition.

changes in his work role. Some of these changes will begin occurring during the nursing education process and continues after the LPN has become an RN, as he takes on the culture of the new RN role. In this stage, the LPN feels somewhat pulled between two worlds: the world of the previous LPN role and the world of the RN role.

In the stabilization stage, the LPN takes on the responsibilities of the RN role. He makes adjustments and minor changes as needed and enjoys the successes of the new role.

Viewing the transition as a challenging opportunity will help prepare you emotionally and mentally for the growth process. An appropriate transition phrase from the movie *Dead Poet's Society* is *carpe diem*, "seize the day." Seize the opportunity the transition offers you. The rewards will be bountiful.

CRITICAL THINKING ACTIVITIES

1. How did you feel when you transitioned into the LPN role? What surprised you the most? What do you wish you had done differently?

2. Identify your present transition phase in becoming an RN and explain your rationale for choosing this phase.

ROLE CONFLICT

Role conflict occurs when a person's role has two or more conflicting or incompatible expectations. From the individual's perspective, the two role expectations seem to conflict with each other, and the person experiences a dilemma in trying to assume both roles.

Role conflicts can be intrapersonal or interpersonal. An example of an intrapersonal conflict is a student who needs to study but feels guilty for not spending more time with significant others, or who struggles to meet school responsibilities and social obligations. Interpersonal conflict occurs when other people's expectations differ or conflict with each other or with one's personal view of the role. An example of an interpersonal conflict is a doctor requesting a nurse to perform a procedure in a manner contrary to a facility's policy. The nurse would have a role conflict between the doctor's expectations and the employer's expectations.

An LPN in an RN program may experience role conflict emotionally and physically. Emotionally the LPN may struggle because he is content as an LPN, yet he is receiving pressure from an employer to become an RN. The LPN may struggle with knowing how to perform a clinical skill but needing to relearn certain methods of doing the procedure to successfully pass the procedure in a lab check-off. If an LPN is working while going to school, the LPN may struggle with being able to perform a procedure as an RN student but not while working as an LPN. The role expectations in each of these situations are incompatible, leading to a potential role conflict. As these conflicts build, the person may develop hypertension, peptic ulcers, or other psychosomatic illnesses.

The LPN student can avoid some of these conflicts by prioritizing tasks, using effective communication skills, and appropriately delegating responsibilities. For example, in dealing with the previously stated conflict between doctor and employer expectations, the nurse uses assertive communication skills. He states that his employer has certain expectations of him in completing the procedure, and, therefore, he will not be able to do the procedure as the doctor has requested.

CRITICAL THINKING ACTIVITY

1. Describe a time when you experienced a role conflict.

THE CHANGE PROCESS

Change is a certainty in life. A **change process** is your response to pressures during various life experiences that cause modifications in behavior. The health care system has undergone and is still experiencing the effects of change with facility mergers and the nursing shortage.

We usually adapt more easily to internal forces than to external forces because the motivation for change starts within us and is not done to us.

Kurt Lewin developed the classic change theory in 1951. Since that time, others have modified the change theory but still use the three stages of Lewin's theory: unfreezing, moving, and refreezing (Figure 2–3). Lewin's theory is based on restraining forces and driving forces (Figure 2–4). Restraining forces are the issues in life or in society that resist change, such as fears, perceived threats, values, and relationships. Driving forces are the motivators to change, such as a desire for a different method or operational norm.

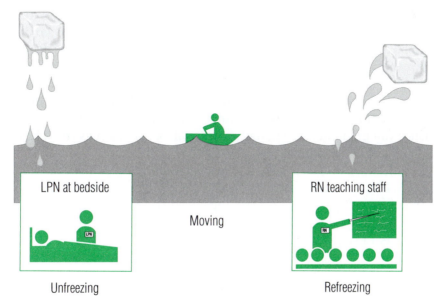

Figure 2–3 Three Stages of Lewin's Change Theory.

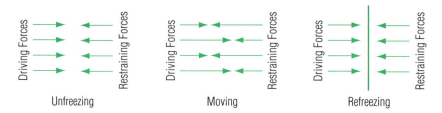

Figure 2–4 Restraining Forces versus Driving Forces.

The unfreezing phase can be an uncomfortable, restless time as a person senses or is told a change is about to occur. If the person desires the change, there is less uneasiness at this time. During the unfreezing phase, there is a struggle between the restraining and driving forces as they jockey to resist or change the status quo. For change to occur, the driving forces must surpass or become more powerful than the restraining forces (12manage, 2009).

In the moving phase, the person has accepted the change and is setting goals to determine the direction of the change. If the change involves several people, it is important to involve all of them during this time. Change is easier if everyone feels they have input and that their input is valued.

In refreezing, equilibrium has been established and the change has become the new status quo. The benefits of the change are emphasized during the refreezing phase.

An example of the change process is your decision to return to school to become an RN. In the unfreezing stage, you went through a process of deciding to return to school. The decision may have been more difficult for some of you than for others. Perhaps you personally made the decision and it affected only you. Or perhaps you made the decision but needed to discuss its ramifications with your family. Perhaps an employer made the decision for you. You may have experienced a time of discomfort or a time of motivation, depending whether the decision was an internal force or an external force. In the moving phase, you had to make goals and plans to accomplish the task of returning to school. In the refreezing phase, your adaptation to student life is (or will be) reinforced and your student role becomes the new status quo. Once you graduate, the change process will occur again as you adapt to the new nursing role and work environment.

12manage, a network of executives that specializes in management techniques, developed a Force Field Diagram that illustrates the driving forces in a change process (see adapted Force Field Diagram in Figure 2–5) (12manage, 2009). They also developed an analysis process (critical thinking process) to evaluate the change process and the driving forces. 12manage suggests 11 steps in analyzing a change process. The 11 steps are:

1. Describe in detail the present situation that you desire to change.
2. Describe in detail the change you desire to see.

3. Explain what will occur if no action or change occurs.

4. Identify and list all the driving forces toward the situation.

5. Identify and list all the restraining forces toward the situation.

6. Discuss and examine all the forces. Are all the forces valid or real? Is it possible to change the forces? What are the crucial forces to examine/address?

7. Rate the strength of the force either numerically or with a Likert scale (strongly agree, agree, neither agree or disagree, disagree, strongly disagree).

8. List the driving forces on the left of the diagram. List the restraining forces on the right of the diagram.

9. Decide if change is possible.

10. What will happen to the change process if the driving and/or restraining forces are increased? Decreased?

11. Keep in mind that as the driving forces increase and decrease, it may affect the strength of the present driving forces or develop new forces that will affect the change (12manage, 2009).

The above list is a critical thinking process that applies to personal and professional situations that would benefit from change. If this process were applied in your decision to continue nursing education, would anything have changed in the process? Would any steps within the process been easier? Would the final result have been the same?

- Describe a current situation that you believe could be improved or changed:
- Describe the change you desire:

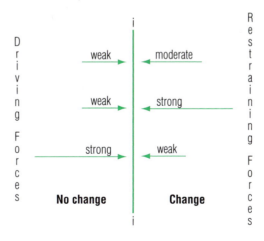

Figure 2–5 Change Process Driving Forces Diagram. Source: Reprinted with permission from 12manage (www.12manage.com). Accessed 9/2009

CRITICAL THINKING ACTIVITY

1. Describe a change process in which you have been involved. What was your role? What were the restraining forces? What were the driving forces? How were others motivated or mobilized in the moving phase?

SUMMARY

When parents take children to a fine-dining restaurant, they expect the children to place their napkin in their lap, use the appropriate fork with the appropriate food, and behave politely. The children are transitioning into a new socialization process.

To a degree, that dining experience is somewhat like the transition from LPN to RN. The RN's role includes a set of expectations in behavior and analytical thinking that is broken down into specific functional components. An LPN has completed certain aspects of these expectations, but in becoming an RN, the role expectations are expanded. A socialization process occurs, and the LPN internalizes the values of an RN and takes on a new identity.

Adults entering an educational experience also have certain expectations. They are self-directed and desire to be an integral part of the educational experience. Faculty members will model critical thinking skills and competence in assessing the client's health status. The LPN will learn the critical thinking skills and clinical expertise needed to function as a competent, decisive, caring nurse.

Transitioning and socialization are change processes. The LPN may experience many interpersonal and intrapersonal emotions and conflicts. He will relearn some nursing procedures, refine his thinking, expand his nursing concepts, and his self-confidence will grow. As the LPN moves through the change process from unfreezing to refreezing, he is equipping himself to move through these steps again and again throughout his nursing career.

CHAPTER REFLECTIONS

1. After reading the chapter, do you feel that you can be an advocate, researcher, mentor, collaborator, and change agent? Were you already doing these things as a nursing assistant, QMA, and/or LPN?

2. Describe the role differences between LPN and RN. Really stop and think about it. What changes can you anticipate as you become an RN?

3. Is this change in your life happening because of an external force or an internal force? Why do you want to become an RN? What stage of Lewin's change theory are you now experiencing?

THEORY TO PRACTICE

1. Develop critical thinking skills that you will use as an RN and analyze the driving and restraining forces of a change issue (see Figure 2–5). Think of a situation that you would like to change. Identify, list, and diagram the driving forces and the restraining forces in the situation using the following diagram. Rate the strength of the forces (weak, moderately strong, strong) and darken and lengthen the lines according to their strength. What could be done to make the change process occur? Describe how the change will be affected if the driving forces or restraining forces increase. Keep in mind that as the driving forces increase and decrease, it may affect the strength of the present driving forces or develop new forces.

CHANGE PROCESS DRIVING FORCES DIAGRAM

- Describe the present situation.
- Describe the change you desire.
- Explain what will occur if no action or change occurs.
- Identify, list, and diagram the driving forces and the restraining forces in the situation. Rate the strength of the forces (weak, moderately strong, strong) and darken and lengthen the lines according to their strength (Figure 2–6).
- Describe a current situation that you believe could be improved or changed:

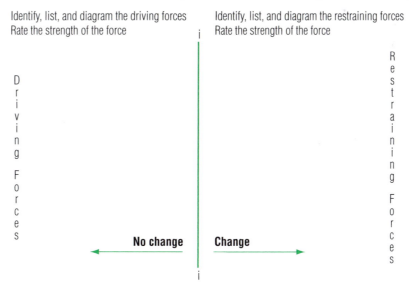

Figure 2–6 Theory to Practice Change Process Driving Forces Diagram. Source: Reprinted with permission from 12manage (www.12manage.com). Accessed 9/2009

- Discuss and examine all the forces. Are all the forces valid or real? Is it possible to change the forces? What are the crucial forces to examine/address?
- Is change possible?
- What will happen to the change process if the driving and/or restraining forces are increased? Decreased?

Keep in mind that as the driving forces increase and decrease, it may affect the strength of the present driving forces or develop new forces that will affect the change (12manage, 2009).

2. a) Develop questions you would like to ask three RNs about their transition from LPN to RN or their RN role.
   b) Interview three RNs with a variety of experiences and backgrounds using the questions you developed. Summarize the interviews.
   c) How can you relate the interview information to your own practice in relationship to professional and personal growth?
   d) What lessons can you take from the RNs you interviewed and transition their experiences into your practice?
3. Send an email to a legislator expressing your concern about an issue that affects nursing in your area or the nation.

Journaling Your Journey

Think about your past experiences as an LPN, your present experiences as a nursing student, and your future as an RN.

1. Describe your current role as an LPN.
2. Describe a role conflict you are experiencing in the role of an LPN/VN and the role of a student. What can you do to alleviate this conflict?
3. Describe what you believe and understand to be the role of the RN.
4. Describe your current strengths as an LPN/VN that will assist you in transitioning to the role of an RN?
5. How do you plan/anticipate to function differently and maybe the same?
6. What nursing roles/functions might you maintain and what do you plan to enhance or improve?

℘ ℘ ℘

My Story...

My hardest adjustment was definitely role conflict! It was hard finding enough time between work, school, and two very active children. I usually coped by studying everywhere I had a chance. I also knew my limitations and had to realize that I was not superhuman and I refused to try.

Taking on more responsibility for my patients was a transition. I continue to do what is right for my patients and cover myself completely. Instead of being under the responsibility of another more educated professional, I am now the one responsible. It is scary . . . I just want to do a really good job and to provide patient care to the best of my ability.

Kyan DiVita, RN

REFERENCES

Abrams, R. (2003). Processing the process of change. USA Today. Retrieved on 3/21/09 at www.uastoday.com/money/smallbusiness/columnist/abrams/2003-11-20-change_x.h

Amos, D. (2001). An evaluation of staff nurse role transition. *Nursing Standard, 16*(3), 36–45.

Brunkhorst, S. (2006). Adapting to change: 5 essential life skills. Ezine @rticle. Retrieved on 3/21/09 at http://exinearticles.com/?Adapting-to-Change:-5-Essential-Life-Skills&id=194914&opt=pr

BusinessDictionary. (2009). *Role*. Retrieved on 3/21/09 at www.businessdictionary.com/definition/role.html

Dickenson-Hazard, N. (2000). Every nurse is a leader. *Nursing, 30*(11), 8–9.

Hood, L., & Leddy, S. (2005). *Leddy and Pepper's Conceptual bases of professional nursing* (6th ed.). Philadelphia: Lippincott Williams & Williams.

Lawler, P. (1991). *The keys to adult learning: Theory and practical strategies*. Philadelphia: Research for Better Schools.

Lewin, K. (1951). *Field theory in social science.* New York: Harper & Row.

Merriam-Webster Online Dictionary. (2009). *Role*. Retrieved on 3/21/09 at www.merriam-webster.com/dictionary/role

Nicholson, N., & West, M. (1988). *Managerial job change: Men and women in transition.* Cambridge, England: Cambridge University Press.

Sendelback, S. (2008). Evidence-based practice: Then and now. American Journal of Nursing, 108(10), p. 75–76. Retrieved on 3/21/09 at journals.lww.com/ajnonline/Fulltext/2008/10000/Evidence_Based_Practice__Then_and_Now.33.aspx

Summers, S. (2008). What is Magnet status and how's that whole thing going? The Center for Nursing Advocacy. Retrieved on 3/21/09 at www.nursingadvocacy.org/cgi-bin/print_article.cgi?article_url

Throwe, A., & Fought, S. (1987). Landmarks in the socialization process from RN to BSN. *Nurse Educator, 12,* 16–17.

12manage. (2009). Force field analysis (Lewin). Retrieved on 3/18/09 at www.12manage.com/methods_lewin_force_field_analysis.html

SUGGESTED RESOURCES

Bacal, R. (2008a). Understanding the cycle of change, and how people react to it. Retrieved on 3/18/09 at http://work911.com; search for *Change Management*.

Bacal, R. (2008b). Understanding the cycle of change, and how people react to iSeven dynamics of change. Retrieved on3/18/09 at http://work911.com; search for *Change Management*.

Bacal, R. (2009). Understanding the change process – How individuals change. Retrieved on 3/18/09 at http://work911.com; search for *Change Management*.

Stefancyk, A. (2009). Transforming care at the bedside. *American Journal of Nursing*, 109(3), p. 68–69.

Chapter 3
Enhancing Assessment Skills

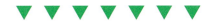

LEARNING OBJECTIVES

By the end of this chapter, you should be able to:

1. Review and enhance assessment skills.
2. Demonstrate therapeutic communication skills when assessing a client.
3. Apply critical thinking skills when analyzing comprehensive client assessment data.
4. Practice a nursing assessment utilizing Gordon's eleven Functional Health Patterns.

KEY TERMS

Gordon's Functional Health Patterns (GFHPs)

Physical assessment

SCENARIO

Jill approaches her 93-year-old female client, who is hard of hearing, and yells "Good-morning!" She proceeds with her assessment, without further explanation, due to the client's poor hearing. Jill completes her routine assessment and gathers good client data. She identifies that the client is alert and oriented to person, place and time; pupils are equal and reactive to light; skin is pink, warm, and dry to touch with pitting edema in both lower extremities; respirations are 22 and currently labored with abnormal lung sounds; heart rate is 90 and irregular, bowel sounds are active and present in all four quadrants. IV is intact and patent in right forearm with no redness, swelling, or drainage at the site. Jill notes that the heart and lung sounds have changed from previous assessments but is unable to identify the exact heart rhythm and abnormal lung sounds involved, so she refers to her mentor RN for further discussion and guidance on how to proceed with client's plan of care.

THINK ABOUT IT

1. Is it appropriate to not explain nursing actions due to known hearing deficit?
2. Did Jill complete an appropriate and comprehensive nursing assessment?
3. Is this the type of information that an LPN would normally take to a mentor RN for guidance?

INTRODUCTION

Life-long learning, the journey of nursing education and the development of skills to provide quality client care continue to evolve over time and include many diverse elements. "The role of the nurse is no longer purely the traditional role of caring and supporting the needs of individuals" (West, 2007, p. 161). Nurses today are required to critically think through different situations and circumstances in each client's individualized plan of care. "Nurses use a wide range of cognitive and physical abilities in daily practice making nursing care a complex and demanding experience even for the most seasoned nurses" (Broom, 2007, p. 22). One of the nursing role's diverse elements is the skill of assessment. Assessment is the process of gathering both subjective and objective data to obtain a holistic view of the needs of both the client and their significant support persons in order to provide individualized quality care. The nursing assessment is one reoccurring feature in the nurse's daily routine, roles, and responsibilities (Jones, 2007).

ASSESSMENT AND COMMUNICATION

As the role of nurses continues to grow and expand, assessment and communication become key components in collaboration among the health care team members to provide the highest quality care for today's client. Nurses need to continue to gain competence in the skill of assessment in order to adequately participate in their constantly developing role. Sharp attention to assessment can often identify subtle changes and needs within client care that may otherwise go undetected. As today's client care becomes more dynamic, it has become more important than ever for the health care team members to collaborate in meeting the needs of today's complex and critically ill clients. Collaboration includes a collection of knowledge and actions leading to a common goal that ultimately provides safer, quality patient care (Stein-Parbury & Liaschenko, 2007). Each client's human body has his own "normal" conditions and behaviors. Nurses have a unique close working relationship with their clients. When their norms begin to change, nurses are able to easily notice. Sudden changes indicate a life threatening situation or emergency that needs immediate attention. Competent and consistent nursing assessment routines identify client physical and psychological changes (Acello, 2007). Acello lists signs and symptoms that should be reported to an RN (Table 3–1). Consider how you would handle these issues if they were reported to you in your new role as an RN.

Table 3–1 Signs and Symptoms to Report to an RN

Chest pain	Pain	Change in mental status
Shortness of breath	Nausea or vomiting	Excessive thirst
Difficulty breathing	Diarrhea	Lethargy
Weakness or dizziness	Cough	Unusual drainage from a wound or body cavity
Headache	Cyanosis or change in color	Changes in vital signs

System or Problem	Observation to Report
Signs/Symptoms of Infection	Elevated temperature
	Rapid pulse, rapid or noisy respirations
	Sweating
	Chills
	Skin hot or cold to touch
	Skin flushed, red, gray, or blue
	Inflammation of skin as evidenced by redness, edema, heat, or pain
	Drainage from wounds or body cavities
	Any unusual body discharge, such as mucus or pus

System or Problem	Observation to Report
Evidence of Pain	Chest pain
	Pain that radiates
	Pain upon movement
	Pain during urination
	Pain when having a bowel movement
	Splinting an area upon movement
	Grimacing, or facial expressions suggesting pain
	Body language suggesting pain
	Moaning or sighing
	Acute headache
	Complaints of binding pain or sensation around forehead
	"Splitting" headache
	Unrelieved pain after pain medication has been given
	Pain is not normal; all complaints of pain should be reported to the RN
Cardiovascular System	Abnormal pulse below 60 or above 100
	Pulse Irregular, weak, or bounding
	Blood pressure below 100/60 or above 140/90
	Unable to palpate pulse or hear blood pressure
	Chest pain
	Chest pain that radiates to neck, jaw, or arm

Table 3–1 (continued)

System or Problem	Observation to Report
Cardiovascular System	Shortness of breath
	Headache, dizziness, weakness, vomiting
	Cold, blue, or gray appearance
	Cold, blue, painful feet or hands
	Shortness of breath, dyspnea, or abnormal respirations
	Blue color of lips, nail beds, or mucous membranes
Respiratory System	Respiratory rate below 12 or above 20
	Irregular respirations
	Noisy, labored respirations
	Dyspnea or Cheyne-Stokes respirations
	Shortness of breath
	Gasping for breath
	Wheezing
	Coughing
	Retractions
	Blue color of lips, nail beds, or mucous membranes
Integumentary System	Skin very dry or very oily
	Rash
	Redness
	Redness in the skin that does not go away within 30 minutes after pressure is relieved
	In dark- or yellow-skinned patients, spots or areas that are darker in appearance than normal skin color
	Pressure ulcers
	Irritation
	Bruises
	Skin discoloration
	Swelling
	Lumps
	Abnormal sweating
	Excessive heat or coolness to touch
	Open areas/skin breakdown
	Drainage
	Foul odor
	Complaints such as numbness, burning, tingling, itching
	Signs of infection

Table 3–1 (continued)

System or Problem	Observation to Report
Integumentary System	Unusual skin color, such as blue or gray color of the skin, lips, nail beds, roof of mouth, or mucous membranes
	Skin growths
	Poor skin turgor/Tenting of skin
	Sunken, dark appearance around eyes
	Cuts, abrasions, skin tears, or other injuries
	Dry, chapped lips
	Dry mucous membranes inside mouth
Gastrointestinal System	Sores or ulcers inside the mouth
	Difficulty chewing or swallowing food
	Unusual or abnormal color or appearance of bowel movement
	Blood, mucus, or other unusual substances in stool
	Hard stool, difficulty passing stool
	Complaints of pain, constipation, diarrhea, bleeding
	Frequent belching
	Changes in appetite
	Excessive thirst
	Fruity smell to breath
	Complaints of indigestion or excessive gas
	Nausea, vomiting
	Choking
	Abdominal pain
	Abdominal distention
	Coffee-ground appearance of emesis or stool
	Oral or rectal bleeding
	Abnormal condition of mouth or teeth, such as ulcerations; dental caries; pain; drainage; lesions on lips or inside mouth; abscesses; cracked, broken, or loose teeth; abnormalities such as bad breath or worn teeth
	Loose dentures or other denture problem
	Dry, chapped lips
	Dry mucous membranes inside mouth
Genitourinary System	Urinary output too low
	Oral intake too low
	Fluid intake and output not balanced
	Abnormal appearance of urine: dark, concentrated, red, cloudy
	Unusual material in urine: blood, pus, particles

Table 3–1 (continued)

System or Problem	Observation to Report
Genitourinary System	Complaints of difficulty urinating or inability to urinate
	Complaints of pain, burning, urgency, frequency, pain in lower back
	Urinating frequently in small amounts
	Sudden-onset incontinence
	Edema
	Sudden weight loss or gain
	Respiratory distress
	Change in mental status
Nervous System	Change in level of consciousness, orientation, awareness, or alertness
	Increasing mental confusion
	Progressive lethargy
	Loss of sensation
	Numbness, tingling
	Change in pupil size; unequal pupils
	Abnormal or involuntary motor function
	Loss of ability to move a body part
	Poor coordination
	Weakness
Musculoskeletal System	Pain
	Obvious deformity
	Edema
	Immobility
	Inability to move arms and legs
	Inability to move one or more joints
	Limited/abnormal range of motion
	Jerking or shaky movements
	Weakness
	Sensory changes
	Changes in ability to sit, stand, move, or walk
	Pain upon movement
	Decreased, unequal, or absent distal extremity pulses
Mental Status	Change in level of consciousness, awareness, or alertness
	Changes in mood or behavior
	Change in ability to express self or communicate
	Mental confusion

Table 3–1 (continued)

System or Problem	Observation to Report
Mental Status	Changes in orientation to person, place, time, season
	Excessive drowsiness
	Sleepiness for no apparent reason
	Sudden onset of mental confusion
	Threats of harm to self or others

Activity	Observations to Report
Activities of Daily Living	Loss of ability to perform an ADL independently
	Increasing need for assistance (note how much assistance, type of assistance)
	Inability to tolerate activity (does patient become fatigued, short of breath, etc.)
	Reduced tolerance to activity
	Weakness
	Pain during certain activities
	Lack of motivation, refusals of care
Dressing and Grooming	Increasing need for assistance
	Need for special services, such as shampoo, cutting of fingernails or toenails, dental services, podiatry services
Walking	Difficulty standing or sitting
	Need for an assistive device, such as a cane or walker
	Unsafe use of an assistive device
	Poor safety awareness
	Gait unsteady, shuffling, rigid, and so on
	Abnormal posture (leaning, pain)
	Sudden onset of falls, weakness, difficulty balancing
Position, Movement	Loss of ability to sit, stand, move, or walk
	Inability to position or reposition self
	Need for special positioning aids
	Presence of contractures, stiffness, or rigidity
	Deformity, edema
	Abnormal range of motion
	Loss of ability to move part or all of body
	Movements shaky, jerking, tremors, muscle spasms, other
	Spasticity (sudden, frequent, involuntary muscle contractions that impair function)
	Presence of pain upon movement
	Splinting, grimacing, or other body language suggesting pain on movement

Table 3–1 (continued)

Activity	Observations to Report
Eating	Food likes and dislikes, refusals
	Lack of adherence to therapeutic diet
	Need for feeding assistance (note how much assistance, type of assistance needed)
	Consumed less than 75 percent of meal
	Difficulty chewing or swallowing, coughing, choking
Drinking	Inability to take a drink at will without assistance
	Inability to drink from straw, cup; need for special device
	Refuses water, if offered (note beverage preferences)
	Inadequate fluid intake
	Difficulty swallowing liquids, coughing, choking
Sleeping	Inability to sleep
	Sleeps constantly
	Sleeps during day, awake at night
	Difficult to awaken
	Needs to be repositioned by staff
	Need to be awakened for toileting
	Safety awareness upon awakening; does patient call for assistance before rising?
	Need for one or more side rails for positioning
	Need for other positioning aids

(From *Advanced Skills for Health Care Providers, 2nd* ed., by B. Acello, 2007, Clifton Park, NY: Delmar/Cengage Learning.)

CRITICAL THINKING ACTIVITY

As you transition into your new role, the signs and symptoms presented in Acello's table, will be brought to you and you as an RN will make nursing judgments and decisions that affect client care and expected outcomes.

1. What resources might you as an RN use to address these questions?

2. Why do we expect the RN to have these answers?

3. Is it expected that the RN will always know the answer?

Gordon's Functional Health Patterns

As you are transitioning in your nursing career, it is generally understood and recognized that as an LPN, you are experienced in completing head-to-toe assessments and are competent in performing accurate and thorough basic assessments. Many LPN to RN students are credited for this experience and knowledge and therefore do not repeat a health assessment or fundamentals type class. As you become a registered nursing student, it is important to take advantage of opportunities to further develop and enhance your assessment skills. Take time to critically think through the rationales of your actions and their ramifications. One way to refine nursing assessment skills is by learning about or reviewing **Gordon's Functional Health Patterns (GFHPs)**. This assessment method provides a thorough client history and physical assessment. It also assists in adapting client assessments to nursing care plans and the nursing process. We will briefly review GFHPs and then provide you with some "real world" or "theory to practice" scenarios that will encourage the use of critical thinking skills, which will assist you in your transition from LPN to RN.

A physical assessment is the gathering of objective data from the nurse's observations, diagnostic procedures, and health record information that together reviews a client's physical state. The nursing heath history focuses on the client's response to illness. This data involves the client's perceptions, feelings, beliefs, and other input from the client and their significant support persons (Gordon, 2008). A nurse utilizes a health history to provide individualized care, to determine the impact the illness has on the client and the family, to determine health teaching needs, and to begin discharge planning.

Margory Gordon (2006) identified eleven functional health patterns to clearly determine what to assess, provide structure for organizing data, guide data collection, and aid in client problem identification. The functional assessment focuses on the psychosocial, physical, and environmental needs and abilities of clients. It determines the abilities of clients to care for themselves. It includes assessment of activities of daily living (ADLs), such as dressing, toileting, and eating. Other aspects of functional assessment include determination of ability to cook, manage finances, and maintain social relationships, along with assessment of self-concept and coping abilities. Gordon's 11 functional health patterns include assessment of:

1. Health perception/health management
2. Nutritional/metabolic status
3. Elimination
4. Activity/exercise
5. Sleep/rest

6. Cognitive/perceptual ability

7. Self-perception/self-concept

8. Role relationships

9. Sexual/reproductive ability

10. Coping/stress tolerance

11. Values/beliefs

The functional assessment explores how individuals adjust and acclimate to their present environment. Throughout the performance of a functional assessment, the interviewer's questions focus on the norms and usual environment of the client. These questions assist in establishing what is normal or purposeful to each individual person. The functional assessment establishes the holistic identification of the client's life and lifestyle.

Topics for questions the nurse can ask within each of the 11 functional health patterns are listed and described in the Guide Sheet for Nursing Assessment (Table 3–2). Through use of the topics in the table, the nurse performs both a health history and a physical examination that results in a thorough and complete nursing assessment.

To perform the physical assessment, the nurse may use either a body systems format or a head-to-toe format. When utilizing a body systems approach, the nurse assesses all pertinent information related to a particular body system: for example, the neurological, cardiovascular, or respiratory system. The body system format can be difficult to remember, whereas in the head-to-toe format the client's body provides a reminder of what should be systematically assessed from head to toe. The physical exam column in Table 3–2 does not follow a head-to-toe approach. Rather, the data acquired in the head-to-toe assessment are grouped under specific health patterns to aid in the identification of client problems and nursing diagnoses.

When incorporating a health history within a head-to-toe assessment, the nurse must remember to include answers to questions about the client's habits or usual patterns along with the physical data collected in the assessment. Functional assessment is best done within the framework of the physical assessment because the environment in which each client resides and participates becomes a part of the physical assessment. The functional assessment brings the client's living environment and physical needs together to establish a holistic picture.

Table 3–2 Guide Sheet for Nursing Assessment

Health History	Physical Exam
Health Perception/Health Management	

• Health perception
  (1) Statement from patient about how patient views overall health
  (2) Statement from patient about why patient is hospitalized
• Lifestyle—Lives:
  Alone or specify with whom
  Type of home
  Nursing home
  No known residence
• Health maintenance:
  Habits: Use of alcohol: none, type and amount per day, week, or month
  Use of tobacco: none, quit date, pipe, cigar, chewing tobacco, cigarettes
    <1 pack per day, 1–2 packs per day,
    >2 packs per day
  Other Recreational or OTC Drugs:
    No, yes
    Type
  Preventive Health Behaviors:
  Breast or testicular self-examination: yes or no
  Date of last physical examination
  Date of last dental examination
• Problems that could contribute to falls or accidents:
  Age 65 or over
  Confused and disoriented, hallucinating
  History of falls
  Recent history of loss of consciousness, seizure disorder
  Unsteady on feet/physical limitations
  Poor eyesight
  Poor hearing
  Drug or alcohol problem
  Post-op condition/sedated
	• General appearance:
	  Race: Caucasian, African American, Hispanic, Asian, other
	  Gender: male, female
	  Age Group: child, teenager, young adult (age), middle aged, elderly
	  Body Build: small, average, large
	  Stature (comparison of height and weight): emaciated, obese, stout, stocky, robust, cachectic, rotund
	  Grooming
	• Signs of distress:
	  Any grossly abnormal signs
	  In acute distress: describe
	  In no acute distress
	• Mental status

Table 3–2 (continued)

Health History	Physical Exam
Health Perception/Health Management (continued)	

Language barrier
Attitude (resistant, belligerent, combative, fearful)
Postural hypotension
• Family history—Risk factors

Nutritional/Metabolic

Health History	Physical Exam
• Previous dietary intake:	• Height and weight:
Diet: Regular, no added salt, ADA, soft, low cholesterol, high fiber, low residue, clear liquids, NPO, list other	• Body temperature:
Vitamins or Supplements: Name	• Skin:
Food Preferences: List	Color: Light pink to dark pink or light brown to dark brown
Appetite: Normal, increased, decreased, presence of nausea or vomiting, decreased taste sensation	Pallor, flushed, cyanotic, ashen, glossy, jaundiced
• Nutritional impairment:	Color Variations: Erythema, ecchymosis/contusion, petechiae, vitiligo, pigmented
Inability to swallow (dysphagia): none, to solids or liquids	Lesions: Macule, patch
Inability to chew	Papule, plaque, nodule, tumor, wheal, verruca, nevus
Inability to feed self	Vesicle, bulla, pustule, furuncle
• Weight fluctuations last 6 months:	Erosion, ulcer, fissure
None, pounds. Gained/Lost	Crust, scab
• Dentures: Upper (partial/full), lower (partial /full)	Excoriation, abrasion, laceration, incisions
Usage—describe	Texture: Smooth, soft, rough, thick, scaling
• Allergies: List, NKDA	Turgor: Returns immediate/returns > 30 seconds
• Skin:	Temperature and Moisture: Warm, dry, extremely cool, extremely warm, wet, oily
History of Skin/Healing Problems: None, abnormal healing, rash, dryness, pruritus, excess perspiration/diaphoresis	Edema: Absent/0, or 1+, 2+, 3+, 4+
Usual Hygiene Practices: Bath/shower, give frequency	• Hair:
Skin-Care Aids: List	Color: Describe
	Length: Describe
	Texture: Fine, coarse, pliant, brittle, dull, shiny, lustrous, glossy
	Amount: Thick, thin, normal
	Distribution: Even, alopecia, hirsutism, sparse
	• Nails:
	Color: Pink, pale, cyanotic splinter, hemorrhages, poor capillary return
	Shape: Beau's lines, clubbing, spooned
	Texture: Smooth, hard, jagged, soft
	Nail Bed: Smooth, firm, pink, inflamed

Table 3–2 (continued)

Health History	Physical Exam
	Nutritional/Metabolic (continued)

- Decubitus risk factor: Calculate and give score
- Mouth:
  Mucous Membranes:
  Color: Pink, pale. cyanotic, reddened
  Consistency: Smooth, moist, dry, bleeding, ulcers, presence of white patches, describe lesions
  Teeth:
  Number: Within normal limits, edentulous
  Position/condition: Stable fixation, smooth surfaces and edges, loose or broken teeth, jagged edges, dental caries, sordes, crooked, protruding, crowded, irregular, broken
  Color: Pearly white and shiny, darkened, brown discoloration
  Gums: Pink, pale, reddened, moist, clearly defined margins, dry, firm, edematous, tenderness, bleeding, ulcers, white patches, receding, shrunken
  Tongue: Symmetry/texture: Moist, papillae present, symmetrical appearance, midline fissures, dry, nodules/ulcers present, papillae or fissures absent, asymmetrical, coated, swollen
- Dietary intake: Regular, no added salt, ADA, soft, low cholesterol, high fiber, low residue, clear liquids, NPO, list other
  Amount Eaten:
  50% or less = poor
  50–75% = fair
  75–100% = good
- Fluid intake during care:
  Oral: give in mL's
  IV: give in mL's

Table 3–2 (continued)

Health History	Physical Exam
	Elimination

Elimination

Health History	Physical Exam

• Previous Urinary Pattern:
 Frequency of voiding: every____ hours or ____ times/day
 Problems: Presence of incontinence, dysuria, hematuria, nocturia, urgency, hesitancy
 • Previous Bowel Pattern:
     Number of BMs/day, constipation, diarrhea, incontinence, presence of ostomy
     Use of laxatives, enemas, suppositories
     Last bowel movement
 • Presence of heavy perspiration/diaphoresis
	• Urinary:
	 Mode: Indwelling catheter, external catheter, incontinence
	 Color: Pale to dark yellow, straw-colored, amber
	 Characteristics: Clear, cloudy, hazy, sediment, aromatic
	 • Bowel/Stool:
	     Bowel Sounds: Audible, hyperactive, hypoactive, inaudible, present, active, not present equally in all quadrants
	     Abdominal Appearance
	     Contour: Rounded, flat, distended, rotund, scaphoid, enlarged, protruding, hard, rigid, relaxed, taut, pendulous, tympanites
	     Symmetry: Symmetrical, asymmetrical
	     Surface motion: no movement, bounding peristalsis, bounding pulsations
	 • Feces:
	     Color: Dark brown, medium brown, mustard yellow, green, dark red/bright red, black, tarry, clay-colored
	     Amount: Small, medium, large
	     Consistency: Soft, semisolid, formed, hard, loose
	     Characteristics: Mucoid, foul-smelling, aromatic, pencil-like, bulky, pasty
	 • Drainage:
	     Amount: Give in mL's, describe size on dressing
	     Color: Pink, red, green, brown, white, yellow
	     Odor: Aromatic, unique, strong
	     Consistency: Thick, mucoid, watery, thin, frothy, tenacious
	     Characteristics: Purulent, suppurative, mucopurulent, sanguineous, blood-tinged, serosanguineous, serous
	 • Emesis:
	     Hematemesis, bile-colored, amount, contents
	 • Fluid output during care:
	     Categorize each type in mL's, then total

Table 3–2 (continued)

Health History	Physical Exam
Activity/Exercise	

- Previous pattern of activity:

  Eating/drinking, bathing, dressing/grooming, toileting, bed mobility, transferring, ambulating, stair climbing, shopping, cooking, home maintenance

  Rate as independent, use of assistive device, assistance from others, assistance from person and equipment, dependent/unable

- History of tolerance limitations:

  Pain, stiffness, dyspnea, fatigue, frequent pauses in activity to rest, dizziness

- Mobility aids:

  Crutches, bedside commode, walker, cane, splint/brace, wheelchair, other

- Exercise pattern/wellness activities:

  Type, frequency, length

- Limitations in ability:

  Missing limbs, paralysis, deformities, casts

- Vital sign ranges:

  Either since hospitalization or verbal from patient

- Use of diversional activities

- Present pattern of activity:

  Eating/drinking, bathing, dressing/grooming, toileting, bed mobility, transferring, ambulating, stair climbing, shopping, cooking, home maintenance.

  Rate as independent, use of assistive device, assistance from others, assistance from person and equipment, dependent/unable

- Musculoskeletal:

  Posture: Relaxed, shoulders back, tense, rigid, slumped, asymmetrical posture, kyphosis, lordosis

  Muscle Tone: Slight resistance, spasticity, rigidity, flaccidity

  Muscle Strength: Rate all major muscle groups according to the following scale—

  0 = No muscular contraction

  1 = Barely flicker of contraction

  2 = Active movement with gravity removed

  3 = Active movement against gravity

  4 = Active movement against gravity and some resistance

  5 = Active movement against full resistance with no fatigue

  Gait: Spastic hemiparesis, scissors, steppage, sensory ataxia, cerebellar ataxia, Parkinsonism

  Balance: Steady, unsteady

  Range of Motion: Unlimited, full, limited with crepitation or pain, immobile, decreased, restricted

  Weight Bearing: Give in percentages—ability to stand on left/right heels/toes, weakness, inability to use either extremity

- Cardiorespiratory:

  Lungs:

  Breath sounds: Clear, crackles, rhonchi, wheezes

  Rate: Apneic, eupneic, tachypneic, bradypneic

  Rhythm: Regular, irregular

  Depth: Deep, shallow

Table 3–2 (continued)

Health History	Physical Exam
	Activity/Exercise (continued)

Health History	Physical Exam
	Cough: Continuous, persistent, frequent, productive, nonproductive, spasmodic, paroxysmal, tight, loose, deep, dry, hacking, harsh, painful, rasping, exhaustive
	Use of O_2: Flow rate and method of delivery—mask, nasal cannula
	Heart:
	Rate: Give in numerical value, tachycardic, bradycardic
	Rhythm: Regular, irregular, regularly irregular, irregularly irregular
	Peripheral Vascular:
	BP
	Peripheral pulses: Strong, equal, bounding, thready, imperceptible, weak asymmetrical, absent, 1+, 2+, 3+, 4+
	Sensation: Nontender, can identify light and deep touch, paresthesia, tenderness, pain, tingling, burning, stinging, prickling, numb
	Motor: Hand grasps and foot movement: equal, strong, weakness, paralysis
	• Present tolerance for activity:
	Pain, stiffness, dyspnea, fatigue, frequent pauses in activity to rest, dizziness
	Sleep/Rest
• Sleep patterns: Bedtime, hours slept	• Observe appearance: Pale, puffy eyes, dark circles
Routine: AM nap, PM nap, work night shifts, --variable shift work	• Observe behavior:
• Sleep aids used:	Yawning, dozing, irritable, short attention span
Medication, food, rituals	
• Position of comfort	
• Problems:	
None, early waking, insomnia, nightmares	

Table 3–2 (continued)

Health History	Physical Exam
Cognitive/Perceptual	

Health History

- Knowledge level
- Educational level achieved
- Primary language spoken
- Developmental level
- Past history of cognitive/perceptual illness
- Past history of sensory perception:
  Heat, cold, taste, smell, touch, vertigo, hearing, sight
- Pain assessment:
  Location, intensity, duration, quality, predisposing factors, grade on 0–10 scale

Physical Exam

- Memory:
  Long term: Intact, impaired; give example
  Short term: Intact, impaired; give example
- Speech:
  Paralanguage: Qualities of speech—pitch, intonation, rate of speaking, voice volume, words that are stressed or accented
  Articulation: Articulate, not articulate: describe
  Sequencing: Logical, illogical: describe
  Appropriateness of Content: Appropriate, inappropriate
  Ability to Express Self Verbally: Words or types of expression used
  Ability to Follow Verbal/Written Instructions: Yes; if no, explain
- Neurological:
  Orientation: Person, place, time
  Pupil Reaction: Sluggish, brisk, PERRLA
  Grasp Strength:
  Level of Consciousness: Comatose, unresponsive to verbal or painful stimuli, semiconscious, stuporous, drowsy, lethargic, alert, responsive
- Perceptual—Cognitive:
  Hallucination: Absent, present
  Delusions: Absent, present
  Attention Span: Intact, not intact: describe
- Sensory:
  Visual Impairment: Absent, present; describe
  Visual Aids: Absent, present: glasses, contacts, prosthesis
  Auditory Impairment: Absent, present: describe— impaired, deaf, tinnitus
  Auditory Aid: Absent, present
  Other Sensory Impairments: Absent, present: describe

Table 3–2 (continued)

Health History	Physical Exam
Self-perception/Self-concept	

• Developmental stage of life:
  Give supporting data
• Ability to accomplish age level tasks:
  Describe
• Present health goals:
  Ask the patient: "How would you describe yourself?"
  "What do you consider to be your strengths?"
  Are the goals and responses age related?
• Body image
	• Posture
	• Eye contact:
	  Present, absent: describe
	• Facial expression (affect):
	  Animated, sad, fixed: describe
	• Grooming:
	  Hair groomed: yes, no
	  Hygiene: good, poor: describe
	  Makeup: present, absent
	  Shaven: yes, no
	  Dress: neat, not neat: describe
	• Attitude: Describe
	• Appropriateness of behavior:
	  Appropriate, inappropriate: describe
	• Mood: Describe
	• Self-derogatory comments:
	  Present, absent: describe
	• Self-affirmative comments:
	  Present, absent: describe
	• Powerlessness:
	  Present, absent: describe
	• Hopelessness:
	  Present, absent: describe
	• Low self-esteem:
	  Present, absent: describe

Role Relationship	

• Patterns of relating to others
• Identification of own role
• Response to authority, peers, subordinates
• Age, marital status, occupation
• Perceptions of responsibilities in life:
  Situation at home, work, and in the community
	• Observe patient's interaction with others:
	  Verbal, nonverbal communication: describe
	  Does patient have visitors?

Table 3–2 (continued)

Health History	Physical Exam
Sexuality/Reproductive	
• Number of living children, abortions, miscarriages, stillbirths	• Breasts:
• Sexual: self-feelings toward sex, role self-concept	Round, pendulous, sagging, equal, pink with/without presence of striae
• Effect of illness or impairment on sexuality	Areola: Pink to dark brown, round oval, everted, presence of discharge
• Present sexual activity	• Genitalia:
• Use of birth control	Presence and distribution of pubic hair, sexually mature, visible lesions, odor, drainage
• Age of onset of menses, menopause	
• Last Pap, mammogram	
Coping/Stress Tolerance	
• Coping patterns:	• Behavior patterns:
Use of counseling, usual methods of problem solving	Abusive to self or others
	Nervous, relaxed, controlled, agitate, mood swings: describe
• Support system	• Appearance
• Recent loss or change in life situation	• Affect
• Presence of stress-related disorders	• Ability to reason and make sound decisions:
	Able, unable: describe
Value/Belief	
• Health/illness beliefs	• Symbols of faith:
• Spiritual, cultural, ethnic heritage, and pattern of participation in	Present, absent: describe
• Concern with meaning of life/death:	• Current religious/cultural ties:
Present, absent: describe	Present, absent: describe (praying, meditation, reading religious materials, clutching religious artifacts, wearing religious jewelry)
• Concern with meaning of suffering:	• Visits from clergy
Present, absent: describe	
• Anger toward God/religion:	
Present, absent: describe	

(Courtesy: University of Saint Francis, Ft. Wayne, IN)

Barkauskas, V., Stoltenberg-Allen, K., Baumann, L .& Darling-Fisher, C. (1994). *Health and physical assessment,* St. Louis, Mosby.

Bates, B. (1995). *A guide to physical examination and history taking.* (Sixth ed). Philadelphia: J. B. Lippincott.

Carpenito, L. (1993). *Nursing diagnosis: Application to clinical practice.* (Fifth ed). Philadelphia: J. B. Lippincott.

Cox, H., Hinz, M., Lubno, M., Newfield, S., Ridenour, N., Slater, M., & Sridaromont, K. (1993). *Clinical applications of nursing diagnosis: Adult, child, women's, mental health, gerontic, and home health considerations.* (Second ed). Philadelphia: F. A. Davis.

Taylor, C., Lillis, C., & LeMone, P. (1993). *Fundamentals of nursing: The art and science of nursing care.* (Second ed). Philadelphia: J. B. Lippincott.

From *Medical surgical nursing: An integrated approach,* by L. White, and G. Duncan, Clifton Park, NY: Thomson Delmar Learning.

CRITICAL THINKING ACTIVITY

1. Identify and list the advantages of using GFHPs.
2. Are there any disadvantages of using GFHPs?
3. Compare using GFHPs to your present assessment method.

SUMMARY

As stated in the opening of this chapter, most LPNs have a strong sense of assessment at this point in their career and have earned recognition for assessment skills. It is also imperative to recognize the value and impact of one's ability to fully assess and care for each individual client. Nursing care is a dynamic process that involves critical thinking and application to unique client situations. What an awesome opportunity for nurses to participate in providing individualized client care. The goal of this quick review of nursing assessment re-establishes the importance and value of what nurses do in their reoccurring, every day routine. Assess with a purpose and communicate well with all appropriate members of the health care team and each individual client and their support persons.

CHAPTER REFLECTIONS

1. Analyze your therapeutic communication skills.
2. Compare GFHPs to your present assessment method.

Journaling Your Journey

Take time now to reflect on your assessment skills.

1. How were your assessment skills in the beginning of your nursing career compared to today's practice routine? Do you remember the first clients you assessed? Describe the most recent clients for whom you cared and your assessment of them?

2. Have you ever had a situation where you identified something in your assessment that has ultimately changed the care or outcome for your client in a positive manner? Describe these scenarios.

3. How might you still improve your current assessment skills? Are you aware of areas that could be stronger? How do you plan to enhance your assessment skills?

ↁ   ↁ   ↁ

THEORY TO PRACTICE

The following ten role playing activities are designed for independent student participation or as a faculty guided activity. Have ten students volunteer to be the client and ten students complete the assessment on the clients. A few of the client scenarios have significant support persons who play important roles in the assessment. Where appropriate have students play the significant support persons' roles.

1. Nurse with a client who speaks a different language—complete your assessment.

2. Nurse with an elderly client who is hard of hearing, appears malnourished, unkempt appearance, and hiding leg ulcer with what appears to be an overly protective and very involved daughter at the bedside—complete your assessment.

3. Nurse (male) with female Muslim client who does not make eye contact and has her husband at bedside at all times to converse and answer any questions—complete your assessment.

4. Nurse with a client who is a retired nurse—complete your assessment.

5. Nurse with terminally ill client that is currently offering little information or conversation and has a family member at side who is a nurse with many questions—complete your assessment.

6. Nurse with a single mother as a client with two young children running around room—complete your assessment.

7. Nurse with client who is the CEO of that facility or the mayor of that city—complete your assessment.

8. Nurse with client who is homeless and has known history of drug and alcohol abuse, possibly HIV positive—complete your assessment.

9. Nurse with client who is actively vomiting and having diarrhea—complete your assessment.

10. Nurse with client of opposite sex who is flirting during the assessment process—complete your assessment.

Next, depending on the roles you played, either pair up with another nurse and report off duty on the client you assessed or meet as a group with all of the clients and their significant support persons when applicable and share your experiences as the clients being assessed.

Return together as a group/class and share your experiences.

1. Were you able to complete your assessment?

2. Did you use a systems approach or head-to-toe?

3. Do you feel your assessment was thorough and complete? Did you address all 11 of GFHPs?

4. Did you use active listening skills and pay attention to verbal and non-verbal communication shared during the assessment?

5. Did you feel comfortable and confident?

6. How did you greet your client—their name and yours? (Any nicknames noted?)

7. What went well and what did not?

8. Did your clients variations impact the assessment?

9. Any feedback you would offer your peers at this time that may help them develop in their assessment and communication skills?

10. Do you feel culturally competent and able to meet the needs of diverse client populations?

11. Identify three ways that you might improve or change your assessment routine as you transition from LPN to RN.

My Story...

I feel that transitioning from an LPN to RN is a wonderful but challenging journey. It was not easy for me to think as an RN. I underestimated the RN program because I felt that I knew a lot and had practiced as an LPN for two years. I discovered that the RN program was much more in-depth. I had to enhance my critical thinking and team leader skills. It was challenging for me to learn to identify client problems. I learned to do a more thorough assessment. There were times that I felt like quitting, because it was challenging to juggle a nursing career, family, bills, school, and other stressors. But the instructors motivated me and encouraged me to continue. Going through the RN program allowed me to gain great respect from family, friends, colleagues, and other students. I would not trade this experience for the world. Because I am an RN, I have the opportunity of advancement. I now am learning to become a charge nurse. It is gratifying when I hear my patients say: "You are a great nurse." Although clinical days seemed long, intense, and tiring, they enhanced my overall growth as a nurse. I have learned the importance of hard work, dedication, education, and time management.

Monique Myles, RN

REFERENCES

Acello, B. (2007). *Advanced skills for health care providers. (2nd Ed.)* Thomson Delmar Learning: New York.

Broom, M. (2007). Exploring the assessment process. *Paediatric Nursing,* 19 (4), 22–25.

Gordon, M. (1995). *Manual of nursing diagnoses 1995–1996 (7th ed.).* St. Louis: Mosby–year Book.

Gordon, M. (2006). *Manual of nursing diagnoses Eleventh Edition. (11th ed.).* Boston: Jones & Bartlet.

Gordon, M. (2008). *Assess notes: nursing assessment & diagnostic reasoning.* FA Davis Company: Philadelphia.

Jones, A. (2007). Admitting hospital patients: a qualitative study of an everyday nursing task. *Nursing Inquiry,* 14(3), 212–223.

Stein-Parbury, J. & Liaschenko, J. (2007). Understanding collaboration between nurses and physicians as knowledge at work. *American Journal of Critical Care,* 16(5), 470–477.

West, S. (2007). Physical assessment: whose role is it anyway? *Journal of British Association of Critical Care Nurses,* 11 (4), 161–166.

Chapter 4
LPN and RN Knowledge and Roles

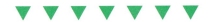

SCENARIO

Kimberly has been an LPN for the last 15 years, and, in that time, she has functioned in many capacities. She was taught many different skills: inserting IVs, caring for central venous lines, blood draws, special dressing changes, and inserting nutritional supplements into feeding tubes of all sizes. She is a very skillful nurse. She also began functioning in a leadership role after being an LPN for just one year, supervising a building of 100 clients, 24 of them in a skilled bed and another 20 on a special unit with Alzheimer's. She was responsible for guiding and directing approximately 30 employees. She organized their work assignments and coordinated their responsibilities throughout the shift. Kimberly dealt with family concerns and client crises as she assisted in reaching a solution to problems. When asked for the reason she is returning to school, Kimberly responds, "Hey, I'm already doing everything the RNs are doing. I might as well get the title and pay along with the work."

THINK ABOUT IT

1. Compare the job descriptions of an LPN and an RN. Are you aware of the Nurse Practice Act for the state in which you practice? Review what you are doing in your current role. Is it within the nurse practice guidelines?

2. Is there a difference between RN and LPN thinking and problem solving? Do you find that an LPN reports to and is guided through difficult situations by an RN mentor?

3. How do you think Kimberly's perception of her role in nursing will change as she transitions into the RN role?

INTRODUCTION

At this point you may be asking yourself, So what *is* the difference between the LPN and the RN? LPN to RN students often perceive their continued education as redundant, instead of looking at it as an opportunity for enrichment and growth. The chapter gives a comparison and contrast of the roles, responsibilities, and knowledge levels of the LPN and the RN. Similarities and differences between the LPN and RN are examined and candidly discussed. Together, we will gain respect for and learn to value the roles and competencies of both the LPN and the RN.

NATIONAL NURSING ORGANIZATIONS' DEFINITIONS OF NURSING ROLES

The national licensing organizations and national nursing organizations defining statements for LPNs and RNs are based on data, research studies, and councils of nurses. These organizations established a valid difference between the LPN and RN.

In 1988 Kane and Colton conducted a job analysis of newly licensed LPNs to establish the entry-level practices of LPNs. Using their data, the National Council of State Boards of Nursing (NCSBN) developed the National Council Licensure Examination for Practical Nurses (NCLEX-PN). In 1993, Chornick, Yocom, and Jacobson conducted a job analysis study similar to the previous LPN study to establish the entry-level practices for RNs. From this study, the National Council Licensure Examination for Registered Nurses (NCLEX-RN) was designed. Cognitive abilities tested on both the LPN and the RN exams are *knowledge, comprehension,* and *application.* The main testing difference between the LPN and the RN exams is that the RN exam has an *analysis* component. A knowledge level question tests the facts; for example, What is the kidney bean–shaped organ in the lower back? Comprehension tests the understanding of the facts; for example, Describe the function of the kidney. Application questions apply facts or put the facts to use; for example, What could an elevated blood urea nitrogen (BUN) indicate? The analysis component of the RN exam is the ability to break down the facts and give the rationale for using or applying the facts; for example, What nursing actions are required when a client's lab report has an elevated BUN? According to the revised Bloom's *Taxonomy of Educational Objectives* (Anderson & Krathwohl, 2001), analysis is a higher level of cognitive thinking than knowledge, comprehension, and application. Analysis requires the RN to use a higher level of critical thinking in making a judgment about the facts or information (see Table 4–1).

In 1989 and 1990, the National League for Nursing (NLN) established roles and responsibilities for practical and associate degree nursing programs as detailed in Table 4–2. The **LPN roles** are detailed as "provider of care," supervised by an RN and "member of the discipline" (Claytor, 1993, p. 228). The **LPN responsibilities** listed under the role *provider of care* are assistance with client assessments and nursing care plans; provision of nursing care; performance of procedures and medication administration; communication with clients, client families, and health care team members; and documentation. The LPN works under the direction of the RN. The LPN responsibilities listed under the role *member of the discipline* are recognition of personal strengths and weakness in relationship to continued educational needs, potential career mobility, and ethical and legal guidelines. The **RN roles** are "provider of care, manager of care, and member of the profession" (Claytor, 1993, p. 228). The **RN responsibilities** listed under the role *provider of care* are initiation, updating, and completion of nursing assessment and nursing care plans, provision of safe nursing care, initiation and completion of discharge planning, utilization of communication techniques including client teaching plans, and documentation. The RN responsibilities listed under *manager of care* are supervision of client assignments and staff, coordination of client conferences, and maintenance of communication with the health care team. The RN responsibilities listed under *member of profession* are maintenance of personal and professional self-development and self-evaluation; maintenance of ethical and legal standards; and participation in research, organizational change process, and quality control measures.

Table 4–1 Distribution of Content for the NCLEX-PN and NCLEX-RN Test Plan. The green font on the chart represents the LPN/VN test content and the black font the RN test content.

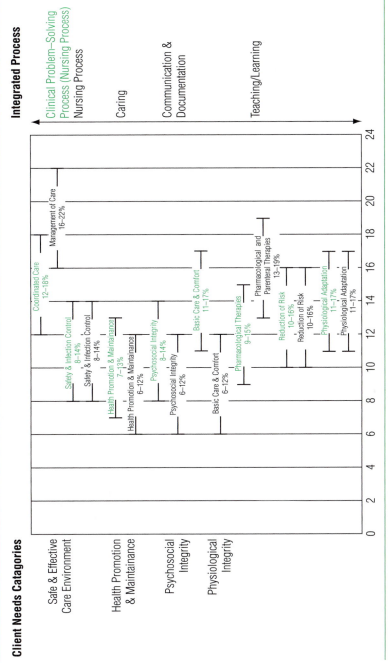

Reproduced from the NCSBN test plans for NCLEX-RN® and NCLEX-PN® and used with permission from the National Council of State Boards of Nursing (NCSBN), Chicago, IL, copyright 2000.

Table 4–2 LPN and RN Roles and Responsibilities

Licensed Practical Nurses	Registered Nurses
Provider of Care	**Provider of Care**
• Assists in client assessment.	• Initiates and/or completes nursing assessment, interview, & history of client.
• Assists with the development, evaluation, & modifications of nursing care plans.	• Initiates & updates written nursing care plans.
• Prioritizes nursing care.	• Implements medical & nursing care plans for clients.
• Gives direct personal care to clients.	• Evaluates & revises nursing care plan through continual assessment.
• Performs technical & nontechnical procedures.	
• Administers medications & monitors IV fluids.	• Provides & participates in comprehensive, safe nursing care to clients.
• Assists clients to prepare for diagnostic tests.	• Initiates client discharge planning.
• Establishes & maintains therapeutic relationship with clients, families, & significant others.	• Makes referrals for continued care after discharge.
	• Assesses verbal & nonverbal communication of clients, families, & significant others.
• Receives information from RN.	• Utilizes communication techniques to assist client in coping with and resolving problems.
• Keeps RN informed.	
• Communicates as appropriate with other health team members.	• Explains nursing care to clients & nonprofessional personnel.
• Documents nursing observations & interventions.	• Implements teaching plans specific to client's level of development, knowledge, & learning needs.
	• Documents nursing care via the nursing process.
Manager of Care Role Not Delineated for LPNs	**Role Not Delineated for LPNs**
• Supervises no one.	• Prepares client care assignments.
• Works under the direction of an RN.	• Assists in evaluation of auxiliary personnel performance.
	• Assists in orientation of new personnel.
	• Supervises employees when in charge of client care.
	• Incorporates cost-effective & environmental safety factors into nursing care plan.
	• Plans, directs, and coordinates nursing care of a group of clients.
	• Initiates, leads, and/or participates in client-centered conferences.
	• Maintains communication & coordination with health care team members.

Table 4–2 (continued)

Licensed Practical Nurses	Registered Nurses
Member of the Discipline	Member of the Profession
• Seeks out learning opportunities and continuing education.	• Assumes responsibility for self-development & self-evaluation.
• Practices within the ethical/legal frame-work of nursing.	• Practices within the ethical/legal framework of nursing.
• Identifies personal potential & considers career mobility options.	• Serves as a role model to members of the nursing team.
• Identifies personal strengths & weaknesses to improve own performance.	• Values nursing as a career.
	• Participates in research (e.g., gathers data).
	• Works within the organizational framework to facilitate change.
	• Assists in quality control measures & procedures.
	• Supports peers in delivery of health care.
	• Utilizes current literature to provide safe care.

(From "Working Effectively with LPN-RN Orientees," by K. Claytor, 1993, *The Journal of Continuing Education in Nursing,* 12 [5], pp. 227–231.)

LPN AND RN ROLES COMPARED WITH THE RN CORE COMPONENTS AND COMPETENCIES

The NLN's detailed LPN and RN roles and responsibilities and RN graduate core components and competencies can be used to compare the nursing roles of the LPN and RN. The NLN-defined LPN and RN responsibilities are embedded in the expected graduate core components and competencies. The discussion of these two tools leads to an understanding of the similarities and differences between the LPN and the RN roles, responsibilities, and knowledge base.

In 2000, the Council of Associate Degree Nursing Competencies Task Force and the National League for Nursing, with the support of the National Organization of Associate Degree Nursing, wrote *Educational Competencies for Graduates of Associate Degree Nursing Programs* (Coxwell & Gillerman). This document defines the competency expectations of associate degree nurses upon graduation. The core components break down the main functions of a nurse, and the competencies describe the expected abilities, skills, or expertise of a graduate associate degree nurse. This document delineates the **core components and competencies** of the associate degree RN as "professional behaviors, communication, assessment, clinical decision making, caring interventions, teaching and learning, collaboration, and managing care" (Coxwell & Gillerman, 2000, pp. 7–11).

Nurses with BSN degrees and advanced practice nurses can expect competencies to expand and include evidence-based practice research, community based nursing, leadership, and management. RNs with higher degrees state that their education experiences improve self-confidence client assessments, critical thinking, collaboration among the health care team, decision making and intervention plans (Phillipchuk, 2007).

Professional Behaviors

In the *Educational Competencies for Graduates of Associate Degree Nursing Programs* (Coxwell & Gillerman, 2000), the definition of **professional behaviors** states that the nurse "adheres to standards of professional practice, is accountable for her/his own actions and behaviors, and practices nursing within legal, ethical, and regulatory frameworks . . . including a concern for others, as demonstrated by caring, valuing the profession of nursing, and participating in ongoing professional development" (p. 7). According to the 1989 description of LPN roles and responsibilities (National League for Nursing, 1989), the LPN demonstrates professional behaviors by seeking continuing education opportunities.

The LPN and the RN have professional behavioral similarities. They both practice within a legal and ethical framework according to their level of practice. Both value caring by providing nursing care to clients and seeking out continuing education opportunities to keep current in nursing practice and knowledge. The RN evaluates personal learning needs and assumes responsibility for continuing education and personal development.

The RN has opportunities to contribute to the profession by gathering research data, facilitating change in the organizational structure, and analyzing and evaluating quality control measures. The RN gathers research data individually or as part of a team by distributing, collecting, and analyzing surveys or conducting interviews. She facilitates changes within an organization by following the change process of analyzing a situation, determining the needed change, recommending desired change to administration, and communicating desired change to colleagues. The RN assists with quality-control measures by participating on committees that develop facility goals, set goal criteria for the facility to meet, and then evaluate how the facility meets the established criteria. Some of the criteria the quality-control committee evaluates are charting, provision of care, and medication administration. Refer to Box 4–1 to see some suggested activities that will expand your knowledge of and appreciation of the RN role.

Box 4–1 Opportunities for Professional Growth

Professional Growth Activities

1. Observe an RN collecting data for a research project.
2. Attend a nurse management meeting to observe ways change is implemented within an organization.
3. Observe an RN conducting quality control within a hospital facility.

Communication

The competencies also define **communication** in nursing as "an interactive process through which there is an exchange of information that may occur verbally, non-verbally, in writing, or through information technology" (Coxwell & Gillerman, 2000, p. 7). "Therapeutic communication is an interactive verbal and non-verbal process between the nurse and client that assists the client to cope with change, develop more satisfying interpersonal relationships, and integrate new knowledge and skills" (p. 7). The LPN has the basic skills to communicate with health care team members and clients. The RN's education and knowledge base give her the ability to assess and analyze verbal and nonverbal communication between clients and family members, clients and health care team members, and among health care team members. The RN also utilizes therapeutic communication techniques to assist clients in coping with problems and to solve problems. Both the LPN and the RN communicate with health care team members, but the RN coordinates communication and activities with clients, family members, and various health care team members.

Assessment

The competencies define **assessment** as "the collection, analysis, and synthesis of relevant data for the purpose of appraising the client's health status. Comprehensive assessment provides a holistic view of the client which includes dimensions of physical, developmental, emotional, psychosocial, cultural, spiritual, and functional status" (Coxwell & Gillerman, 2000, p. 8). The LPN gathers basic data on each of the previously mentioned assessment dimensions and contributes information for the nursing process (Figure 4–1). The RN does an in-depth assessment, analyzes and synthesizes the information, and utilizes the nursing

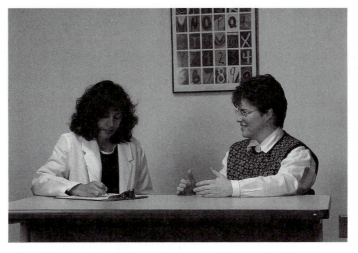

Figure 4–1 Nurse interviewing client.

process steps of goal setting, planning, and interventions to address the client needs. In-depth general education and social science classes equip the RN to assess how each human dimension influences and affects the client.

Clinical Decision Making

The competencies state that **clinical decision making** "encompasses the performance of accurate assessments, the use of multiple methods to access information, and the analysis and integration of knowledge and information to formulate clinical judgments" (Coxwell & Gillerman, 2000, p. 8). The LPN assists in client assessments and works under the direction of the RN. The RN performs more comprehensive, in-depth assessments obtained from multiple sources and then applies critical thinking to determine the best client care approach and rationale.

Caring Interventions

The competencies define **caring interventions** as "those nursing behaviors and actions that assist clients in meeting their needs . . . based on a knowledge and understanding of the natural sciences, behavioral sciences, nursing theory, nursing research, and past nursing experiences. . . . Caring behaviors are nurturing, protective, compassionate, and person-centered" (Coxwell & Gillerman, 2000, p. 9). Both LPNs and RNs provide excellent caring interventions to clients. The RN has more educational background in natural sciences, behavioral sciences, nursing theory, and nursing research that enables her to have a more holistic view with in-depth psychological insight of the client.

Teaching and Learning

The competencies state that **teaching** "encompasses the provision of health education to promote and facilitate informed decision making, achieve positive outcomes, and support self-care activities. Integral components of the teaching process include the transmission of information, evaluation of the response to teaching, and modification of teaching based on identified responses" (Coxwell & Gillerman, 2000, pp. 9–10). The competencies also state that **learning** "involves the assimilation of information to expand knowledge and change behavior" (Coxwell & Gillerman, 2000, p. 10). An RN would fulfill these responsibilities by assessing the needs of the client and then developing an individualized client teaching plan (Figure 4–2).

Learning outcomes are set for the client and then the RN evaluates the client's progress toward those learning outcomes. The RN modifies the teaching plan according to the client's progress in expanded knowledge and observed changed behaviors. Teaching responsibilities of the LPN are not mentioned in the 1989 competencies. However, the LPN assists with some client teaching under the direction of the RN. The depth of teaching increases as the nurse obtains more education.

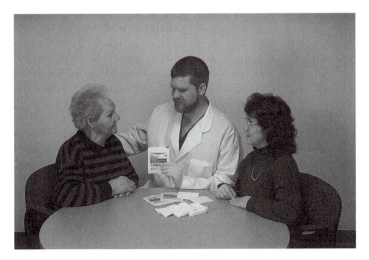

Figure 4–2 Nurse teaching client.

Collaboration

The competencies define **collaboration** as "the shared planning, decision making, problem solving, goal setting, and assumption of responsibilities by those who work together cooperatively, with open professional communication" (Coxwell & Gillerman, 2000, p. 10). The LPN is part of the collaborating team, but the RN initiates and directs the planning, decision making, problem solving, and goal setting of the collaborative process. The LPN assists with the planning, decision making, problem solving, and goal setting.

Managing Care

The competencies define **managing care** as "the efficient, effective use of human, physical, financial, and technological resources to meet client needs and support organizational outcomes" (Coxwell & Gillerman, 2000, p. 10). According to the NLN's LPN roles and responsibilities, the LPN's managing care consists of assisting with client assessments and the development, evaluation, and modification of nursing care plans; prioritizing nursing care; and giving direct client care. The LPN works under the direction of an RN and supervises certified nursing assistants. The RN initiates and completes the nursing assessment including the client interview and history; initiates, evaluates, and revises written nursing care plans; and initiates discharge planning. The RN includes community resources in the discharge planning according to the assessed physical, psychosocial, and financial needs of the client. The RN completes client care assignments; orients, supervises, and evaluates staff performance; is in charge of client care; coordinates care for a group of clients; includes safety and cost-effective factors in the clients' care plans; and leads individualized client conferences.

CRITICAL THINKING ACTIVITY

1. Compare and contrast the roles and responsibilities as well as the core competencies to your current nursing position.
2. Reflect on the performances of LPNs and RNs from your experience. Identify at least three key roles or competencies seen in the LPN and RN.
3. Do you believe the current nursing education levels lead to conflict and confusion in our roles and responsibilities? Why or why not?

SUMMARY

In transitioning from LPN to RN, it is necessary for the LPN to rethink the concept that the LPN does everything the RN does. The LPN does perform some of the same procedures as the RN; the difference between the LPN and the RN is the rationale for performing a procedure in a certain way. The rationale is based on knowledge and critical thinking skills gained through the educational experience of the RN. In other words, the reason a procedure varies slightly between one client and another is determined by nursing judgment and critical thinking based on in-depth scientific principles and psychological and social issues involving the client. These skills are gained from the general education and social science classes required in the RN program. There are many similarities in the procedures that LPNs and RNs perform; the differences are rooted in the knowledge base and critical thinking skills that include analysis, modification, assimilation, synthesis, problem solving, and evaluation.

Critical thinking skills will be developed in the next few semesters. Maria Gomez, as a new LPN to RN graduate, said her toughest transition to the RN role "was accepting the autonomy and authority of an RN" (personal communication, May 13, 2003).

"The greatest impediment to future success in a new role is inability to relinquish your old one" (Porter-O'Grady, 1999, p. 8). Take the opportunity to transition into the RN role with higher levels of performance and reasoning.

CRITICAL THINKING ACTIVITY

1. Observe an RN performing each of the following role components. Record what you observe as the main differences in the LPN role and the RN role.
   - Professional behaviors
   - Communication
   - Assessment
   - Clinical decision making
   - Caring interventions
   - Teaching and learning
   - Collaboration
   - Managing care

CHAPTER REFLECTIONS

1. What nursing practices do you expect to change as you become an RN? You may want to consider concepts such as professional behaviors, communication, assessment, decision making, client teaching and client learning, collaboration, and managing care.

2. How do you think your education and role as an RN will assist in making decisions related to client care?

3. Describe the RN you most admire. What qualities does this person possess that you want to make part of your own nursing practice? How do these qualities differ from your current nursing behavior?

THEORY TO PRACTICE

1. Make arrangements to spend approximately 20–30 minutes interviewing the following individuals:

   - A current upper classman in your RN program
   - RN with six months to one year experience
   - RN with three to five years experience
   - RN with ten years or more experience

   Some of the questions you might want to ask are:

   - Why did you become an RN?
   - Describe your roles and responsibilities.
   - Do you plan to continue on in your nursing education? Why or why not?
   - What are the differences between RNs and LPN/VNs?

   Summarize the key points you learned from these RN interviews and share with your peers in class discussions.

2. Go to the state board of nursing website and review your scope of practice for both LPNs and RNs. Are there any other resources or organizations that help a nurse learn the roles and responsibilities as they transition into this new role? What can you share about these two roles from these resources?

3. Do an online search for blogs and other discussions on roles and responsibilities for RNs and LPNs. Summarize what you found and how it makes you feel. Is it a positive, professional reflection of nurses? Are RNs and LPN/VNs mutually respectful of one another? Will our public discussions make others want to join the profession? Will our discussions make those under our care and supervision feel safer?

Journaling Your Journey

1. Describe your experience with nursing roles and responsibilities to date. What have you seen, heard, witnessed, or experienced in relationship to roles and responsibilities?

2. What do you anticipate will change the most in terms of your roles and responsibilities as you transition from LPN/VN to RN? Are you prepared to deal with those changes? What do you find the most exciting and the most intimidating about transitioning into the new roles and responsibilities?

ɔ ɔ ɔ

My Story...

I have always had a positive attitude but going to school and balancing family responsibilities gave me more confidence. Even though I was an LPN and currently working as a nurse, what surprised me the most during the transition process was there was still a lot to learn. Classes were not as easy as I had anticipated, and I found that I had to study much more than I had originally expected.

The biggest difference between LPN and RN are the actual responsibilities you have on a day-to-day basis. For instance there are some medications and treatments that you just cannot do as an LPN. Another example is the LPN works with the least threatening conditions in the emergency room, and the RNs work with trauma cases and with clients experiencing heart attacks and strokes.

Heather Kongar, RN

REFERENCES

Anderson, L., & Krathwohl, D. (2001). *A taxonomy for learning, teaching and assessing: A revision of Bloom's taxonomy of educational objectives.* New York: Longman.

Chornick, N., Yocom, C., & Jacobson, J. (1993). *1993 job analysis study of newly licensed entry-level registered nurses.* Chicago: National Council of State Boards of Nursing.

Claytor, K. (1993). Working effectively with LPN-RN orientees. *The Journal of Continuing Education in Nursing, 12*(5), 227–231.

Coxwell, G., and Gillerman, H. (Eds.). (2000). *Educational competencies for graduates of associate degree nursing programs.* Sudbury, MA: Jones and Bartlett Publishers.

Kane, M., & Colton, D. (1988). *Job analysis of newly licensed practical/vocational nurses: 1986–87.* Chicago: National Council of State Boards of Nursing.

National Council of State Boards of Nursing. (2000). *NCSBN testplans for NCLEX-RN® and NCLEX-PN®.* Chicago: Author.

National Council of State Boards of Nursing (NCSBN). (2007). *2007 NCEX-RN® detailed test plan.* Retrieved 5/5/09 at http://ncsbn.org

National Council of State Boards of Nursing (NCSBN). (2008). *2007 NCEX-PN® detailed test plan.* Retrieved 5/5/09 at http://ncsbn.org

National League for Nursing: Council of Practical Nursing Programs. (1989). *Entry-level competencies of graduates of educational programs in practical nursing.* New York: Author.

National League for Nursing. (1990). *Educational outcomes of associate degree nursing programs: Roles and competencies.* New York: Author.

Phillipchuk, D. (2007). The time has come; describing and shaping RN practice. *Alberta RN, 63*(2), 6–7.

Porter-O'Grady, T. (1999). Technology demands quick-change nursing roles. *Nursing Management, 30*(5), 7–8.

SUGGESTED RESOURCES

Boblin, S., Baxter, P., Alvarado, K., Baumann, A., & Akntar-Danesh, N. (2008). Registered nurses and licensed/registered practical nurse: a description and comparison of their decision-making process. *Nursing Leadership, 21*(4), 56–72.

Hallin, K. & Danielson, E. (2008). Registered nurses' perceptions of their work and professional development. *Journal of Advanced Nursing, 61*(1), 62–70.

Oelke, N., White, D., Besner, J., Doran, D., Hall, L., & Giovannetti, P. (2008). Nursing workforce utilization: An examination of facilitators and barriers on scope of practice. *Canadian Journal of Nursing Leadership, 21*(1), 58–71.

Pope, B. (2002). The synergy match-up. *Nursing Management, 33*(5), 38–41.

Rick, C. (2003). Differentiated practice: Get beyond the fear factor. *Nursing Management, 34*(1), 11–12.

Chapter 5
Communication

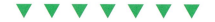

LEARNING OBJECTIVES

By the end of this chapter, you should be able to:
1. Describe communication development factors.
2. Describe communication structure.
3. Describe communication barriers.
4. Describe therapeutic communication techniques.
5. Implement basic effective communication techniques.
6. Describe effective crisis communication techniques.
7. Describe techniques to improve communication with team members.

KEY TERMS

Action language

Communication

Communication barriers

Intrapersonal communication

Metacommunication

Nonverbal communication

Nurse-client communication

Perception

Social communication

Somatic language

Therapeutic communication

Verbal communication

SCENARIO

Nicole is a new RN who is paired with a mentor while orienting to a medical floor. Her mentor is teaching a diabetic client that is frequently admitted for complications from noncompliance with her treatment plan. The mentor's arms are folded across her chest during the exchange and her tone is terse. The mentor informs the client and her husband that they have had diabetic teaching several times already. The husband looks down at the floor during the exchange.

THINK ABOUT IT

1. What does the term *therapeutic communication* mean to you?
2. In your experience, what type of barriers occur to prevent effective communication with clients?
3. Identify your own personal communication style. Do your own thoughts and opinions come out in discussions with others? Do you allow others to finish their thoughts before you speak? Do you really listen to what the other person is saying?

INTRODUCTION

Clients are more knowledgeable about disease conditions and health options, and they are not as intimidated about entering the health care system as they once were. Even though the nurse-client relationship is an involuntary relationship, clients rely on nurses for guidance, teaching, and assistance to regain or maintain health. Nurses can accomplish these tasks with effective communication skills.

Our view of the client determines our communication style. If we see clients as dependent on us, we may approach them with a one-upmanship manner or, possibly, in a patronizing manner. If we see them as intelligent clients who desire input and partnering in their health care choices, we will communicate with them as equals. We will see ourselves as mentors and guides to assist them with their health issues.

Communication is the essential element in establishing interpersonal relationships and nurse-client relationships. In this chapter we focus on effectively communicating interpersonally with others—therapeutically with a client, interventionally in a crisis, and competently with other health care team members. We will also briefly discuss developmental factors that affect communication.

DEVELOPMENTAL CONSIDERATIONS

Infants express themselves verbally and nonverbally. They cry when hungry or uncomfortable, thus expressing personal desires with verbal communication. Chitty & Black (2007) describes an infant's nonverbal communication of kicking, turning red in the face, and making facial gestures as **somatic language**.

As the infant progresses into the toddler stage, verbal communication develops by repeating words and then phrases. The toddler also communicates nonverbally with **action language**, such as looking at or pointing to desired objects or holding out a hand for food (Chitty and Black, 2007).

Verbal communication continues to develop as family members verbally stimulate the child. If the child's family is quiet, verbal communication may develop more slowly or inadequately. Nonverbal communication also develops within the environmental setting as the child observes nonverbal communication such as kisses, hugs, and hand gestures (Chitty and Black, 2007). Children take on the observed behaviors and spoken language of their exemplars.

Cultural influences affect communication in words, speed of speech, and gestures. Culture determines distance between individuals during conversation. Some cultures also determine who can speak to whom based on gender or social status.

Communication begins in infancy and is influenced by family and cultural environments. Communication techniques continue to develop from infancy through adulthood. Refer to Table 5–1 for Jean Piaget's Theory of Language Development. Effective communication skills are learned depending on desire and practice.

Table 5–1 Piaget's Theory of Language Development

Stage/Age	Piaget's Cognitive Stages
1. **Infancy**	Sensorimotor (birth to 2 years): begins to acquire language
Birth to 1 year	Task: Object permanence
2. **Toddler**	Sensorimotor continues
1 to 3 years	Preoperational (2 to 7 years): begins: use of representational thought
	Task: Use language and mental images to think and communicate
3. **Preschool**	Preoperational continues
3 to 6 years	
4. **School Age**	Preoperational continues
6 to 12 years	Concrete Operations (7 to 12 years) begins: engage in inductive reasoning and concrete problem solving
	Task: Learn concepts of conservation and reversibility
5. **Adolescence**	Formal Operations (12 years to adulthood): engage in abstract reasoning and analytical problem solving
12 to 18 years	Task: Develop a workable philosophy of life

(Source: *Health Assessment and Physical Examination* 3rd ed., by M. Estes, 2006, Clifton Park, NY: Delmar/Cengage Learning.)

INTERPERSONAL COMMUNICATION

Communication is the "dynamic interaction between two or more persons in which ideas, goals, beliefs and values, feelings, and feelings about feelings are exchanged" (Hood & Leddy, 2003, p. 453). Communication is the nucleus of relationships and the mechanism by which we influence others (see Figure 5–1). Communication techniques may either develop or fracture personal relationships and nurse-client relationships.

It is vital for nurses to grasp the components of communication and experience the dynamics of effective communication. It is imperative that nurses learn effective communication techniques to develop helping relationships with clients. "The quality of communication between the nurse and the client is an essential determinant of the success of the professional relationship" (Hood & Leddy, 2003, p. 452). Quality relationships with clients determine our influence in assisting the client to a healthier lifestyle.

According to Rowe (1999) the majority of formal complaints at a community health council stemmed from a lack of communication, personnel attitudes, and inappropriate communication of unpleasant news. These communication issues are inappropriate behaviors for caring nurses. Communication consists not only of the spoken word (**verbal communication**) but also of the unspoken word (**nonverbal communication**). Attitude is communicated in the verbal and the nonverbal message. Attitude also is revealed in the timing, place, and way in which unpleasant news is shared. Caring and communicating are inseparably linked—you cannot hope to communicate effectively if you do not care about the person on the receiving end (Rowe).

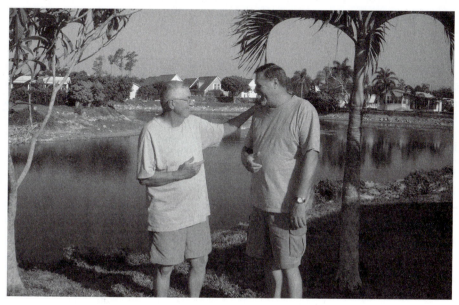

Figure 5–1 Communication is the core of relationships.

CRITICAL THINKING ACTIVITIES

1. Write about a time when a client's attitude hindered the communication process with the health care staff.
2. Write about a time when your attitude affected your communication with a client.

Communication Structure

For communication to occur, there must be a message sender and a message receiver. When we communicate face-to-face, two messages are sent. One is the verbal message of thought and feelings expressed in words influenced by voice volume, inflection, and speech rate. The other message is the nonverbal message or unspoken word expressed with eye movements, gestures, facial expressions, and body movements. Some nonverbal communication needs no spoken word, such as rolling your eyes upward or giving a warm smile.

The sender of a message determines the desired message and encodes the words and gestures with thoughts and feelings. To interpret the message the receiver has to decode the thoughts and feelings in the sender's verbal and nonverbal message. After determining the perceived meaning of the message, the receiver responds to the message by encoding a message with personal thoughts and feelings expressed in words and/or gestures. An interaction occurs between sender and receiver simultaneously. While the sender is sending a message she is interpreting the receiver's message, and as the receiver receives the message she is interpreting and sending a message (Balzer-Riley, 2008).

To interpret a message, a person analyzes two parts of the message: the message content, and the message's perceived meaning. The message content is what is literally expressed verbally or nonverbally. The message **perception** is how the content is interpreted and how the relationship between the message sender and the message receiver is perceived or emotionally interpreted. To put perceptual meaning to a message is to put meaning to the sensed emotions of the message. Taylor (1997) views perception as something that people learn from their individual socialization experience. Therefore, each person interprets messages according to her learned perceptual ability, causing message interpretation to vary.

Metacommunication

Metacommunication is the message perception of verbal and nonverbal communication. Hood and Leddy (2003) state, "The nurse searches for the content theme (the central underlying idea or links), the mood theme (the emotion communicated—the how of the message), and the interaction theme (the dynamics between the communicating participants)" (p. 457). To communicate effectively, the nurse must comprehend the content of the message, the emotions of the message, and the emotional relationship of the communicators. The nurse must understand the content or key idea that the communicator is attempting to communicate. If the key idea is missed, then communication is misinterpreted by all parties involved. An example of this is the classic Abbott and Costello baseball routine, "Who's on first?"

The nurse needs to be attuned to the manner or emotions in which the message is communicated. For example, she needs to perceive the communicator's anxiety, negativity, excitement, frustration, or fear. The emotions are displayed by voice fluctuation (voice elevation or a soft, fading voice) and nonverbal communication (looking down, avoiding eye contact, and rolling the eyes).

The emotional relationship of the communicators may depend on past experiences, trust, respect, and cultural practices. If the nurse is attuned to the content of the message, the emotions of the message, and the emotional relationship of the communicators, she communicates more effectively. Keep in mind that this type of communication will not occur overnight. Communication is a lifelong process and a major component of nursing. Your educational experience in the next few semesters will assist you in identifying the components of communication.

Factors Influencing Message Interpretation

Factors other than the content and emotional aspects of metacommunication can affect communication. Some of these factors influence the sent messages and the interpretation of the messages (see Figure 5–2). Balzer-Riley (2008) has suggested six factors that influence message interpretation:

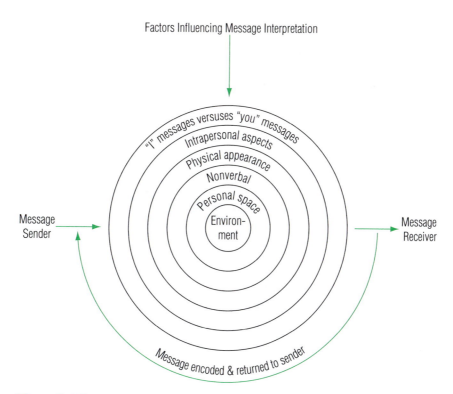

Figure 5–2 Factors that influence the interpretation of messages.

1. Environment—temperature, distance between people (across the room or at opposite ends of the table), furniture placement, formal and informal atmosphere.
2. Personal space—rank, position, seating arrangement, physical build (height and weight), touching (see Figure 5–3).
3. Nonverbal—eye movements, gestures, body language, eye contact, crossed arms.
4. Physical appearance—body profile, hair, body movements and gestures, age, gender, posture, body art and piercing.
5. Intrapersonal aspects—speech, values, self-concept, thinking processes, learning styles.
6. "I" messages verses "you" messages.

An example of factors that interfere with message interpretation relating to environment, personal space, and nonverbal communication is a nurse's standing in the doorway with her arms crossed and talking to a client rather than approaching the client's bedside, pulling up a chair, or placing a hand on her arm when talking about the client's concern (Figure 5–4). Most people find the nurse's moving closer to the bed very comforting and conducive to a more positive nurse-client relationship. However, each individual's personal space varies. All health care providers should acknowledge and respect an individual's personal space.

Another situation in which a personal space factor may interfere with message interpretation is a formal atmosphere where a client may hesitate to ask the nurse manager a health-related question due to her position. The client may also hesitate to ask the health question

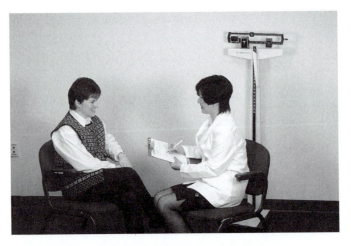

Figure 5–3 Personal space effects communication.
(Source: *Health Assessment and Physical Examination* 3rd ed., by M. Estes, 2006, Clifton Park, NY: Delmar/Cengage Learning.)

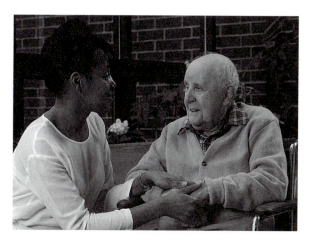

Figure 5–4 Both verbal and nonverbal communication are important in the nurse-client relationship.

because she does not want to bother the nurse manager or ask her to do something that she does not feel is her responsibility.

Other examples of nonverbal factors are a client's being distracted when a nurse uses excessive hand movements or is overly dramatic when talking. Some clients become uncomfortable with prolonged eye contact or avoidance of eye contact.

Physical appearance may interfere with message interpretation in a variety of ways. Clients respond very differently to the physical appearance and gender of the nurse. A female client may or may not be open with a male nurse. The nurse's white uniform may comfort some clients and intimidate others.

Intrapersonal aspects are other factors interfering with message interpretation. The self-concept of a nurse or a client can be expressed in a pleasing or intimidating manner that enhances or interferes with communication. It is important to recognize that each individual's learning style varies and affects the way a nurse communicates with a client. A nurse with a concrete learning style might list steps when explaining a procedure or give more specific directions that seem demanding, whereas a nurse with an abstract learning style might give more descriptive examples when explaining concepts. The nurse with an abstract learning style might take more care with the decorations in a client's room, such as placing cards on a bulletin board or watering the client's flowers.

"I" messages attempt to keep communication open. "You" messages may put a person on the defense. I messages give an individual freedom to express feelings without blaming others. For example, "I am not sure I see it that way" versus "You are wrong."

It is important that we carefully select the correct words to convey our desired meaning. Messages are often incorrectly interpreted or misunderstood. If we do not understand a message or are not clear as to what is being said or related, we need to validate the meaning of the message with the receiver. Asking "Are you saying . . . ?" or "Do you mean . . . ?" clarifies the message.

The techniques used in interpersonal relationships will assist you as you communicate with clients. Other communication techniques discussed later in the chapter also improve nurse-client relationships.

CRITICAL THINKING ACTIVITY

1. Concentrate on your interactions with others for two days, focusing especially on the content of the message, the emotions of the message, and the emotional relationship of the communicators. Review Riley's six factors that influence communication and determine ways those factors influenced your interactions with others. Complete the following communication chart to analyze two conversations you have with others.

Conversation	Content	Emotions	Emotional relationship	Factors that influenced message interpretation	Perception enhancement/ interference

COMMUNICATION WITH CLIENTS

Nurse-client communication is the therapeutic interaction between a nurse and a client that improves the client's health physically, emotionally, and/or spiritually. Before we discuss effective communication techniques to improve nurse-client communication, let's review some barriers to effective communication.

Communication Barriers

Communication barriers are ineffective phrases or behaviors that damage personal interactions and should be avoided when communicating with clients. Hood and Leddy (2003) refer to these as noncaring communication behaviors. Some of these barriers are responding defensively, blaming, giving advice or opinions, changing the subject, questioning the client, giving judgmental responses, and patronizing (Coordinating Council for Continuing Education in Health Care, 1990; Daniels, 2010).

Box 5–1 Barriers to Communication

Blaming statements

Giving advice

Changing the subject or topic

Why questions

Judgmental statements

Patronizing statements

Falsely reassuring statements

Failure to listen

Blaming Statements

Examples of blaming statements are "You made me drop this" or "That is a stupid question you put on this exam. You tried to trick me." No one likes to be blamed for a situation, and a blaming statement places the blame on another person. Blaming statements may cause an individual to respond defensively and in anger. A defensive response is an attempt to protect oneself from a negative opinion. It also denies individuals the right to express their view or opinion of a situation (Hood & Leddy, 2003). It attempts to deflect the statement. Rather than responding defensively with a blaming statement, a person could approach an error, difficult situation, or hurt feelings with an "I" statement or by saying, "How can we handle or repair this situation?"

Giving Advice

If a nurse gives advice or shares her opinion, the client may assume the nurse knows the best option. In essence, the nurse is saying that the client does not have the ability to make wise decisions. An example of giving advice is a scenario in which an elderly client is ready for discharge from the hospital. The physician and family think it is best for the client to be admitted to a nursing home. The client asks the nurse what she thinks. The nurse says, "I think you are capable of caring for yourself at home, especially if you have a home care nurse visit you once a week." The nurse has expressed an opinion and given advice that will confuse the discharge issues.

If a client asks a nurse a question, the nurse's ideal response would be to explore various options with the client and assist the client in making her own decision. In this case, the nurse shows the client she believes that the client is capable of making sound decisions.

Changing the Subject or Topic

A client with cancer says, "I feel like I am getting weaker every day. I wonder if the chemotherapy is working." The nurse responds, "Isn't it beautiful outside today?" This type of nontherapeutic communication is called changing the subject or topic. A nurse may change the topic when the client is sharing personal feelings or thoughts about a subject that make the nurse uncomfortable. When a client is talking and the nurse purposely changes the topic, the client's impression is that the nurse is in charge of discussion topics. Changing the client's topic also negates the importance or value of the client.

Why Questions

A client in a nursing home states, "I don't think you like me." "Now *why* would you think that?" replies the nurse. "Why" statements or questions tend to put the other person on the defensive. The client may think the nurse is probing for more information or questioning her thinking.

Judgmental Statements

When a nurse uses a judgmental statement, she passes judgment on the client or the client's statements. This type of statement judges the client's values and indicates a value difference between nurse and client. The statement implies that the nurse's values, standards, or perceptions are better than the client's. If a client consistently is given judgmental statements, a dependent relationship is fostered because the client begins to think that her opinion has no value and that the other person has all the appropriate knowledge or correct thinking.

Patronizing Statements

A patronizing statement is a demeaning, condescending statement made to another. For example, a nurse may say to a client, "You just don't understand. We always use EKGs in this type of situation." When a nurse uses a patronizing statement, the client receives the impression that the nurse is superior or arrogant and that the nurse and the client are not in an equal position or on an equal playing field. The nurse's communication implies contempt toward the client.

A nurse may fall into the trap of using this type of communication when she has worked in the same place for a long time, has become very knowledgeable, and feels that she knows what is best for the client. If a nurse is in a hurry, she may give a quick, demeaning response instead of giving the client the explanation she is seeking. Instead of assisting the client in understanding, the nurse belittles the client because she does not understand.

Another environment where a nurse might use patronizing communication is communicating with clients who are experiencing changes in mental status, such as someone having an emotional breakdown or in a state of depression. When a client is not thinking as quickly as she used to think or as quickly as we expect her to, the patronizing nurse simply determines the client's needs without involving her in the process. Sometimes as a client ages and becomes more dependent on the health care provider for her activities of daily living, the nurse assumes that her mental capacity has also become reduced, making her more dependent on the nurse. The nurse cuts the client short and gives a quick response to what she thinks the client is attempting to say.

Falsely Reassuring Statements

An example of a falsely reassuring statement is, "Oh, everything will be all right. You have the best doctor in town." This negates the client's concerns and fears and makes her hesitant to share other feelings with the nurse. The nurse is failing to assist the client in exploring personal thoughts and feelings. A nurse may use false reassurance when communicating in difficult situations with a grim prognosis, or if she does not recognize the anxiety in a client's statement or question.

Failure to Listen

Failing to listen is the most noncaring communication a nurse can demonstrate (Hood & Leddy, 2003). By failing to listen to the client, the nurse is saying that the client's needs are not important. She may even be implying that her own needs are more important than the client's. This is the behavior of a noncaring nurse. The most valuable tangible action one individual can give to another is to listen to what that individual is saying.

Hood and Leddy (2003) suggest that nurses who use nontherapeutic communication have a need to act in a regressive or retreating manner. "This need, accompanied by increasing anxiety, sometimes leads to nurses seeing themselves as superior, and is expressed in negative actions such as moralizing, rejecting, or reacting with hostility" (pp. 475–476). Learning to communicate therapeutically encourages an individual to look inward as well as learn to listen and respond in a caring, effective way. Communication involves personal analysis, attentive and active listening skills, and meaningful, caring responses.

Therapeutic Communication

Therapeutic communication and social communication are not the same. We use **social communication** in everyday life. Social communication is communication in a less formal environment when we are discussing less personal or serious issues. Social communication is spontaneous and does not have specific goals.

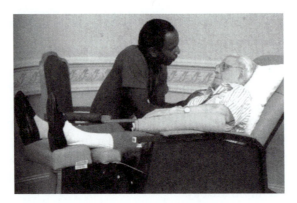

Figure 5–5 Therapeutic communication enhances client communication. (Source: *Health Assessment and Physical Examination* 3rd ed., by M. Estes, 2006, Clifton Park, NY: Delmar/Cengage Learning.)

A nurse uses **therapeutic communication** in nurse-client relationships. Therapeutic communication has the client's best interests at heart and is goal oriented. The purpose of therapeutic communication is to enhance and improve communication with clients. Nurses use therapeutic communication in a specific, focused manner to obtain information to meet the client's health care concerns and needs (Estes, 2006). The nurse's therapeutic communication goals are to assist a client to formulate ideas, express those ideas more clearly, and sort through issues to find a solution (see Figure 5–5). Therapeutic communication can also be very effective with other nurses, other health care workers, and even family members.

Nurses demonstrate caring behaviors by avoiding communication barriers and effectively using techniques to improve communication with clients. Some therapeutic communication techniques are broad open-ended statements or questions, reflection, clarification, silence, reassurance, summarization, and acknowledgement (Coordinating Council for Continuing Education in Health Care, 1990; Estes, 2006).

Box 5–2 Therapeutic Communication Techniques

> Broad open-ended statements or questions
>
> Reflection
>
> Clarification
>
> Silence
>
> Reassurance
>
> Summarization
>
> Acknowledgment

Broad Open-Ended Statements or Questions

A nurse effectively communicates with the client when she uses broad open-ended state-ments or questions. An example of an open-ended statement is, "Tell me more about . . ." or "Can you explain that to me in another way?" Open-ended statements offer the client an op-portunity to guide the direction of the conversation. They allow the client to choose the topic focus and proceed with the conversation. This type of statement shows the client that the nurse is personally interested in her and what she is saying. It also does not put the client on the defensive as a "why," "what," or "how" question does.

Reflection

The nurse uses a reflection statement by restating or rephrasing the client's statement to show interest in the client's concerns and have the client expand on an idea. A client says, "I wish my children would call me. They have been on vacation for two weeks." The nurse would use a re-flective statement by saying, "You're missing your children and would like to receive a call from them?" or "You are worried about your children because they're on vacation and you haven't heard from them since they left?" Reflection also allows the nurse to say, "I'm listening. Keep going." This statement reassures the client of the nurse's interest in the client's statements.

Clarification

Clarification is attempting to make the client's meaning clear. With clarification, the nurse usually explains to the client that she desires clarification. The nurse may say, "I want to make sure I understand you correctly. Did you mean. . . ?" Or the nurse could simply say, "You are saying. . . ."

Silence

At times there is no need for verbal communication between client and nurse. The nurse shows client acceptance by silently remaining with the client when she is receiving distressing news (Hood & Leddy, 2003). This way, the nurse is nonverbally indicating a desire to be with the client. Even if she says nothing, the nurse desires to share the moment with the client.

The nurse might use silence when a client receives disappointing news such as a terminal diagnosis or a family death. By remaining at the client's side silently and perhaps holding her hand, the nurse uses silence effectively.

Reassurance

A client has expressed concern about the length of time it is taking to get results from a test. If the nurse were to say, "This is the typical length of time for the test results to be processed," she would be giving the client verbal reassurance. The nurse is not falsely reassuring the client but, rather, giving the client accurate, positive affirmation to ease her concerns.

Summarization

Summarization may be used after a nurse-client teaching session to recap the main points. The nurse also uses summarization after detailed instructions are given to review the main facts. A nurse's summarization statement could be, "Now I would like to summarize the things we have discussed."

Acknowledgment

The client feels valued when the nurse acknowledges and addresses her concerns. "I understand you would like to talk with the doctor this morning" is an example of acknowledgment.

To use any of these techniques requires the nurse to listen attentively and actively to the client and to desire to communicate with the client. To be an effective communicator, there must be desire and practice—desire to become an effective communicator, and consistent practice in effectively using the techniques.

CRITICAL THINKING ACTIVITY

1. Write about a professional situation when you experienced any of the following barriers in communicating with a client. Then write how that situation could have been different if you had used any of the following communication techniques.

Barrier to communication	How did the barrier occur?	What was the effect on the communication?
Giving advice		
Changing the subject or topic		
Why questions		
Judgmental statements		
Patronizing statements		
Falsely reassuring statements		
Failure to listen		

Therapeutic communication technique	How did you use the technique?	What was accomplished?
Broad open-ended statements or questions		
Reflection		
Clarification		
Silence		
Reassurance		
Summarization		
Acknowledgment		

CRISIS COMMUNICATION

Hood and Leddy (2003) state, "Anxiety is the tension state resulting from the actual or antici-pated negative appraisal of the significant other in the communication process." Anxiety is communicated to the other by voice and nonverbal body language. A client may be anxious if she is anticipating negative news or test results. It is important for the nurse to sense the client's tension and not respond to the situation with personal anxiety. If both parties com-municate anxiety, the tension will only escalate.

Anxiety causes the client to ineffectively use energy that is needed to solve a problem or act appropriately (Hood & Leddy, 2003). It is important for both the nurse and the cli-ent to channel energy into positive actions. Sullivan (1953) stated that anxiety in limited amounts and duration could lead to increased alertness and energy needed to take appro-priate action to reduce tension. If the anxiety is not limited, there may be a decrease in the effectiveness of handling situations. Mild anxiety allows a person to focus on the situa-tion at hand. Moderate anxiety limits an individual's focus and twists reality for her. Severe anxiety does not allow an individual to focus her energy on the real issues and, therefore, limits her problem-solving and decision-making abilities. It is important for the nurse to recognize both her own and the client's anxiety levels to effectively assist in problem solv-ing and decision making. For the client or the nurse to utilize their energy most effectively, anxiety must be decreased. Nurses can learn, use, and share stress-reduction techniques with clients.

Assess a client's anxiety level before starting a teaching session. If the client's anxiety level is moderate to severe, her learning ability is limited. The use of therapeutic communication techniques reduces the client's anxiety level.

An example of effective therapeutic communication techniques with an anxious client is demonstrated in the scenario in Box 5–3.

Box 5–3 Therapeutic Communication Scenario

> *Client:* "I just don't think I can give myself the insulin injection. I have always been afraid of needles. Even when I was a child, I would become very anxious and scream with injections."
>
> *Nurse:* "I can see that you are very anxious and it sounds like you have been afraid of needles for a long time. Is there something specific about a needle that scares you?
>
> *Client:* "I don't like the pain when I get a shot."
>
> *Nurse:* "Can you compare the pain from an insulin injection to the pain from other injections you have had?"
>
> *Client:* "I guess the insulin injection really doesn't hurt as bad as the other injections I have had, like antibiotics and pain medication."
>
> *Nurse:* "Do you think that if you were in control of the injection, rather than a nurse, you could handle the situation better?"
>
> *Client:* "Now, I hadn't thought of that idea. I actually can be in control of the insulin injection."
>
> *Nurse:* (after a slight pause) "Do you feel comfortable trying the injection now?"

COMMUNICATING AS A TEAM MEMBER

We have discussed interpersonal communication techniques, therapeutic communication techniques, and nontherapeutic communication techniques. Nurses must communicate effectively not only with clients but also with members of the health care team. Many of the same techniques we use in interpersonal communication and therapeutic communication can be used with team members. A judicious nurse does not drop the effective communication skills at the client's bedside but continues to apply them in interacting with health care team members (Chitty and Black, 2007).

Some communication enhancement techniques the nurse could use with team members are active listening, respect of others, spacing and distance, attention to nonverbal communication cues, "I" messages, and avoidance of communication "barriers." The nurse is not attempting to accomplish the same goals of therapeutic communication with team members that are accomplished in nurse-client interactions. However, effective communication techniques used with clients can be carried over into conversation with team members (see Figure 5–6). Communicating in concise, well thought-out, simple messages enhances communication personally and professionally.

Trust and support are vital for a smooth, efficient working environment. Effective communication can provide these encouraging factors. As team members sense trust and support, they feel free to share creative ideas and suggestions for change. In an accepting environment, employees gain job satisfaction and blossom.

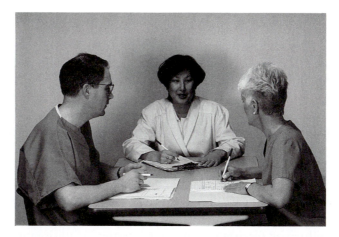

Figure 5–6 Effective communication improves the health care team's quality of care. (Source: *Nursing Fundamentals: Caring and Clinical Decision Making*, 2nd ed. Daniels, R. 2010. Clifton Park, NY: Delmar/Cengage Learning.)

The nursing shortage and early hospital discharges add more stress to the clinical environment. Effective communication skills such as clarification, reflection, and reassurance decrease tension in stressful situations.

Self-Talk

Self-assessment, self-worth, and self-talk has a definite effect on team member communication. Kearney-Nunnery (2008) calls communicating with one's self or self-talk **intrapersonal communication**. How a person feels about self determines the portrayal of self to others in appearance, body carriage, gestures, and expression. If a nurse has a negative encounter with a manager, the nurse's thoughts and talk may tend to take on a negative air. It is important at that point to assess personal accountability for the encounter candidly and make amends as needed. Self-talk is also important to instill positive input back into self. The self-talk will influence future interactions with other team members that could be negatively or positively influenced by the self-talk (Kearney-Nunnery, 2008).

Body Language

Ineffective body language that affects communication is crossing the arms, indicating rejection or closed-mindedness; biting fingernails, signifying nervousness; and turning the body away from the other person, representing boredom, rejection, or conflict. Portraying a relaxed attitude and demeanor is generally positive (Kearney-Nunnery, 2008). It is also important to be genuine.

Team Interactions

For several years nurses used the phrase, "Nurses eat their young" implying that older or experienced nurses thought the younger less experienced nurses should jump through some difficult "hoops" in the profession as previous nurses had done. Sometimes the "hoops" were disrespectful and aggressive. Recently, literature has focused on verbal abuse in the medical profession with a focus on the importance of communicating assertively and openly in attempts to break the "eating young" cycle. A study by the Institute for Safe Medication Practices (ISMP) (2004) found 7 percent of 2,095 health care professionals were involved in medication errors because they felt intimidated by another person. Not only does the survey indicate disruptive behavior in the health care system, but the actions jeopardize client safety. Rosenstein and O'Daniel (2005) surveyed 675 nurses finding verbal abuse mostly involves physicians to nurses (86 percent reported abusive situations) and then nurses to nurses (72 percent witnessed disruptive behaviors by nurses) with one in five of the nurses and physicians stating these incidents occurred on a weekly basis. Verbal abuse is not effective or therapeutic communication and displays a lack of respect of others.

As nurses learn effective communication skills, disruptive behaviors such as verbal abuse will decrease or be eliminated. Nurses can learn productive reactions to verbal abuse that makes them assertive and points out the abusive behavior to the perpetrator. If the nurse learns appropriate communication responses, her reactions in the heat of the situation protects her and gives the inflictor of abuse an opportunity to change and respond respectfully.

According to Johnson, DeMass Martin, and Markle-Elder (2007), the first step in stopping verbal abuse is to react appropriately in the moment of disruptive behavior. Often the nurse is shocked, taken aback, and humiliated making it difficult to respond with effective communication skills in a quick manner. Johnson, et al., suggest the nurse respond immediately with an appropriate statement such as, "I can't answer you while you are yelling. If you lower your voice, I can respond" or "Your behavior is unacceptable for a professional" (p. 32). These statements do not attack the offender but draw a line for unacceptable abusive behavior. It draws attention to the behavior and gives the offender an opportunity to personally grow, apologize, and change future responses.

Johnson, et al., recommend the nurse be firm in expecting a response from the offender. She can do this by stating, "You owe me an apology for the way you spoke to me." Johnson, et al. relate the situation of a nurse responding to a physician yelling at her with the statement, "You're not talking to me. I know you're not talking to me because I don't allow anyone to yell at me. Now, if you can calmly tell me what you need, I can help you" (p. 34). By making this type of statement, the nurse is stating that disruptive behavior is not the expected role of being a nurse; it is not part of the nursing package. Assertive statements do not demean the offender but show the offender her inappropriate actions or statements and does not permit continued abuse in the future. Assertive statements compel respect from the co-worker, for self, and, essentially, provide quality client care.

THEORY TO PRACTICE

A co-worker has a heavy assignment of critically ill clients. Shift report lasted longer than usual and has set her even more behind schedule. When she starts to administer medications, some of the medications are not available because pharmacy has not re-stocked her cart. A physician arrives on the floor and asks her questions that she does not know about the client because this is her first day of caring for the client. You reach for the glucoscan to monitor your client's blood sugar. Your co-worker reaches for the glucoscan at approximately the same time, but you retrieve the glucoscan first. She yells at you, "Give me that glucoscan. You have an easy assignment and I don't. I need the glucoscan now."

1. How would you handle her aggression?

2. What could you say to defuse the situation and address her aggressive statement?

Team Communication Technique

Personal interactions are not only affected by ineffective communication skills, but long-range effects ripple from the communiqué. In clinical situations, ineffective communication can have devastating effects on client care and safety. These situations occur when inadequate information is given to a person, lack of information is handed off to another caregiver, receiver of information is not listening, and one caregiver acts on his perception of the situation when another caregiver thinks another action would be more beneficial and does not relate those actions (Groff and Augello, 2003).

Dr. Michael Leonard states we have a "historical mindset" of thinking each person is educated as an expert and can handle any situation alone. With more effort, more willpower, more sacrifice, we think we can handle the situation (Groff and Augello, 2003). This thinking hinders teamwork and team communication. The care environment has become so complex one person cannot keep track of all the needed details and handle all the details of care. In order to work as a team and provide client safety, an effective communication method is needed.

Dr. Leonard addresses four limitations that affect caregivers: multi-tasking, short-term memory, fatigue, and stress. In our daily lives, we attempt to be all and in contact with all every moment of every day. We are constantly bombarded with cell phone calls, cell phone messages, emails, instant messages, and personal interactions. Multi-tasking is good, but only to a level of safe productivity.

There are limitations on our short-term memories and how much our brains can process. A person mentally can only hold five pieces of information. Think of a typical minute in a nurse's clinical day. She answers the phone, receives orders, processes orders as needed, answers a call light, consoles a client, gives a medication, and documents. Her brain is on overload. We are "constantly exceeding the ability of our brains to manage and capture all that information" (Groff and Augello, 2003, p.10).

Fatigue impacts our ability to process information and perform effectively and safely. Yet, we attempt to work an 8-hour job and then go to another facility and work 6-8 more hours. Or, a nurse works 12 hours shifts for three or four days in a row. The nurse becomes exhausted. According to Dawson, 24 hours without sleep is equal to a blood alcohol level of 0.10 (Dawson, 1997). Perhaps the scheduling of nurses and other health care personnel needs re-evaluating for client safety.

Mild to moderate stress for a short time increases alertness and productivity. However, moderate to high intensity stress decreases accurate performance. A routine action done correctly many times a day can, in a stressful situation, make the error factor increase 25 percent (Groff and Augello, 2003). Nurses and other health care personnel find themselves in extremely stressful situations many times throughout the day depending on the clinical unit.

These facts make us fully aware that we need not get in the mindset that we can handle it all. Just getting up one more hour, just staying awake two more hours, just working faster, is not always the best solution. In these situations, one misinterpretation of communication, one fact omitted, one person not listening to all the facts, one incorrect view of a client's condition, may have a devastating effect on a client.

Dr. Leonard states nurses and physicians are educated to communicate differently. Nurses communicate in a very descriptive, detailed narrative and physicians communicate with brief statements that get to the facts and the solution (Groff and Augello, 2005).

Since effective, correct communication is so vital, Dr. Leonard developed a communication tool to improve communication between nurses and physicians that is also effective in communication with other health care providers, co-workers, and in personal communication. The tool is the Situational Briefing model or Situation, Background, Assessment, and Recommendation (SBAR) as shown in Figure 5–7. The nurse explains the present situation, describes the background, shares present assessment findings, and her recommendation for solving the problem. Box 5–4 gives an example of SBAR that a nurse uses to report information to the physician.

SBAR REPORT TO A PHYSICIAN

BEFORE CALLING THE PHYSICIAN

1. Assess the patient
2. Review the chart for the appropriate physician to call
3. Know the admitting diagnosis
4. Read the most recent Progress Notes and the assessment from the nurse of the prior shift.
5. Have *available* when speaking with the physician:

Chart, Allergies, Meds, IV fluids, Labs / Results

SITUATION

State your **name and unit**
I am calling about: **(Patient Name & Room Number)**
The **problem** I am calling about is:

BACKGROUND

State the **admission diagnosis and date of admission**
State the pertinent **medical history**
A Brief Synopsis of the **treatment to date**

ASSESSMENT

Most recent vital signs:

BP_____ Pulse_____ Respirations_____ Temperature_____

The patient ❏ **is** or ❏ **is not an oxygen**
Any changes from prior assessments, such as:

Mental Status	Respiratory rate/quality	Retractions / use of accessory muscles
Skin Color	Pulse/BP rate/quality	Rhythm changes
Neuro changes	Pain	Wound drainage
Musculoskeletal (joint deformity, weakness)	GI/GU (Nausea / Vomiting / Diarrhea / Output)	

RECOMMENDATION

Do you think we should: (State what you would like to see done)
  ❏ Transfer the patient to ICU or PICU?
  ❏ Come to see the patient at this time?
  ❏ Talk to the patient and/or family about the code status?
  ❏ Ask for a consultant to see the patient now?
      ❏ Other suggestion?

Are any tests needed?
  ❏ Do you need any tests like ❏ CXR ❏ ABG ❏ EKG ❏ CBC ❏ BNP
      ❏ Others? _____

If a change in treatment is ordered, then ask:
  ❏ How often do you want vital signs? _____
  ❏ If there the patient does not improve, when would you want us to call again?

DOCUMENT THE CHANGE IN CONDITION &
THE PHYSICIAN NOTIFICATION

Figure 5–7 SBAR communication tool. © Haig, K.M., Sutton, S. and Whittington, J. "SBAR: A Shared Mental Model for Improving Communication between Clinicians." Joint Commission Journal on Quality and Patient Safety. Volume 32: page 172, 2006. Reprinted with permission.

Box 5–4: SBAR Communication with Example

Situation—State present situation or what has caused the need for communication.
    Example: For the last two weeks I have not had the 9:00 A.M. medications to
    administer to the clients.

Background: Explain the background that has lead to the present situation. Give the
    context of the situation to the listener or reader.
    Example: Previously the pharmacy stocked medications before 7:00 A.M., but
    in the last two weeks the computer medication drawers on our unit are not
    stocked until around 11:30 A.M. Therefore, I do not have the 9:00 A.M. medica-
    tions for the clients. I called the pharmacy department three times and they
    say they are running late.

Assessment—What from your perspective is the problem?
    Example: The late medication administration affects the client's medication
    blood levels and puts me behind schedule.

Recommendation—State your suggestion for solving the problem.
    Example: Perhaps a representative could meet with the pharmacy department
    director and see if the medication drawers could be stocked before 7:00 A.M.

Adapted from Haig, K., Sutton, S., and Whittington, J. (2003). SBAR Communication. Journal on Quality
and Patient Safety, 32(3), 167–175.

The SBAR tool provides a person an assertive method of addressing a situation that needs
reporting.

THEORY TO PRACTICE

1. Use the SBAR tool to address a personal problem.

    Situation:

    Background:

    Assessment:

    Recommendation:

2. Use the SBAR tool to address a clinical situation.

    Situation:

    Background:

    Assessment:

    Recommendation:

3. Share your thoughts about using the SBAR tool. What are the advantages of using the tool? What are the disadvantages?

4. How did the SBAR tool make you a more effective communicator?

CRITICAL THINKING ACTIVITY

1. Relate two interactions with a team member when you and/or other team members implemented at least two communication techniques. How did the communication techniques hinder or improve the communication?

First interaction	Communication technique implemented	Communication technique's effect on the interaction
Second interaction	Communication technique implemented	Communication technique's effect on the interaction

SUMMARY

Communication dramatically affects personal and professional relationships. Communication is not only the words you speak, but also how you express the words verbally and nonverbally. As nurses, our communication skills are important in everything we do. Our professional role often elicits an automatic respect or trust from clients. We must be responsible in that role and always strive to communicate in a therapeutic manner. It is important for us to evaluate how we communicate with others, to change what is not effective, and to develop and implement effective communication techniques.

CHAPTER REFLECTIONS

1. What is the mentor's nonverbal communication saying in the chapter scenario?
2. Is therapeutic conversation occurring between the mentor and the client's husband?
3. What are some of the barriers to therapeutic communication in the scenario?
4. Do you think that this communication interaction with the client and her husband will promote compliance? Why or why not?

Journaling Your Journey

1. Describe current strengths and weaknesses in your personal communication skills.
2. Describe communication skills that you admire and/or dislike in others.

3. Describe changes you would like to make in your personal and professional communication techniques.

4. Share steps you plan to take to improve your communication skills.

ಌ   ಌ   ಌ

My Story...

I worked in various long-term care facilities, assisted living facilities, and at local hospital for 10 years before I decided to return to school. I felt I had become comfortable in my job skills, but also was eager for a new challenge. I knew I was limited as an LPN, but with an RN license, many opportunities opened for me. I was a bit nervous about returning to school, not because I was older, but because I felt "safe" as an LPN. I was accustomed to having supervision and registered nurses around to give me direction. After I graduated, I didn't "feel" like an RN. After graduation, I left the hospital and became a school nurse. I found myself completely on my own. The school was just opening and had no policies or guidelines for their nursing clinic. I was in charge of it all. After the panic subsided, I began to organize myself and realized that I was the RN now. I was the one expected to make decisions, I was the one who was to advise the staff on health issues, and educate the staff about caring for our special needs students. I learned to become confident in myself and my skills as an RN.

Katrina Evans, RN

REFERENCES

Balzer-Riley, J. (2008). *Communication in nursing* (6th ed.). St. Louis, MO: Mosby.

Chitty, K. and Black, B. (2007). *Professional nursing: concepts and challenges* (5th ed.). Philadelphia: W.B. Saunders Company.

Coordinating Council for Continuing Education in Health Care. (1990). *Barriers and bridges on the road to better communication* [Motion picture]. University Park, PA: Pennsylvania State University.

Daniels, R., Grendell, R., Wilkins, F. (2010). *Nursing fundamentals: Caring and clinical decision making.* (2nd ed.). Clifton Park, NY: Delmar-Cengage Learning.

Dawson, D. and Reid, K. (1997). Fatigue, alcohol and performance impairment. *Nature,* 388, 235.

Estes, M. (2006). *Health assessment and physical examination.* (3rd ed.). Clifton Park, NY: Thomson Delmar Learning.

Groff, H., and Augello, T. (2003). From theory to practice: An interview with Dr. Michael Leonard. Forum, 10–13.

Haig, K., Sutton, S. and Whittington, J. (2006). SBAR: A shared mental model for improving communication between clinicians. *Journal on Quality and Patient Safety,* 32(3), 167–175.

Hood, L., & Leddy, S. (2003). *Leddy and Pepper's conceptual bases of professional nursing* (5th ed.). Philadelphia: Lippincott Williams & Wilkins.

Institute for Safe Medication Practices. (2004). *Results from ISMP survey on workplace intimidation.* The Institute. Retrieved on 4/25/09 at www.ism.org/Survey/surveyresults/Survey0311asp

Johnson, C., DeMass Martin, S., & Markle-Elder, S. (2007). Stopping verbal abuse in the workplace. *American Journal of Nursing, 107*(4), 32–34.

Kearney-Nunnery, R. (2008). *Advancing your career: Concepts of professional nursing.* (4th ed.). Philadelphia: F.A. Davis Company.

Rosenstein, A. & O'Daniel, M. (2005). Disruptive behavior and clinical outcomes: Perceptions of nurses and physicians. *American Journal of Nursing, 105*(1), 54–64.

Rowe, J. (1999, November 10–16). Self-awareness: Improving nurse-client interactions. *Nursing Standard* [On-line]. Available: 80-proquest.umi.com

Schuster, P. (2000). *Communication: The key to the therapeutic relationship.* Philadelphia: F.A. Davis.

Sullivan, H. (1953). *The interpersonal theory of psychiatry.* New York: Norton.

Taylor, A. (1997). *Communicating.* Englewood Cliffs, NJ: Prentice Hall.

SUGGESTED RESOURCES

Chant, S. (2002). Communication skills: Some problems in nursing education and practice. *Journal of Clinical Nursing, 11*(1), 12–21 [Online]. Available: lore.inspire.net

Communicating and managerial effectiveness. (2003). *Nursing Management, 9*(9), 30–35.

Dixon, N. (2004). Does you organization have an asking problem? *Knowledge Management Review, 7*(3), 18–23.

Meadows, G., & Chaiken, B. (2003). Using IT to improve clinical teamwork and communication. *Nursing Economics, 21*(1), 33–35.

Chapter 6
Caring: The Soul of Nursing

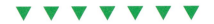

LEARNING OBJECTIVES

By the end of this chapter, you should be able to:

1. Define caring.
2. Explain the relationship of caring to nursing practice.
3. List some goals of nursing practice.

KEY TERM

Caring

SCENARIO

Kerry, a 22-year-old male, is one day post-op from an ileostomy for the treatment of Crohn's disease. He is feeling anxious and has many questions about care of the ileostomy and the lifestyle changes that he will have to make. He has total parenteral nutrition (TPN) infusing through his central line, a patient-controlled analgesia (PCA) pump, a Jackson-Pratt (JP) drain, and a new ileostomy and its appliance. The alarm has just gone off on the intravenous (IV) pump, and Kerry is experiencing increased pain at the stoma site.

Jamie, a cheerful young nurse, enters Kerry's room with a smile. While offering support and encouragement, she attempts to determine the problem with the IV. She finds the alarm silence button but is unable to restart the IV, affecting the administration of both the TPN and pain control. When Kerry groans with pain, the nurse begins to assess him; she finds a discoloration in the stoma and recognizes that the physician needs to be notified. Unsure of what else to do to correct the problem, Jamie tells Kerry she will need to get assistance. She returns shortly with her mentor nurse, Jack. He does not smile or speak to Kerry but quickly attends to the technical equipment. Then he checks the stoma, again without speaking or making any connection with the client. He tends to all of Kerry's needs in a timely manner. Jack is obviously very technically competent and knowledgeable about the post-op care of a new ostomy client.

THINK ABOUT IT

1. Compare and contrast the care provided by the two nurses, Jamie and Jack, in the preceding scenario.
2. Which nurse would you prefer to have care for you? Why?
3. Define *caring* as it relates to nursing.

INTRODUCTION

Caring has been described as the very heart of nursing practice since the beginning of nursing. Khademian and Vizeshfar (2007) believe that caring is commonly accepted as the essence of nursing. With the advances in technology and changes in nursing roles, do you think the personal touch has been diminished or lost in nursing practice? When you think of nurses that you most admire and classify as "good" nurses, do you include the concept of caring in the list of characteristics or behaviors that best describe them? A nurse has the opportunity to combine the knowledge and skills they have developed with the human connection of caring at a very crucial time in different clients and their family's lives. Chauhan (2009) reminds readers that nursing is not just about treating others as you would want to be treated yourself, but also about treating others as they want and expect to be treated—this is even more important. It allows caring nurses to treat individuals as unique and valued human beings with competent care, compassion, dignity, and respect resulting in enhanced, high quality client care. Reeder (2002) quotes theorist Martha Rogers as describing nursing practice as: "the heart that understands and the hand that soothes" (see Figure 6–1). In this chapter, we will discuss the relationship of caring and nursing practice and list goals of nursing practice as they relate to caring.

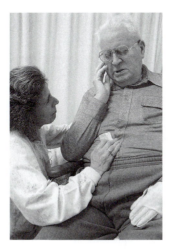

Figure 6–1 "The heart that understands and the hand that soothes" (Martha Rogers). (Source: *Nursing Fundamentals: Caring and Clinical Decision Making*, 2nd ed. Daniels, R. 2010. Clifton Park, NY: Delmar/Cengage Learning.)

Complete the caring survey in Figure 6–2 to examine your thoughts on caring and nursing.

CARING EFFICACY SCALE*

INSTRUCTIONS: When you are completing these items, think of your recent work with patients/clients in clinical settings. Circle the number that best expresses your opinion.

Rating Scale:

−3 Strongly disagree   +1 Slightly agree

−2 Moderately disagree   +2 Moderately agree

−1 Slightly dissagree   +3 Strongly agree

	Strongly disagree			Strongly agree		
1. I do not feel confident in my ability to express a sense of caring to my clients/patients.	−3	−2	−1	+1	+2	+3
2. If I am not relating well to a client/patient, I try to analyze what I can do to reach him/her.	−3	−2	−1	+1	+2	+3
3. I feel comfortable in touching my clients/patients in the course of caregiving.	−3	−2	−1	+1	+2	+3
4. I convey a sense of personal strength to my clients/patients.	−3	−2	−1	+1	+2	+3
5. Clients/patients can tell me most anything and I won't be shocked.	−3	−2	−1	+1	+2	+3
6. I have an ability to introduce a sense of normalcy in stressful conditions.	−3	−2	−1	+1	+2	+3
7. It is easy for me to consider the multifacets of a client's/patient's care, at the same time as I am listening to them.	−3	−2	−1	+1	+2	+3
8. I have difficulty in suspending my personal beliefs and biases in order to hear and accept a client/patient as a person.	−3	−2	−1	+1	+2	+3
9. I can walk into a room with a presence of serenity and energy that makes clients/patients feel better.	−3	−2	−1	+1	+2	+3
10. I am able to tune into a particular client/patient and forget my personal concerns.	−3	−2	−1	+1	+2	+3
11. I can usually create some way to relate to most any client/patient.	−3	−2	−1	+1	+2	+3
12. I lack confidence in my ability to talk to clients/patients from backgrounds different from my own.	−3	−2	−1	+1	+2	+3
13. I feel if I talk to clients/patients on an individual, personal basis, things might get out of control.	−3	−2	−1	+1	+2	+3
14. I use what I learn in conversations with clients/patients to provide more individualized care.	−3	−2	−1	+1	+2	+3

Figure 6–2 Caring Efficacy Scale. (continues)

		Strongly disagree				Strongly agree	
15. I don't feel strong enough to listen to the fears and concerns of my clients/patients.	−3	−2	−1	+1	+2	+3
16. Even when I'm feeling self-confident about most things, I still seem to be unable to relate to clients/patients.	−3	−2	−1	+1	+2	+3
17. I seem to have trouble relating to clients/patients.	−3	−2	−1	+1	+2	+3
18. I can usually establish a close relationship with my clients/patients.	−3	−2	−1	+1	+2	+3
19. I can usually get patients/clients to like me.	−3	−2	−1	+1	+2	+3
20. I often find it hard to get my point of view across to patients/clients when I need to.	−3	−2	−1	+1	+2	+3
21. When trying to resolve a conflict with a client/patient, I usually make it worse.	−3	−2	−1	+1	+2	+3
22. If I think a client/patient is uneasy or may need some help, I approach that person.	−3	−2	−1	+1	+2	+3
23. If I find it hard to relate to a client/patient, I'll stop trying to work with that person.	−3	−2	−1	+1	+2	+3
24. I often find it hard to relate to clients/patients from a different culture than mine.	−3	−2	−1	+1	+2	+3
25. I have helped many clients/patients through my ability to develop close, meaningful relationships.	−3	−2	−1	+1	+2	+3
26. I often find it difficult to express empathy with clients/patients.	−3	−2	−1	+1	+2	+3
27. I often become overwhelmed by the nature of the problems clients/patients are experiencing.	−3	−2	−1	+1	+2	+3
28. When a client/patient is having difficulty communicating with me, I am able to adjust to his/her level.	−3	−2	−1	+1	+2	+3
29. Even when I really try, I can't get through to difficult clients/patients.	−3	−2	−1	+1	+2	+3
30. I don't use creative or unusual ways to express caring to my clients/patients.	−3	−2	−1	+1	+2	+3

Figure 6–2 (continued)

CRITICAL THINKING ACTIVITY

1. What new concepts of caring as a nurse did you discover as you completed the caring survey?

CARING

Kearney-Nunnery (2008) states that the concept of caring is not new. Rather, caring has been discussed as a part of nursing since the days of Florence Nightingale and has a direct link associated between nursing and service to others. Research identified a theme in patient feedback regarding caring nurses that explores the concept of nurses meeting patients needs without being asked and going above and beyond to make sure the patient's needs were met (Finch, 2008). While there are a variety of reasons for becoming a nurse, very often when nursing students are surveyed about their motivation in pursuing a nursing degree, their response is "to help others." This response only partially defines caring because caring cannot occur if others are not involved; it is important to note that caring requires both a giver and a receiver. The literature becomes diverse when attempting to commit to one common definition or description of caring and rather displays a wide array of potential caring behaviors. Chauhan (2009) identifies some important caring behaviors and includes such actions as: right skills and positive attitude, nurses who challenge poor practice, nurses who are generally kind and compassionate about what they are doing, good communicators, and nurses who involve clients in their planning of care.

Caring is a deep-seated involvement in the lives of others; a commitment to provide quality care, to assist the client to a quality state of health, or a presence as the client dies with dignity. Caring is a complex, observable fact and experience.

Caring as the Core of Nursing

Several theorists have developed conceptual models based on caring. They include Dorthea Orem's Self-Care Deficit Model (2001), Jean Watson's Human Science and Human Care Model (2007), and Leininger and McFarland's Culture Care Diversity and Universality (2006). Orem believes that all individuals desire to care for and meet their personal care needs and that each person has varied abilities to participate in meeting his personal self-care needs. The nurse attempts to meet the client's self-care needs in an effort to reduce the client's self-care deficits. Watson believes that caring is a moral ideal and that nursing is a caring art and science. The client is the center of human caring. Leininger believes that nursing is a learned art focused on caring in accord with an individual's culture. To these theorists, caring definitely is an element of nursing.

Nursing research indicates that nurses and clients identify different concepts when defining *caring* in the provision of care. To Bertero (1999) caring includes "all aspects of delivering nursing care to patients" (p. 414). Caring is the heart and unifying core of nursing. Theorist Leininger proposes that caring is the trademark of nursing practice: "Care is the essence and the central unifying and dominant domain to characterize nursing. Care has also been postulated to be an essential human need for the full development, health maintenance, and survival of human beings in all world cultures" (1988,

p. 3). These statements imply that caring is the very essence of nursing care and at the core of nursing practice.

Caring also is a basic human need that must be fulfilled if an individual is to obtain his full potential. Nurses can meet a client's needs when providing nursing care. "Caring is a commitment by the nurse to become involved, and its character is relational. Nurses enter this relationship with their whole being" (Bertero, 1999, p. 415).

"The nurse's role is 'being with' rather than 'doing to' a patient" (Bertero, 1999, p. 415). Clients expect competence in performing procedures. Nurses provide competent and safe care when they adeptly perform procedures and are "with" the client relationally during the procedure. The nurse can also be with or "connected to" the client when the client needs to talk or share intimate personal feelings. "Caring means connecting with clients by listening to their thoughts and fears, and communicating concern" (p. 415). Caring is more than a physical presence, it is a relational concern for the other's well-being.

Caring Defined by Caring Experiences

A research project analyzed the narrative writing of 68 nursing students as they described caring experiences (Schaefer, 2002). From the study, five themes were identified:

1. Nurses need to care for themselves to care for others.
2. Emotional attachment has dangers.
3. Caring involves a moral responsibility.
4. Reflections on care teach about caring.
5. Reflection engages one in defining caring. (p. 293)

In the first theme, the students identified their need to receive care in order to prepare them to care for others. As the students experienced caring in personal situations, they learned the value of receiving care and also acquired a desire to meet others' needs by caring for them. The caring process is a continuous, ongoing process. An individual receives care, then gives care to another, who learns about care and then gives care to another. Our life experiences in which we receive care prepare us for future caring opportunities. In this way, nurses who receive care learn and are equipped to give care.

The second theme, that emotional attachment has dangers, is described (Schaefer, 2002) in a situation in which a client started to cry, causing an emotional response from the student that led to the student's bursting into tears. The student was then incapable of meeting the physical or emotional needs of his client. Nurses walk a tightrope between caring and tempering their emotions to provide competent care. Emotional attachment spurs caring, but emotional attachment can be painful, difficult, and a hindrance to adequate care. Nurses learn to balance these emotions with experience and growth.

The third theme emphasizes that caring is a moral responsibility. As nurses become aware of the needs of others, they have to make a choice. Do they meet the need, or do they ignore the need? In that decision lies the moral choice or responsibility. Hopefully, in becoming aware of another's need, the nurse comprehends and has an emotional response to the client's situation and is motivated to respond with conscious, caring, appropriate actions to address the client's situation. The choice to respond with caring actions is self-giving and will cost the nurse something—time, energy, or possibly convenience—but responding positively to a moral choice is a self-satisfying, personal decision.

The fourth theme supports the idea that as we reflect on caring experiences, we learn about caring. As the students pondered their client caring experiences, one student realized that she had cared for a client for several days but had not really gotten to know her particular likes and dislikes. The author recently observed a similar situation, in which a nurse offered a client a nutrition tray with the regular tea provided by the facility, but another nurse who had taken the time to get to know the client was aware that the client preferred a special tea she had stored in her bedside drawer. Other personal stories where caring was defined by experiences include the following. Debra Sturdy (2008), an RN, shares her story of dealing with death from a personal perspective for the first time when her father died, versus her experiences in less connected times with death as a nurse. She reminds readers that one does not totally understand how the experience of death feels until they have actually experienced it themselves. She reminds us of the importance of remembering the loved ones left behind by the empty bed. She believes that assisting clients and their families through the experience of death is one of the "most skilled acts of caring" in which nurses participate. She identifies this as one of the last things a nurse can do for their client and their family and that "nurses have only one chance to do it right" (p. 14).

Olson (2005), an advanced practice nurse, shares a similar story from when his mother was ill and hospitalized. He identified nurses who kept his mother clean and safe, allowed her individual need to be useful in her own way, respected her dignity, showed compassion through a caring touch, and included the family members in their acts of caring. Olson believes the acts of caring eased the process of death for his mother and the family. Olson challenges all nurses to remember the importance of and power of caring at the bedside and believes very strongly that is part of the nursing role and responsibilities.

Waters (2009) shares from his interview with Lord Mancroft in the UK this powerful quote: "When you go into the hospital and you feel vulnerable, lonely and in pain or distressed, you want someone to . . . give that human touch. It is about making people feel comfortable, loved and secure. And if a patient is feeling distressed, spend time with them. You can train someone to be brilliant technically, but if they do not care about the people there just is no point to it" (p. 18). One student stated that her caring experience could be labeled "caring, patient advocacy, or simply my job" (Schaefer, 2002, p. 290) How would the environment of a facility change if all nurses provided genuine care because caring was "simply my job?"

CRITICAL THINKING ACTIVITY

1. Describe a time when you showed caring in your role as a nurse. Describe the events leading to the interaction, your interaction with the client, and the result of the interaction (Schaefer, 2002).

2. After writing about your caring experience, share what you learned about caring with your classmates.

Acts of Caring

Bertero (1999) conducted a qualitative research study of nurses' sharing their experiences in situations when caring was given and was not given to a client. The theme that emerged from the nurses' sharing their caring experiences was the development and maintenance of a "helping-trusting interpersonal relationship" (p. 416). This relationship was maintained in five ways, or subthemes:

1. Creation of an interaction with the client and next of kin.
2. Actions to satisfy the needs of the client and next of kin.
3. Feelings of frustration in the caring role.
4. Influence of time constraints.
5. Development of self and gaining insight (Bertero, 1999).

The first subtheme, creating an interaction with the client and next of kin, included verbal and nonverbal communication and touch. The interactions could include eye contact that says "I know" or "I care," or compassionately placing a hand on the client's forearm to say "I care." "Creating interaction is not just a task: It is making contact, relating and being present with the patients and their next of kin" (Bertero, 1999, p. 417). Caring is seen not as a duty but as an actual giving of self to establish a relationship with another. When have you given of yourself to establish a professional relationship with a client? This emotional interaction can be extremely rewarding.

The second subtheme, acting to satisfy the needs of the client and next of kin, includes recognizing and anticipating the client's physical, emotional, social, and spiritual needs. These are actions of competence, service, presence, and respect for the client and next of kin.

Frustrating feelings in the caring role, the third subtheme, were experienced when unclear, unrealistic, or false information was given to the client and next of kin. The nurses also experienced frustration when they could do nothing to save the client's life. It was then that the client was assisted with a comforting, peaceful, and dignified death.

In the fourth subtheme, nurses felt that time constraints influenced their ability to care for a client. They also felt limited by the brevity of some lives and attempted to improve quality in the time frame available. Quality could take the form of fluffing a pillow for comfort, attentively listening to a client's sharing past experiences with children, or assisting a client in forgiving a past hurt.

The fifth subtheme was nurses' experiencing self-development and gaining insight. "The nurses stated that when they viewed themselves as competent in caring and obtaining satisfaction from the patient, they developed their sense of self and improved their self-esteem" (Bertero, 1999, p. 419). The nurses felt that they gained insight from client interactions and viewing clients' life experiences. Caring is truly a two-way, relational experience. It is a complex experience involving personal interaction and competence in skilled techniques.

Hayes & Tyler-Ball (2007) shared details from a research study that looked at the perception of trauma clients and the ideas of caring behaviors identified below in Box 6–1. This study has shown some very specific behaviors that can enhance the care that nurses give and the care that clients are feeling in return.

Box 6–1 Caring Behaviors

Emotional/spiritual well-being	Saving lives
Patient dignity	Patient safety
Self-control	Comfort
Individuality	A trusting relationship
Physical assistance in healing	Social support

(Adapted from Hayes, J. & Tyler-Ball, S. (2007). Perceptions of nurses' caring behaviors by trauma patients. *Journal of Trauma Nursing 14(4), 187–190.*)

THEORY TO PRACTICE

Nursing care goes beyond disease processes and technical skills. Nurses are growing daily and developing their skills and responses with every nursing experience. Take time to think about each experience and how it has impacted you and your belief system or practice routines. It is important to think about the theory and textbook knowledge versus the real world experiences. To help you reflect on these details, think about each of the following questions, and then answer them as best you can.

1. Share a personal experience when you:
   - Interacted with a client and her next of kin.
   - Acted to satisfy the needs of a client and her next of kin.
   - Felt frustrated in the caring role.
   - Felt the influence of time constraints when caring for a client.
   - Developed your sense of self and gained personal insight.
2. What were the dynamics that made the interaction a positive experience?
3. How could the experience have been improved?

CRITICAL THINKING ACTIVITY

1. What does it mean to care?
2. What are ways you might improve your caring behaviors?

GOALS OF NURSING PRACTICE

To some nurses, nursing provides financial reward. To others, nursing provides self-satisfaction or self-fulfillment. To still others, nursing defines who they are. Nursing, to a professional, is a career plan, a central part of his core being; and caring is the behavioral outcome.

Most nurses would agree that attitude is a powerful driving force on any nursing unit and that the impact of strong role models has the ability to make a difference in many situations. Soldwisch & Lockhart (2003) decided to set the standard by developing service ambassadors from individuals who they considered strong role models that could lead by example and ensure high quality care. They believed that if the standard was set and individuals were held accountable, a more respectful, collaborative and supportive working environment would not only become the expected standard, but the new norm.

Brown, Holcomb, Maloney, Naranjo, Gibson & Russell (2005) became concerned about cutbacks and downsizing in the 1990s and its impact on nursing care. They decided to explore a new position on nursing units called patient care facilitator (PCF) that was much like the case manager role. The PCF would enhance caring practices and provide more continuity in care, which clients would experience as more caring. They felt this role could provide more continuity in care, which patients would experience as more caring. The role of the PCFs allowed stronger relationships to develop and the passion for nursing to resurface. In this experience, they found strong themes of love, care giving, and emotional connection. Having a nurse in this lead role enhanced the unit teamwork as well as caring behaviors. Patients interpreted this as individualized care and enjoyed getting their own needs met in a timely manner.

Communication was occurring in a respectful, caring manner and enhanced the experience for all involved. Brown et al., stressed the importance of choosing PCFs from clinically competent, caring staff who have the ability to work well with the entire health care team. They decided to have PCFs as a permanent part of their staff to enhance caring when providing client care. See Figure 6–3 for a positive interaction between nurses.

According to Ryan (2005), Meleis stated that "an established nursing theory would strengthen practice by providing structure and languages to describe, explain, support, and guide the professional nursing practice" (p. 26). She explored the experience of implementing one nursing theorist's theory, Watson's Caring Theory, into the working practice on her unit and found it to be very successful. As Watson did, she called for "high touch along with high technology" when practicing nursing. Ryan challenged nurses to go above and beyond the scientific clinical aspects of nursing and to remember to include the humanitarian and moral side as well. In Ryan's process of implementing this on her nursing unit, some questioned whether there was really time for nurses to practice the caring approach, but what they soon learned was that indeed there was time and that professional nurses are doing this every day in spite of the busy nursing routines as shown in Figure 6–4.

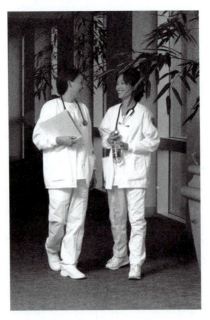

Figure 6–3 Caring does not stop with clients; it carries over into respectful caring interactions between nurses.
Source: DeLaune, S.C. and Ladner, P.K. *Fundamentals of Nursing, Standards and Practice, 3e.* Cengage/Delmar. 2006.

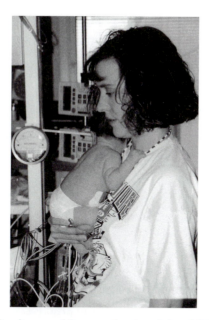

Figure 6–4 Nursing provides a caring touch in a high tech world
(Source: *Nursing Fundamentals: Caring and Clinical Decision
Making*, Second Edition. Daniels, R. 2010. Clifton Park, NY: Delmar/
Cengage Learning.)

The concepts of essential relationships and self-reward may comprise care of others and
care of self. Service to others provides a meaningful life purpose. Service gives the individual
feelings of competence in the ability to perform a task. Service is the link between concern for
others and action in response to concern (Hood & Leddy, 2006).

SUMMARY

The goals of nursing practice combine knowledge, self-care, and competent technical skills.
Caring is providing competent physical, emotional, and spiritual care; interacting verbally
and nonverbally with clients and their families; satisfying the needs of clients and their
families; and experiencing self-development and gaining personal insight. Nursing is "caring from the heart . . . and the head." Nurses should "exercise their intellectual skills to provide the best care possible. . . . Nurses who constantly think, as well as feel for their patients,
are the best nurses." The best nurses are those "who are smart critical thinkers, who are
constantly questioning what is best for the patient, what is best for the organization, is there
a better way?" (Curran, 1999, p. 73). The union of caring and competence are the goals of
nursing practice. Nursing is defined as an art and a science. Nursing is the "science of caring"
(Huch, 2003, p. 82). Finch (2008) states that "patients are well aware of and able to
articulate the types of interactions they prefer to have with nurses and the behaviors that

specifically convey caring to them" (p. 31). Caring is an important part of quality nursing care and a desirable characteristic expected from all nurses.

CRITICAL THINKING ACTIVITY

After reading this chapter, write your own definitions of the terms *nursing practice, caring,* and *competence.*

1. Nursing practice
2. Caring
3. Competence

CHAPTER REFLECTIONS

1. We have said that the goals of nursing practice are a combination of knowledge, caring, and competent technical skills. List your personal goals of nursing practice.
2. What role does caring have in your nursing practice?

Journaling Your Journey

1. Describe times personally and professionally when you showed caring to others.
2. Describe times when you were the recipient of caring.
3. How did the identified caring experiences make you "feel"?
4. How did the caring experience impact the interaction with others?

My Story...

I worked as an LPN for 2 years when I decided to go back to school to become a registered nurse. It was a lot of work, but becoming an RN was one of the best decisions I have ever made. In my journey, I learned two very important things about myself and about nursing in general. First, getting a nursing education does not provide a nurse with all of the answers that you will need when you graduate and start your RN career. It is only the beginning of life-long learning. There is no way you can learn everything about every disease, medication, or treatment; and passing an exam does not make you an expert. What RN students need to understand is that at first, "you don't know what you don't know." Education is not only about learning, but also about stimulating thinking. Hopefully you will not leave a class satisfied that you now are the expert about the topic of the day, but leave class knowing that there is always more to know, always unanswered questions. Excellent nurses have self-awareness that they do not have all the answers, don't pretend they do, and have the desire to always learn more. For me, education has led to more questions about things than answers.

The second important thing that I learned throughout my education and nursing career is that some things will not automatically change about an individual because of more education. Caring, for example, won't change without self-awareness and practice, regardless of how many letters you have behind your name. Think about the nurses in your class, or nurses with whom you work. Who are the most caring? Who are the least caring? What were the initials behind their name? I have found there are LPNs and RNs in each category. Consider your caring skills. Caring is the essence of nursing practice; how will your education prepare you to care not only for your patients, but about your patients?

Kim Penland, PhD (c), FNP-BC

REFERENCES

Bertero, C. (1999). Caring for and about cancer patients: Identifying the meaning of the phenomenon "caring" through narratives. *Cancer Nursing, 22*(6), 414–420.

Brown, C., Holcomb, L., Maloney, J., Naranjo, J., Gibson C. & Russell, P. (2005). Caring in action: The patient care facilitator role. *International Journal of Human Caring, 9*(3), 51–58.

Coates, C. (2002). Caring Efficacy Scale. In J. Watson, *Assessing and measuring caring in nursing and health science* (pp. 171–173). New York: Springer Publishing Company.

Chauhan, R. (2009). Timely reminder of care standards—but is the message strong enough? *Nursing Standard, 23*(28), 12–13.

Curran, C. (1999). Caring from the heart . . . and the head. *Nursing Economics, 17*(2), 73.

Finch, L. (2008). Development of a substantive theory of nurse caring. *International Journal of Human Caring 12*(1), 25–32.

Hayes, J. & Tyler-Ball, S. (2007). Perceptions of nurses' caring behaviors by trauma patients. *Journal of Trauma Nursing, 14(4), 187–190.*

Hood, L., & Leddy, S. (2006). *Leddy and Pepper's conceptual bases of professional nursing* (6th ed.). Philadelphia: Lippincott.

Huch, M. (2003). The many facets of caring. *Nursing Science Quarterly, 16*(1), 82–83.

Kearney-Nunnery, R. (2008). *Advancing your career: Concepts of professional nursing,* (4th ed.). Philadelphia: F.A. Davis Company.

Khademian, Z. & Vizeshfar, F. (2007). Nursing students' perceptions of the importance of caring behaviors. *Journal of Advanced Nursing, 61*(4), 456–462.

Leininger, M. (1988). *Care: The essence of nursing and health.* Detroit, MI: Wayne State University Press.

Leininger, M. (1995). *Transcultural nursing* (2nd ed.). New York: McGraw-Hill.

Leininger, M. & McFarland, M. (2006). Culture care diversity and universality: A worldwide nursing theory (2nd ed.). Boston, MA: Jones and Bartlett Publishers.

Olson, T. (2005). Searching for care: A personal journey. *Nursing Forum 40*(2), 58–59.

Orem, D. (2001). *Nursing: Concepts of practice* (6th ed.). St. Louis: Mosby.

Reeder, F. (2002, March). Remembrances of Martha E. Rogers. *Rogerian* Nursing Science News 1(2).

Ryan, L. (2005). The journey to integrating Watson's Caring Theory with clinical practice. *International Journal of Human Caring 9*(3), 26–30.

Schaefer, K. (2002). Reflections on caring narratives: Enhancing patterns of knowing. *Nursing Education Perspectives, 23,* 286–293.

Soldwisch, S. & Lockhart, C. (2003). In our unit: Accept no less than caring behaviors. *Critical Care Nurse 23*(4), 96,126.

Sturdy, D. (2008). One chance to get it right. *Nursing Older People, 20*(10), 14.

Waters, A. (2009). I did the right thing. *Nursing Standard 23*(25), 16–18.

Watson, J. (2007). *Nursing: Human science and human care: A theory of nursing.* Boston, MA: Jones & Bartlett Publishers.

SUGGESTED RESOURCES

Huffman, D., Lewis, S., & Nelson, M. (2002). Advancing technology, caring, and nursing. *Nursing Science Quarterly, 15*(4), 434–437.

Loxterkamp, D. (2009). The old duffers' club. *Annuals of Family Medicine, 7*(3), 270–272.

Mustard, L. (2002). Caring and competency. *JONA's Healthcare Law, Ethics, and Regulation, 4,* 36–43.

Sitzman, K. (2006). Faculty matters. *Nursing Education Perspectives, 27*(1), 8–9.

Chapter 7
Clinical Decision Making
and the Nursing Process

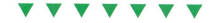

LEARNING OBJECTIVES

By the end of this chapter, you should be able to:

1. Define the stages of clinical judgment.
2. Explain the steps in problem solving.
3. Explain the steps in decision making.
4. Explain the steps in the nursing process.
5. Develop a care plan using the steps in the nursing process.
6. Develop a concept map.

KEY TERMS

Assessment
Clinical judgment
Concept map
Decision making
Decision tree
Diagnosis
Evaluation
Gantt chart
Implementation
Nursing interventions
Nursing process
Outcome identification
PERT chart

Planning nursing care

Problem solving

SCENARIO

Tameka is a new graduate who has worked on a medical surgical unit for three months. Her client experienced left arm pain, nausea, shortness of breath, and diaphoresis three days postoperatively. She medicated the client for pain, but the pain was not relieved by the medication. She sought advice from a more experienced nurse on the unit who had her call the doctor because she was concerned that the client was experiencing symptoms of a myocardial infarction. Tameka feels disappointed in herself that she did not recognize these symptoms. She feels like an incompetent nurse and that maybe she should just quit.

THINK ABOUT IT

1. Should new nurses be expected to determine what is happening with a patient from observed signs and symptoms in all cases?
2. Does seeking advice from a co-worker make you an incompetent nurse?
3. Did Tameka respond in an appropriate manner?

INTRODUCTION

It is critical for nurses to make quick, accurate, and effective decisions. In this chapter the steps in clinical judgment, problem solving, and decision making are discussed. The nursing process is the nursing discipline's method of assisting nurses in making decisions, so the steps of the nursing process are explained in detail with an opportunity for the student to complete a nursing care plan. Concept maps are explained and the student is given an opportunity to develop a concept map.

CLINICAL JUDGMENT

Benner, Tanner, and Chesla (2009) propose that "the clinical judgment of experienced nurses resembles much more . . . engaged practical reasoning . . . than the disengaged, scientific, or theoretical reasoning . . . represented in the nursing process" (p. 1). They suggest that **clinical judgment** progresses from a novice stage to an expert stage. Their theory, known as the five-stage novice-to-expert practice model, is based on inductive studies of clinical practice settings. Benner et al.'s model proposes that an experienced nurse gains understanding of and responds to a person's illness by knowing the client and by having gained proficient clinical knowledge through the experience of caring for many persons in similar situations, rather than by labeling a client with a nursing diagnosis. The experiential clinical knowledge makes the nurse more aware of possible issues and concerns that could occur in other similar clinical situations. Hood and Leddy (2003) state, "this [Benner et al.'s] model is individualized rather than rule based, and emphasizes the integration of nonconscious, nonanalytical aspects of judgment, experience, and reflection on rational critical thinking" (p. 253). Benner et al.'s model encourages the nurse to view the client as an individual with individual issues and concerns instead of applying a set of rules to each client's situation.

It is important to remember that each client's response to a situation will vary and requires a different approach in the care provided. For example, two clients enter the health care setting with pneumonia. The basic treatment for each client is the same, but each client has varying issues and concerns that require different clinical approaches. For instance, one may have good-quality insurance and not be worried about the medical bills, and the other may have postponed seeing a physician because of financial concerns. The clients may vary in age, and the elder require more intensive therapy. Both clients have pneumonia, but one client's is uncomplicated, and the other, elderly client has a history of asthma, and emphysema. The nurse's clinical approach obviously will differ with each of these clients.

As the nurse progresses through the novice to expert stages, she begins to rely on her internal instincts along with her clinical judgment and experience in the critical thinking process. If the nurse is attuned to her instincts, she may sense the client's financial concerns and collaborate with the facilities' social services department. Or she may recall, from previous experience with other seriously ill clients, that advanced directives should be addressed with an elderly client with pneumonia, asthma, and emphysema. Each of these clients may have the same basic nursing diagnoses, but the nurse varies the clinical interventions to meet the client's individual needs.

CRITICAL THINKING ACTIVITY

1. Review the clinical judgment section and identify the key components related to clinical judgment that you think are important. Note the passage quotes from Benner et al. and Hood and Leddy. How will these components change your clinical judgment?

Stages of Clinical Judgment

The five stages of Benner et al.'s model of clinical judgment (2009) are novice, advanced beginner, competent, proficient, and expert.

Novice Stage

The novice stage occurs during the education process (Benner et al., 2009). The novice is presented with tasks that are completed by a standard set of rules or guidelines. The novice focuses on the task and memorizes the rules to complete the task successfully. The context in which the task occurs is not totally seen by the novice at this point. For example, when learning to transfer a stroke client with left-side involvement from the bed to a wheelchair, the novice learns as many rules as possible, such as placing the wheelchair on the client's uninvolved side (in this case, the right side) and locking the wheelchair wheels before transferring the client.

Advanced Beginner Stage

During the advanced beginner stage (Benner et al., 2009), the nurse begins to recognize the surroundings in which tasks are completed. The advanced beginner nurse has gained experience and learned more rules for handling the tasks. She begins to recognize difficult situations when performing tasks and sees the tasks as more difficult. Clinically, the advanced beginner is anxious, perhaps somewhat overwhelmed, and she sees the clinical experience as a list of tasks to complete in an organized, prioritized manner. The advanced beginner has a fragmented view of the situation and is dependent on the knowledge and skills of others. She does not see herself as a participant in the overall situation. She views her clinical practice as a set of external standards or orders that test her personal abilities. She is uncertain of her ability to contribute to the overall clinical situation. For example, consider a new nurse who is caring for a renal dialysis client. She knows the classification, action, side effects, and nursing considerations of the client's medications, but she is uncertain if these medications should be given prior to, during, or following dialysis. She needs to consult with a more experienced RN for guidance in medication administration.

Competent Stage

In the competent stage, the nurse has gained organizational and technical skills and approaches client care with a plan that assists in making decisions about the client's condition. She feels confident and competent in her nursing care. She knows she can no longer function totally by rules and memorized steps but needs to see the client's individual needs and assess the overall physical condition. She then analyzes all of the obtained data and makes a decision or seeks another health care provider's input. In the advanced beginner stage, we used the example of a nurse caring for a renal dialysis client who knew something about the client's medication but was not knowledgeable about administering the medication. In the competent stage, the nurse knows what medications to give and when the medications should be given in relationship to dialysis. She completes thorough assessments of the client and recognizes the rationale behind complications. For example, if a client returned to the floor with slight hypotension, the competent nurse would know why dialysis clients may have hypotension after dialysis but might have difficulty determining when or if to give the hypertensive medication. She might have to refer to a more experienced colleague for advice on when or if to give the hypertensive medication.

Proficient Stage

The proficient nurse intuitively determines the importance of various factors in client situations. The nurse differentiates patterns and anticipates needed actions in client situations. Emotional and reasoned decisions of nursing options in these situations are easier and less stressful, but decisions are still based on rules. The nurse interacts with the clients and families with acquired, wide-ranging skills. An example is a nurse receiving a report from surgery that a client who had a thyroidectomy is returning to the floor. The nurse checks the computer for clinical skills of a post-op thyroidectomy client and then orders a tracheostomy tray to the floor in case of an emergency. The nurse prepares the family prior to bringing the tracheostomy tray into the room so that the family will not become overly concerned.

Expert Stage

The expert nurse uses discernment and critical thinking based on experienced intuition, observations, and non-emotional, practical reasoning. She relies on theory or asks other expert nurses for advice. She sees the big picture and anticipates and responds to potential complications. In the proficient stage example, the nurse used the computer to gather data on caring for a post-op thyroidectomy client. In the expert stage, the nurse in the same situation, without mentally reviewing steps of care, would immediately order the tracheostomy tray to the floor and prepare the family for the client's return to the room.

CRITICAL THINKING ACTIVITY

1. Review the examples presented in each stage of clinical judgment. Do you think the examples in each stage appropriately represent the actions of a nurse in that stage?
2. Determine your placement in the five-stage novice-to-expert practice model. Support your decision by relating appropriate statements from this text to two personal clinical examples.

PROBLEM SOLVING

We are confronted daily with problems and situations in which we have to seek the best solution. **Problem solving** is thoroughly analyzing a problem or situation and looking at multiple options in determining the best solution to the problem. Problem solving involves using critical thinking skills that lead to the most effective solution. According to Tommey (2008), the steps in problem solving (revised) are: identify the problem, generate possible solutions and examine suggested solutions, choose the best solution, implement the chosen solution, and evaluate the effectiveness of the solution and whether the problem has been resolved. These steps can be followed in solving personal, professional, or client problems.

Identify the Problem

Sometimes problems that surface are not the root of the problem, but symptoms of the root. We need to gather all available information by asking questions of and seeking information from several sources. We must be open to all sides of the issue, regardless of the personalities or personal issues involved. The nurse needs to examine personal feelings and thoughts about the issue to make sure that they do not interfere with finding the best solution. These actions allow the nurse to get to the root of the problem. If the root is not defined and addressed, the problem may resurface at a later time.

Generate Possible Solutions and Examine Suggested Solutions

Once you have identified the problem, generate as many solutions as possible. It is important to brainstorm ideas regardless of how irrational or crazy they appear at first. Some of the best solutions are created when we feel free to think outside the box. Explore the future ramifications of all suggested solutions. What will be the potential results of each one? Which solutions are viable, and which ones are not?

Choose the Best Solution

Some decisions are hard to make because the consequences will not be pleasant for all persons involved. The best solution is chosen only after all data and all possible solutions are reviewed. A common scenario for the decision-making process is a family with a terminally ill member. The spouse is no longer physically able to care for the ill family member. The children cannot financially care for their own families if they take time off work to care for their parent, nor do they have the knowledge and nursing skills to do so. None of them wants their family member to be admitted to a long-term care facility. However, after considering all possible solutions, they find that the best solution is placing the family member in a long-term care facility.

Implement the Chosen Solution

After determining the best solution, implement it. Make sure all parties involved are appropriately informed. Keep in mind that change is often difficult, and new issues may arise as the solution is implemented. Address the issues appropriately and adequately, reexamining them in light of the original problem.

Evaluate the Effectiveness of the Solution

Allow an adequate amount of time to pass after implementing the solution, then reevaluate the situation to determine the appropriateness and effectiveness of the solution. Determine whether the root problem has been solved or if the problem needs to be reevaluated.

CRITICAL THINKING ACTIVITY

1. Think of a problem you encountered on the clinical unit. Use each step of the problem-solving process to determine the best solution. Before implementing the chosen solution, share your problem solving example in a group of two other students requesting their input into the problem. Was the group's solution the same as your personal solution to the problem?
   - Identify the Problem
   - Generate Possible Solutions and Examine Suggested Solutions

- Choose the Best Solution
  - Did you review/analyze all data and all possible solutions before choosing this solution?
- Implement the Chosen Solution
  - Explain how you implemented the solution.
  - How did you inform all involved parties? What was their response? Did you encounter any issues?
  - Keep in mind that change is often difficult, and new issues may arise as the solution is implemented. Were the issues addressed appropriately and adequately?
  - Did you refer back to the origin of the problem to see if you were addressing the real issue and if the solution you are implementing addresses the "real" problem.
- Evaluate the Effectiveness of the Solution
  - Was the root problem solved or do you need to reevaluate the problem?
  - Meet again with your group of two other students and evaluate the implementation strategy of each student's problem.
  - Share your problem solving activity with an experienced RN.
  - Share and evaluate her input into your problem solving skills.

DECISION MAKING

Clinical nurses are required to make efficient, sound, and effective decisions. **Decision making** is a process of using critical thinking in choosing the best option from several alternatives to achieve a desired result. The steps for decision making and problem solving are very similar, but decision making is different from problem solving. Decision making does not always solve the problem, but it supplies an immediate solution or action to a situation. Problem solving seeks to find a solution to the problem when the decisions have not solved the problem (Ham, 2002). The following example illustrates the difference between decision making and problem solving. A nursing student owns an older car that has prominent rust spots, uses a quart of oil a week, and has a hole in the tailpipe. At 9 P.M. one night, a bald tire goes flat. The student decides to call a friend to assist in changing the tire. After clinical at midnight a week later, the radiator overheats. The student again makes a decision, to call a friend for a ride home. After having made several decisions to address the situation, the student uses problem solving to review various options and decides to purchase a different car.

Many nursing decisions are based on the decision-making process. At first a nurse may make decisions slowly, working step-by-step through the decision-making process. Experienced nurses probably do not follow each step of the decision-making process as they make every decision; instead, by working through the steps to reach previous decisions they develop critical thinking skills to complete the process quickly and effectively. The decision-making process may be used individually or in groups. Clinical nurses may use the process to solve a problem on the unit, such as scheduling or dispensing medications. When solving a group problem, communication through each step is vital for the success of the decision-making process.

Charts and Graphs for Decision Making

Several charts and graphs have been developed to assist in decision making. They include the decision tree, the Gantt chart, and the PERT (program evaluation and review technique) chart.

Decision Tree

The **decision tree** is a visual diagram of a decision, alternatives, risk factors, and possible outcomes. First, the decision regarding a problem is listed with at least two possible alternatives. The risk factors are listed for each alternative, followed by possible outcomes. It is called a decision tree because the diagram resembles a tree with several branches (see Figure 7–1). By working through the decision tree process, we recognize alternatives to a decision and the potential risks and consequences of each alternative decision (Tommey, 2008). Figure 7–2 is a completed decision tree using the earlier car example.

Gantt Chart

The **Gantt chart** is a grid schedule that lists various tasks needed to complete a project. The chart consists of several columns, including one for the task, one for the person responsible for completing the task, and columns for the time frame for task completion (Figure 7–3). The time frame could be hours, days, months, or years. There is a separate row for each task or responsible person. A line is drawn in the time frame for tasks in progress. An X is placed on the completion point of the time frame. With a Gantt chart, you plan backward from the due date through the needed tasks.

PERT Chart

The **PERT chart** is a detailed graph of multiple tasks needing completion for a multitask project. The graph offers a diagram of projects needing completion before others can be started (Figure 7–4). This gives a visual image of task sequencing. Time frames are established for task completion. The time frames can be broken down into shortest time, for completion with no complications, reasonable time, with usual complications, and longest time, with multiple complications (Tommey, 2008). These time frames are written on the lines between each task.

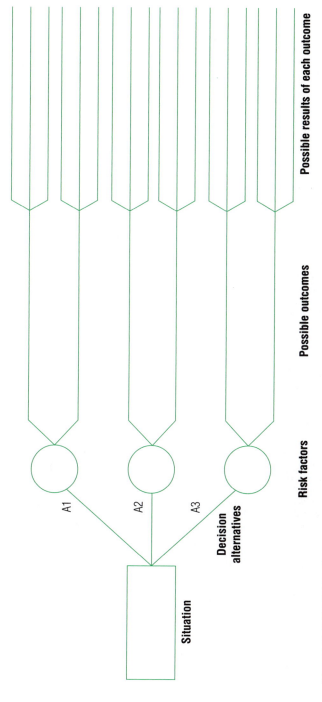

Figure 7–1 Decision Tree.

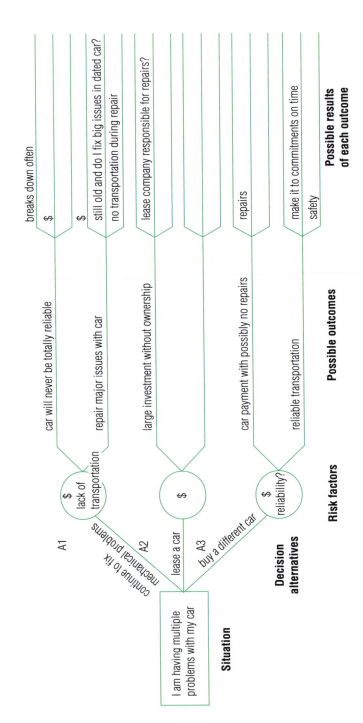

Figure 7–2 Decision Tree Example.

Task	Responsible person	Monday	Tuesday	Wednesday	Thursday	Friday

Figure 7–3 Gantt chart.

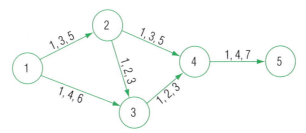

Figure 7–4 PERT chart. The numbers within the circles represent tasks to complete. In this PERT chart, task 1 needs completing before tasks 2 and 3, and task 2 slightly before 3. Tasks 1, 2, and 3 should be completed before task 4, and tasks 1, 2, 3, and 4 before task 5. The smaller numbers on each line represent possible time frames for completion of the task, with the first number being when the task could be completed most quickly, the second number most likely, and the last number the longest amount of time for completion. The arrows indicate the direction of task performance. Each of the numbers inside a circle represent an assigned task; for example, 1 = determine topic for research paper, 2 = obtain literature review.

Using Gantt and PERT Charts

Gantt and PERT charts are used for decision making and for short- and long-term planning. They assist with time management in detailed projects. They help in the decision making and problem solving process of forming the needed steps to make decisions, solve problems, or complete projects. Sequencing tasks or steps in each of these charts develops critical thinking and decision-making skills. The charts also provide a visual method or process of decision making.

CRITICAL THINKING ACTIVITIES

1. Use a decision tree, Gantt chart, or PERT chart to work through a decision or plan a project, term paper, or committee responsibility. Draw the chart of your choice and compare your chart with your classmates.

2. Describe how you think your decision-making skills were developed by making the chart.

THE NURSING PROCESS

It is essential for nurses to make effective decisions in clinical practice. The **nursing process** is a discipline-specific method that provides a logical way for nurses to make decisions and solve problems in providing individualized, holistic, and effective client care. Even though the nursing process is a scientific, rational approach, it is carried out in a caring manner, truly making nursing a science *and* an art (Hood and Leddy, 2005).

In 1953 Fry first used the term *nursing diagnosis*. In 1955 Lydia Hall referred to nursing as a "process," but the term *nursing process* was not widely used until the late 1960s. In 1967 Yura and Walsh defined four steps in the nursing process: assessment, planning, implementation, and evaluation. The North American Nursing Diagnosis Association (NANDA) met for the first time in 1974 and added nursing diagnosis as a step in the nursing process. In 1991 the ANA revised the *Standards of Practice* to include outcome identification as a part of the planning phase (White, Duncan, Baumle, 2009). NANDA, now known as NANDA International, continues to revise and refine nursing diagnoses. The steps in the nursing process are assessment, diagnosis, outcome identification and planning, implementation, and evaluation (ANA, 2009).

A client's condition frequently changes, resulting in the constant need to reassess, re-evaluate, and revise the steps in the client's plan of care as developed through the nursing process. Therefore, these steps are not as linear as they may seem but are both integrated and circular in process as shown in Figure 7–5. The National Council Licensure Examination for Registered Nurses (NCLEX-RN) uses these steps as a method to organize exam questions.

Assessment

The purpose of an assessment is to obtain a database of a client's physical, psychosocial, cultural, and spiritual health status so the nurse can assist in promoting health behaviors and identifying and addressing potential and actual health problems (White, Duncan, & Baumle, 2009). **Assessment** is obtaining a holistic view of a client by means of a thorough physical examination and a history collected through a personal therapeutic client interview, support system input, and a health record review. The steps in the assessment section of the nursing process are listed in Box 7–1.

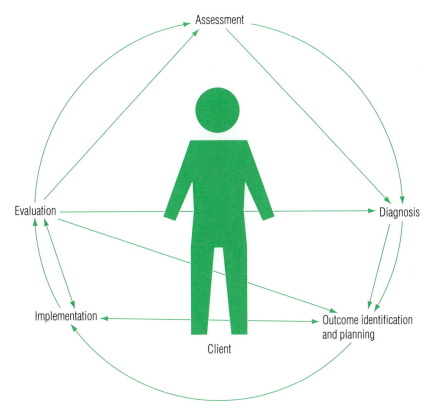

Figure 7–5 The nursing process is integrated and circular.

Box 7–1 Nursing Process Assessment Steps

Data collection

Data validation

Data organization

Data categories or patterns

Drawing data inferences

Data recording and reporting

Adapted from Daniels, Grendell, & Wilkins, 2010, Nursing
Fundamentals: Caring and Clinical Decision Making, Delmar Cengage
Learning.

Data Collection

The assessment step includes data collection that is pertinent to planning and implementing client care. Data is collected as a primary source and secondary sources. The primary source of data is the client and secondary sources of data collection are the client's family members, medical records, diagnostic reports, and other health care providers.

Objective data is measurable and observable data obtained through a physical assessment. A therapeutic interview assists in obtaining subjective data from the client and includes the client's "feelings, perceptions, and concerns" (Daniels, Grendell, & Wilkins, 2010, p. 222). Assessment is an ongoing process with each nurse-client interaction.

Data Validation

The collected data is validated with other sources for accuracy and completeness. This is a particularly important step when assessing a client with cognitive issues, questionable lifestyle habits, or condition denial. Validation of data prevents misunderstandings, omission of data, and incorrect inferences. The thoroughness of the assessment determines the accurate collection of data and the logical, comprehensive conclusions or inferences drawn from the data. Asking questions during this process is important because a valid appropriate, priority nursing diagnosis cannot be identified without considering all available data. See Table 7–1 for examples of critical thinking questions to ask during the nursing process.

Table 7–1 Examples of Critical-Thinking Questions for Use with the Nursing Process

Assessment	Is the data complete? What other data do I need? What are some possible sources of the data? What assumptions or biases do I have in this situation? What is the client's point of view? Are there other points of view?
Diagnosis	What does the data mean? What else could be happening? Are there any gaps in the data? How are these data similar and how are they different? What assumptions or biases do I have in this situation? Have my assumptions affected my interpretation of the data? If so, in what way?
Outcome identification and planning	What are the goals for this client? What do I want to accomplish? How are my goals related to what the client wants to accomplish? What are the expected outcomes for this client? What interventions are to be used? Who is the best-qualified person to perform these interventions? How much involvement can the client and family or significant other have at this time? How much involvement does the client wish to have at this time?
Implementation	What is the client's current status? What are the most critical steps in this intervention? How must I alter the intervention to best meet this client's needs and maintain principles of safety? What is the client's response during and after the intervention? Is there a need to alter the intervention any way? If so, why and how?
Evaluation	Were the interventions successful in assisting the client to achieve the desired goals? How could things have been done differently? What data do I need to make new decisions? Where will I get the data? Were there assumptions, biases, or points of view that I missed that affected the outcomes? What can be done about these assumptions, biases, or points of view?

(From *Fundamentals of Nursing: Standards and Practice*, 3rd ed., by S. Delaune and P. Ladner, 2006, Clifton Park, NY: Thomson Delmar Learning.)

Data Organization

Data is collected using various methods, including a Body Systems approach, Gordon's Functional Health Patterns (Gordon, 2006), Maslow's Hierarchy of Needs, and Orem's Self-care. Most facilities have assessment formats that guide data organization and assist in clustering the information for significance and relevance. Whatever method is used, the data guides nursing care.

Data categories or patterns

As the data is collected, the nurse uses critical thinking to determine the relevance and pertinence of the information. After collecting the data, the nurse organizes it into categories to gain insight into the relationships of the data. The nurse begins to see connected, significant patterns. The related pieces of data are then placed into groups called data clusters. By placing the data into clusters, the nurse separates the significant data from the insignificant data and identifies the client's problems and strengths. Potential gaps in data become evident. The nurse uses critical thinking to determine cause and effect of client factors and symptoms (White, Duncan, Baumle, 2009).

Drawing Data Inferences

The nurse objectively analyzes the clustered data to see what it reveals about the client. Relying on nursing knowledge, the nurse analyzes the data and uses problem solving skills to converge on conclusions and inferences about the collected data. If there are gaps in the data or if the nurse has misunderstood data, errors occur in the drawn inferences.

Data Recording and Reporting

The nurse uses critical thinking to determine data that needs reporting immediately to the clinical manager or physician and what only needs recording or documenting. Abnormal findings, such as a B/P of 200/110 or O_2 saturation of 89, are reported and recorded, but normal findings of regular heart rhythm or temperature of 98.6 need only be recorded. Accurate and thorough documentation serves as an effective communication tool between all health care providers (White, Duncan, and Baumle, 2009).

Diagnosis

After analyzing the data and synthesizing it into a different format, the nurse uses critical thinking and decision making processes to develop a nursing **diagnosis** that is a statement describing the client's health problem. The nursing diagnosis is the foundation of the care plan (ANA, 2009). The nursing diagnosis consists of three parts: 1) the nursing diagnosis, 2) the etiologic phrase—the "related to" statement, and 3) the supporting signs and symptoms or defining characteristics. An example of a three part nursing diagnosis is: Impaired Memory related to neurological disturbances as evidenced by forgetting daily appointments, forgetting to take medications, and inability to recall activities of three days ago. The nursing diagnosis is written according to the NANDA International criteria. The nursing diagnoses are prioritized according to client needs to address first, then second, and then continue through the list of nursing diagnoses.

Outcome Identification and Planning

In **planning nursing care**, the nurse writes client goals or objectives that address client needs and assist the client to an optimal health status. Goals or expected outcomes (**outcome identification**) are written in specific, measurable, time-limited, and realistic terms so they can be evaluated objectively once the nursing interventions are implemented. Ideally the nurse and client together determine the goals, so the client has input into the goals that correspond to his perceived abilities, limitations, and lifestyle (Hood and Leddy, 2005). The nurse writes short term goals and long term goals. Short term goals are obtained within the acute care setting, such as: client will verbalize stressors in his life within one day or client will demonstrate correct insulin injection technique before discharge. Long term goals are accomplished over a period of time, perhaps in another facility. An example of a long term goal for a client who suffered a stroke is: client will ambulate 200 feet with assistance of a walker within three weeks. These goals determine the outcomes of the nursing care and are evaluated for degree of obtainment during the evaluation part of the nursing process.

Implementation

Nursing interventions are the nursing care or activities completed with the client to obtain the goal of optimum health. An example of nursing interventions for a newly diagnosed diabetic are: 1) refer to nutritionist for diabetic diet teaching, 2) teach insulin injection technique, 3) teach insulin safety guidelines, 4) demonstrate insulin injection technique, and 5) teach diabetic foot care. Nursing interventions change as the client's condition changes. **Implementation** of the plan is the nurse's interventions or actions that assist the client to an optimum health state or a quality end of life. Nursing actions assist the client in reaching optimum health goals. These actions require skill, client teaching, communication, and collaboration with various health personnel. The nurse is sensitive to the client's desires and individual needs when completing interventions (Hood and Leddy, 2005). It is important to record the client's condition, specific nursing interventions or nursing actions performed, the client's response to the interventions, and client outcomes (Delaune and Ladner, 2006).

Evaluation

During **evaluation** of the plan, the nurse reviews the client's progress toward the stated goals. The goals are evaluated as goals met, partially met, or not met. An evaluation example is: Goal met as glucose levels remain within normal limits. Or, goal not met as client unable to calculate carbohydrates for insulin coverage. The evaluation phase of the nursing process is continuous and ongoing. Depending on the results of the evaluation, the nurse reassesses the client for goal attainment, reprioritizes the problems, develops new goals, and revises the nursing interventions. If the goals were met, the nurse-client relationship may cease. Each phase of the nursing process is recorded on the client's record.

The steps in the nursing process are presented in a linear form, but the nursing process is interrelated and interdependent in each phase. The cognitive processes of the nursing process are the true form of nursing as a science, and the caring nursing interventions are the art of nursing.

THEORY TO PRACTICE

Using the following case scenario, develop a nursing care plan according to the guidelines in the chapter.

Case Scenario

A. R., a 55-year-old truck driver, is admitted to the emergency room. He states he has a heavy squeezing pressure in his chest. The pain is radiating to his left shoulder. He is diaphoretic, short of breath, and nauseated. He states the chest pain came on suddenly while watching a football game. He was mowing his yard and decided to rest. The emergency physician gives A. R. a nitroglycerin tablet and connects him to an EKG monitor. Cardiac biomarkers and a chest x-ray are requested STAT. Morphine sulfate 2 mg is given intravenously. Oxygen is given by mask at 4 liters/minute. A.R.'s apical pulse is 102 and his blood pressure is 150/88. A cardiac catheterization with fluoroscopy is ordered to determine the patency of the coronary blood vessels and functioning of the heart muscle. Three hours after admission the nurse hears crackles in the lungs. (Case scenario by Gena Duncan in White, Duncan, Baumle, 2009.)

Assessment:

Collect all the client data presented in the scenario.

Subjective data:

1. Even though you cannot interview the client, list the subjective data stated in the scenario.

2. List other data you would ask the client during the assessment interview.

Objective data:

1. List the objective data stated in the scenario.

2. To help you see relationships within the data, place all the data in categories or make data clusters.

3. Draw conclusions/inferences about the cluster data to develop nursing diagnoses.

Nursing diagnosis (ND):

1. Write three nursing diagnoses based on your inferences.

Outcome Identification and Planning:

1. Write a short term goal for the client.

2. Write a long term goal for the client.

3. Plan the needed nursing interventions. Write as many interventions as is appropriate to meet the client's needs.

Implementation:

1. Write the nursing interventions for each of the three nursing diagnosis.

Evaluation:

1. Write evaluation statements that indicate the client goals were met, partially met, not met, or need modification.

APPLICATION

The LPN's role in the nursing process is collecting data, documenting that data, relating the data to the RN, and contributing suggestions to the care plans regarding clients' identified needs. The RN facilitates and oversees the nursing process. She initiates the plan of care by delegating responsibilities to team members according to responsibility and capability levels; for example, nursing assistants bathe and weigh the client and LPNs collect assessment data. The RN performs a complete, thorough assessment by physically assessing the client, interviewing the client, and referring to multiple sources for client information. Together, the RN, the client, and other health care team members set goals for the client's return to a maximum health state. The RN then determines appropriate nursing interventions to address the client's individual health needs. The LPN completes nursing interventions according to the nurse practice act in the state of clinical practice. As the nursing interventions are implemented, the RN, with the LPN's input, determines whether the nursing goals/outcomes are being met. If the nursing interventions are not accomplishing the client's goals/outcomes, the RN, with input from the LPN, determines nursing interventions that will meet the goals/outcomes. If the client's condition changes so that the goals/outcomes are not realistic, the RN rewrites the goals/outcomes and proceeds through the nursing process steps as needed.

CRITICAL THINKING ACTIVITY

1. Using the scenario at the beginning of this chapter, develop a plan of care using the steps of the nursing process.

- Assessment
- Nursing diagnosis
- Outcome Identification/Planning
- Implement the plan (nursing actions)
- Evaluate the plan

Table 7–2 Comparing the Steps of Problem Solving, Decision Making, and the Nursing Process

Problem Solving	Decision Making	Nursing Process
Identify the problem	Address the problem	Assess client needs
Generate possible solutions and examine suggested solutions	Consider the options	Decide on appropriate nursing diagnosis
Choose the best solution	Choose a solution	Plan nursing care
Implement the chosen solution	Implement the choice	Implement nursing action
Evaluate the effectiveness of the solution for the problem and decide if the problem has been resolved	Evaluate the outcome	Evaluate the outcomes

(Source: *Decision-making and Problem-solving models and nursing process: Guide To Nursing Management and Leadership,* 8e; A. Marriner Tomey, © Mosby 2009.)

CONCEPT MAPPING

Nurses use care plans in health care facilities as a means to communicate between all health care providers, to organize a clients' nursing interventions, and to provide holistic, quality, safe care. Nursing education programs develop care plans based on the nursing process and, as an essential part of nursing education, expect students to create care plans for their assigned clients. Concept maps were introduced as another way to present the clients' condition, assessment, and interventions. Kim Lubesnick (2003) calls a concept map a "picture of the care plan" and states that concept maps do not replace nursing care plans but rather show nursing care plan data in a different way (p. 1). A **concept map** is a visual view of the client's pathophysiology, disease process, medical treatment, care needs, and nursing interventions.

A concept map presents key concepts in a pictorial, diagram showing relationships between the concepts (Craig and Hanson, 2005). Concepts include the client's medical diagnoses, assessment, lab tests, nursing diagnosis, client goals, treatments, and other factors of client care. Concept maps are created with a variety of formatting to show relationships between the client's condition and various aspects of client care. A student develops critical thinking skills by prioritizing client needs and analyzing relationships between the data presented in the concept map (Craig and Hanson, 2005). Other benefits of concept mapping are listed in Box 7–2.

Box 7–2 Benefits of Concept Mapping

Organizes a nurse's knowledge to improve application in clinical practice and profession

Integrates previous knowledge with newly acquired knowledge

Improves nurse's critical thinking and clinical judgment

May improve knowledge retention by visual recall

Makes a connection between nursing theory and nursing practice

Ascertains known knowledge about the client's condition and determines unknown factors to learn in caring for client

(Adapted from Craig, G. and Hanson, K. (2005). Concept mapping health care management. Brookings, SD: South Dakota State University College of Nursing. Retrieved on 1/9/09 from learn.sdstate.edu/nursing/ConceptMapModule1.html)

When student nurses use concept maps, they do not memorize content. Instead, they move to a higher cognitive level where they organize, relate, and analyze relationships. These learning techniques encourage the student to see the whole picture of the client's condition and care.

Developing a Concept Map

There is no right or wrong way to create a concept map. Be as creative as you desire. Most concept maps center on one main idea or theme and relate the information on the concept map. Students use pictures, boxes, circles, or just words in concept maps. Keep in mind that the purpose of the concept map is for you to organize your thoughts about complex information, see concept relationships, improve critical thinking and problem solving skills, and provide better overall care to the client.

Create a concept map by first choosing a client, a disease, or main theme around which the concept map is developed. If a client is chosen, then do a complete assessment to collect data that is placed in the concept map. If a disease is chosen, prioritize the main items of the disease, such as pathophysiology, etiology, risk factors, diagnostic tests, signs and symptoms or clinical manifestations, interventions, and medications to treat the condition. Then, prioritize the data and determine what to include in the concept map. Draw a basic diagram including the data headings for content you desire to include. For example, if you choose to represent a disease in a concept map, the headings could be pathophysiology, etiology, risk factors, and other pertinent content. If a client is

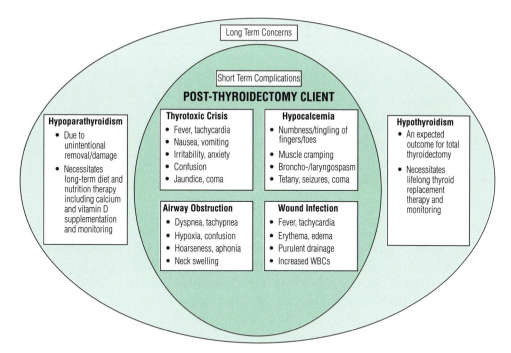

Figure 7–6 Post-thyroidectomy Client Concept Map example. (Courtesy of Vicki Coopmans, Assistant Director, Nurse Anesthesia Program, Barnes-Jewish College of Nursing and Allied Health, St. Louis, MO).

chosen, collect and prioritize the assessment data and relate it to the disease risk factors, her medications, and diagnostic tests. The risk factors, medications, and diagnostic tests, would be the headings of the boxes, circles, or rectangles of the concept map. Rather than shapes, a well-organized concept map of words with lines or arrows showing relationships between the concepts will also work. Again, keep in mind there is no right or wrong way to do a concept map. See Figure 7–6 for an example of a concept map for a post-thyroidectomy client. Be creative!

After the basic diagram is developed, place the data on the concept map in an organized manner. Once all the data is included on the concept map, draw lines to show the relationship between the data. This is the step where you use critical thinking to determine the relationships between the various data. Some learners color code the headings or main concepts to make the concepts and relationships between the concepts more visible. Once all the data is organized either for a client or a disease, develop interventions to address the client's condition or the chosen disease. Problem solving and critical thinking skills are also used in this step. The steps in developing a concept map are listed in Box 7–3.

Box 7–3 Steps in Developing a Concept Map

1. Choose a client, a disease, or main theme around which the concept map is developed.
2. Prioritize the main concepts of the client, disease, or theme.
3. Develop the basic diagram.
4. Place all the data on the concept map in an organized manner.
5. Draw lines to show the relationship between the data.
6. Develop interventions to address the client's condition or the chosen disease.

CRITICAL THINKING ACTIVITIES

The following are guidelines to develop a concept map for A.R. who entered the emergency room with potential myocardial infarction (MI) symptoms (Refer to the Theory to Practice Case Scenario on page 137). You may use pictures, symbols, or words for any of the following steps or you may use the basic concept map for A.R. in Figure 7–7.

1. Describe pathophysiology of an MI.
2. List risk factors for an MI.
3. List textbook symptoms for an MI.
4. List A.R.'s presenting symptoms.
5. List textbook risk lab tests for an MI.
6. List ordered lab tests for A. R.
7. Connect relationships of risk factors to textbook symptoms.
8. Connect relationships of lab tests to symptoms. Write a word or a few words to describe relationship between lab tests and symptoms on the connecting line.
9. Connect relationships of pathophysiology to client symptoms and lab tests.
10. Develop nursing diagnoses for A.R.
11. List nursing interventions for A.R.
12. List discharge teaching for A.R.

Share your concept map with other students. Do all the concept maps have the same design? Describe the uniqueness of each concept map.

Steps 1–6 are basic steps that you are probably very comfortable in completing. Steps 7–9 take the basic facts and challenge you to develop decision making, problem solving skills, and critical thinking as relationships between the basic facts are explored, analyzed, and developed. Steps 7–9 prepare you for increased critical thinking skills that you need as your pursue your goal of becoming an RN.

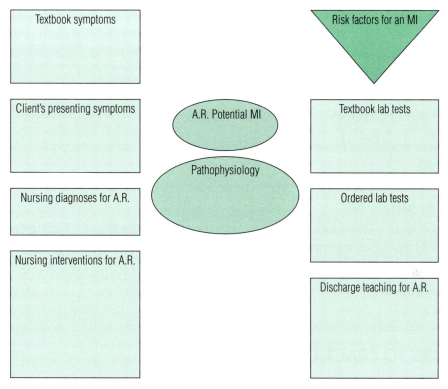

Figure 7–7 Concept map to develop for A.R. with a myocardial infarction.

SUMMARY

Benner et al. (2009) support using intuition based on facts in clinical decision making. The decision-making process is similar to the problem-solving process and the nursing process (see Table 7–2). Each of these processes takes a scientific problem-solving approach. In problem solving, the problem is analyzed thoroughly and multiple solutions or options are reviewed before a decision is made and implemented. Decision making requires critical thinking to choose the best option for the directed action. The nursing process is the nurse's systematic method of clinical decision making.

Sometimes students find working through the nursing process very rigorous, time consuming, and laborious. Yet, the nursing process is one method, or process, of building a stronger knowledge base and connecting aspects of nursing care to develop expert decision making skills. Concept maps offer students an option to create a visual view of data, information, and facts to enhance critical thinking, problem solving, and decision making.

Nurses making sound decisions provide quality care to clients. Effective, sound decisions conserve time, resources, and energy. Develop your critical thinking skills and your decision-making and problem-solving abilities so that you will soon be the facilitator of the nursing process, providing quality care to the client.

CHAPTER REFLECTIONS

1. Where would you place Tameka in Benner et al.'s five-stage novice-to-expert practice model?

2. What skills did Tameka use when she decided to seek advice from a more experienced co-worker?

3. If you were in Tameka's position, would you view yourself as an incompetent nurse? Would this be an appropriate reaction to the situation? Why or why not?

4. Using each of the decision-making steps presented in this chapter, what would you do to address Tameka's client scenario?

THEORY TO PRACTICE

1. Write appropriate nursing diagnoses for the following scenario. C. F., a 32-year-old male, has experienced chest pain three times in the last two weeks. He thinks he is too busy to go to the doctor right now. He works 12 hours a day 7 days a week and has not had a vacation in three years.

2. You notice a colleague has not walked her postop clients for the last three days, but always goes to break and lunch and leaves the unit as soon as possible at the end of the shift. What is your responsibility as an RN in this situation? What actions as an RN would you take?

Journaling Your Journey

1. Choose some of the problems you have identified in your nursing career and describe how you addressed each of them.

2. Describe how you grew in problem solving, decision making, and critical thinking by completing the concept map for A.R.

3. Then, describe ways to improve your problem solving and critical thinking skills.

ↄ ↄ ↄ

My Story…

One day when I was sixty years old, I decided to return to school to prove to myself that I could accomplish my goal of becoming an RN. My biggest transition from LPN to RN was having more responsibilities in coordinating the care of patients.

I found that, with my transition from LPN to RN, I have more confidence in my decisions; I no longer have to seek as much guidance from nurses with higher education. The benefits of being an RN is having a skill set that is combined with knowledge to make appropriate clinical decisions for the patients in my care. In the LPN program, I learned what to do for specific problems and conditions. In the RN program, I learned the "why" of selected specific actions and the ability to evaluate the results of those actions. In other words, it really enhanced my critical thinking skills.

Charles Burd, RN

REFERENCES

American Nurses Association (ANA). (2009). The nursing process: A common thread amongst all nurses. Silver Spring, MD: American Nurses Association, Inc. Retrieved on 1/27/09 from www.nursingworld.org/EspeciallyForYou/StudentNurses/Thenursingprocess.aspx

Benner, P., Tanner, C., & Chesla, C. (2009). *Expertise in nursing practice: Caring, clinical judgment, and ethics* (2nd ed.). New York: Springer Publishing Company.

Craig, G. and Hanson, K. (2005). Concept mapping health care management. Brookings, SD: South Dakota State University College of Nursing. Retrieved on 1/9/09 from learn.sdstate.edu/nursing/ConceptMapModule1.html

Daniels, R., Grendell, R., & Wilkins, F. (2010). Nursing Fundamentals: Caring and Clinical Decision Making, (2nd ed.). Clifton Park, NY: Delmar Cengage Learning.

Delaune, S., & Ladner, P. (2006). *Fundamentals of nursing: Standards and practice* (3rd ed.). Clifton Park, NY: Delmar Cengage Learning.

Gordon, M. (2006). *Manual of nursing diagnosis* (11th ed.). Sudbury, MA: Jones & Bartlett Publishers.

Ham, K. (2002). *From LPN to RN: Bridges for role transitions.* Philadelphia: W. B. Saunders.

Hood, L., & Leddy, S. (2003). *Leddy and Pepper's conceptual bases of professional nursing* (5th ed.). Philadelphia: Lippincott Williams & Wilkins.

Lubesnick, K. (2003). Nursing care plans and mapping: Guidelines for clinical mapping. Des Plaines, IL: Oakton Community College. Retrieved on 1/8/09 from www.oakton.edu/~mikey/nur104/guidelinesformapping.html

Tommey, A. (2008). *Guide to nursing management and leadership* (8th ed.). St. Louis, MO: Mosby.

White, L., Duncan, G., and Baumle, W. (2010). *Foundations of nursing* (3rd ed.). Clifton Park, N.Y.: Delmar Cengage Learning.

SUGGESTED RESOURCES

www3.sdstate.edu/ (Click on Desire2Learn. Next, type *concept map* in the search section and click on SDSU: Karen Hanson.)

Chapter 8
Client Teaching

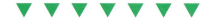

LEARNING OBJECTIVES

By the end of this chapter, you should be able to:

1. Explain the role of the nurse as teacher.
2. List the principles of adult learning.
3. List factors that enhance learning.
4. List factors that interfere with learning.
5. Develop a client teaching plan.

KEY TERMS

Andragogy
Pedagogy
Teach
Teaching-learning

SCENARIO

Carlos, an LPN for one year, has been asked by his RN mentor to complete the discharge teaching plan for his assigned client. He completes the discharge instructions by filling information in the appropriate sections as guided by the form. He returns to the RN to see if the discharge information is accurate and complete. Carlos relies on the RN for the final decision about implementing the discharge teaching.

THINK ABOUT IT

1. Compare your client teaching with Carlos's teaching experience.
2. How do facility policies affect your ability to complete client teaching?

INTRODUCTION

In a research study titled *A Study of Professional Nurses' Perceptions of Patient Education,* 92 percent of the nurses stated that client teaching was "a priority in their nursing care" (Marcum, Ridenour, Shaff, Hammons, & Taylor, 2002, p. 112). The teaching-learning process can be informal or formal. A nurse teaches informally by explaining the action of heparin when giving a heparin injection. Formal teaching usually includes some preparation of a teaching plan to explain a concept to a client, such as preoperative preparation for surgery, diabetic diet instruction, and self-administration of insulin. Because clients are quickly discharged from the hospital and often are expected to continue complex care, teaching is essential to effective health care.

The topics of the nurse as a teacher, principles of adult learning, factors that interfere with teaching-learning situations, and effective methods of teaching clients are discussed in this chapter. There is an opportunity to develop a teaching plan for a client applying the teaching-learning principles presented in the following pages.

THE NURSE AS TEACHER

Teaching is an integral part of nursing. Sandra Cornett (2003) effectively stated the emotional, tangible, and intangible components of teaching when she said, "Teaching is the part of caring that stays with a patient and his or her family long after all physical contact has stopped. The impact of teaching is often delayed and the results are usually not seen by the health care provider while the patient is in the hospital" (p. 1). When a nurse teaches, there are lasting implications.

CRITICAL THINKING ACTIVITY

1. Write two concepts that someone taught you in the past that you are still able to recall.
2. How long has it been since you were taught these concepts?

Nurses not only teach clients, they also teach students and model nursing care for students. These nurses set standards for the next generation of nurses. It is important that nurses be exemplary in their ethical choices, client care, and professional standards. This role modeling is an honor and a responsibility of nurses. Even though nurses are very involved in teaching students, the rest of the chapter presents the nurse as client teacher.

CRITICAL THINKING ACTIVITY

1. List two nurses who have served as your teaching role models. Share your reasons for choosing these nurses.

Teaching Defined

Nurses are the key educators in health care. To **teach** is to effectively share information so that another can learn. The goal of client teaching is to increase knowledge, impart skills, and change behavior. Teaching assists the client in coping with future events related to his condition. Teaching is not restricted to caring for the present condition, but it also includes information to promote a healthy lifestyle. Every nurse-client interaction is a potential teaching-learning opportunity. In these interactions, both the nurse and the client learn from each other.

Informal Teaching

Effective teaching is completed in an efficient, timely manner. As nurses do daily activities, such as ambulating and bathing clients, administering medications, and changing dressings, they can use these opportunities to educate the clients about ambulation techniques, stimulation of circulation with bathing, medication actions and side effects, and dressing-changing procedures. Every interaction is used to improve the client's knowledge of his condition. Teaching clients about tests, procedures, and surgery are other educational opportunities.

CRITICAL THINKING ACTIVITY

1. Relate something you taught a client. What method did you use to teach the client?

Clients in health care settings are more educated today than they were years ago because of new technology advances. Many clients use the internet and other resources to complete their own research before ever consulting with their health care providers. Clients' familiarity with computers offers other effective teaching methods besides one-on-one nurse-client interaction. Independent study worksheets or booklets, videos, and computer instruction assist the nurse in relaying valuable information to the client.

Formal Teaching

Client teaching is not always done informally but can also be very effective in structured teaching-learning situations. In a structured setting, a nurse selects specific content to teach a client and writes specific client-oriented goals for the teaching-learning session. The nurse plans the session content and prepares specific effective methods of communicating the information. After the session, the nurse evaluates the content, presentation, and methods. The nurse and client each should be given an opportunity to evaluate the teaching-learning session.

Chronic illnesses are challenging experiences for clients. By teaching the client about the disease and methods of handling the disease, the nurse assists him in making necessary life changes to deal with the disease condition. The nurse suggests changes to accommodate client care within the home. These suggestions include shower grab bars, elevated toilet seats, and adaptive handles for kitchen utensils. Self-management is the teaching goal for clients with chronic illness (Cornett, 2003).

It is important to listen to what the client and the family say about the information taught to accurately assess the client and family's comprehension. If the nurse has the client repeat the instructions, he reteaches or clarifies misconceptions as needed.

PRINCIPLES OF ADULT LEARNING

Literature supports the theory that adults learn differently than children. Knowles (1980) coined the term **andragogy**, "the art and science of helping adults learn" as opposed to the commonly known term **pedagogy**, "the art and science of teaching children" (p. 43). Knowles was one of the first individuals to propose adult learning principles. Lawler (1991) expanded on Knowles's principles and suggested nine principles of adult learning. Lawler's nine principles of adult learning are:

1. Adults learn best in an environment of mutual respect.
2. Adults like a collaborative style of learning.
3. Adults' educational knowledge builds on life experiences.
4. Adult education should encourage insightful critical thinking.
5. Adults learn from problem-solving situation scenarios.
6. Adults take pleasure in applying their learning in real-life situations.
7. Adults enjoy participating in the learning environment by identifying personal learning needs.
8. Adult learners are empowered through education.
9. Adult education provides and encourages self-directed and independent learning.

Lawler's principles apply adult education in teaching-learning environments. Pamela Schuster (2000) also developed four adult learning principles, but she applied them more directly to client teaching situations. Schuster's four adult learning principles for client teaching are:

1. Build on previous experiences.
2. Focus on immediate concerns first.
3. Adapt teaching to lifestyle.
4. Make [the client] an active participant. (pp. 214–216)

Let's discuss teaching concepts that we can glean from these adult learning principles by Lawler and Schuster.

Develop a Climate of Trust

The nurse encourages and develops a climate of trust and respect with the client. To provide the best client-learning environment, the nurse respects the client and the client's learning desires. The nurse communicates confidence in the client's ability to learn the material verbally and nonverbally. The client also needs to trust and respect the nurse. An informal and relaxed atmosphere provides an environment conducive for teaching-learning. The nurse encourages an effective, trusting, teaching-learning environment by being open, honest, and truly interested in the client's concerns.

Encourage Participation

Encourage the client to list and prioritize learning goals. The written learning goals provide a visual plan of action for both nurse and client. The written goals also provide a record to evaluate progress and achievement. Both client and nurse have a sense of accomplishment as the learning goals are achieved.

Build on Past Experiences

To build on past experiences, Schuster (2000) suggests that nurses determine what the client knows about the subject being taught. Once the client's knowledge base is determined, the nurse builds on that foundation. The nurse ascertains the client's past experience with health, illness, health care, or the behaviors the client may need to change. How a client thinks about these concepts affects what and how a nurse teaches. The nurse addresses the client's fears or misconceptions. The client needs to unlearn incorrect information and relearn new information and techniques. This sequence of steps is part of the unfreezing stage of the change process discussed in Chapter 2. An example of relearning as it relates to the change process is a client who had surgery 10 years ago and was given pain medication by the nurse. He is hospitalized and during his preoperative teaching is told that he can now participate in controlling his pain. After surgery, he will press a button on a patient-controlled analgesia (PCA) pump to receive a small dose of pain medication through his IV without having to wait for a nurse to bring him the medication. He can press the button any time he is experiencing pain. In this situation, the client has to relearn the way to receive pain relief: that he does not have to call a nurse for pain medication but can press a button to control his postoperative pain.

CRITICAL THINKING ACTIVITIES

1. Think of an experience in your life that has occurred more than once and describe how it was different the second time.

2. As an LPN-RN student, do you think you will need to unlearn some nursing concepts previously taught?

3. How can you use your experience of learning to help your clients build on their past experiences?

Address Immediate Concerns

Adults want information for their immediate concerns. The client may have a more pressing and different concern than the nurse. If a client is worried about children at home that are not supervised because of his hospitalization, that need must be met before the client can concentrate on learning how to lower his blood pressure. The nurse uses the therapeutic skills of active listening, clarifying, and summarizing to determine and address the client's concerns before teaching methods of lowering his blood pressure.

Assist in Lifestyle Adjustments

Teaching assists the client in making lifestyle adjustments. For example, if a client works long hours the nurse offers suggestions and assists him in finding ways to fit an exercise routine into his schedule. Some suggestions are taking a walk at lunch, stopping by a gym on the way to work, or purchasing a treadmill or stationary bicycle to use when watching television.

Involvement in the Learning Process

Adult learners like to determine their learning needs and be involved in the learning process. Teaching methods that enhance client involvement are discussion, demonstration with return demonstration, and scenarios with problem-solving situations. These scenarios relate lifelike situations with questions stimulating the client to answer with real life responses. For example, if the nurse is teaching diabetic classes, he could demonstrate insulin administration and ask the client to do a return demonstration. The nurse provides immediate positive reinforcement when the client performs the return demonstration correctly. A problem solving scenario is asking the client how to handle insulin administration correctly if he has the flu. This discussion gives the client an opportunity to gain confidence that he will handle the situation appropriately when it arises outside the teaching environment. These discussions are often more effective than lecture and provide an opportunity to verify whether learning occurred and whether the nurse communicated effectively. Offering the client an opportunity to evaluate the teaching-learning experience provides feedback for the nurse to improve his teaching techniques.

Following the described teaching-learning principles enables the client. Knowledge equips the client to successfully manage individual health concerns and issues.

CRITICAL THINKING ACTIVITY

1. Think of a time you utilized one of the adult learning principles when you were teaching a client. Describe the experience.

INTERFERING FACTORS

In a study by Marcum et al. (2002), nurses listed the three main factors that interfered with teaching clients as time, staffing, and client receptiveness. Three factors nurses identified that could assist them in client teaching were more time to teach, teaching guidance sheets, and available resources. The nursing shortage and client assignment load affect the available time a nurse has to teach clients. Basic teaching sheets routinely used in the facility could make the issue of time less problematic for both nurses and staff. Some examples of these sheets are information on medications that are frequently dispensed, common diagnoses, diagnostic procedures, and basic discharge instructions. A nurse could quickly pick up a pamphlet and share it with a client even on a very busy day. Some hospital units provide access to a library, a computer, or videos, so the client can research health information as desired. Providing these resources frees the nurse for other responsibilities and would be a vital educational tool for the client teaching-learning process (Figure 8–1).

Clients' emotional and/or physiological state, lifestyle, or value system affects their receptiveness to the nurse's teaching. Anxiety about a diagnosis decreases teaching receptivity. Older clients may have memory problems or take a passive role during the teaching session, especially if their children are present. Before teaching a client, assess his openness to being taught (Figure 8–2).

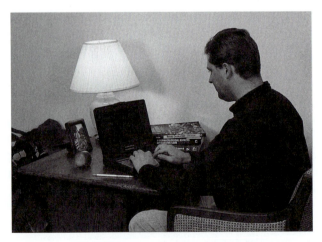

Figure 8–1 Encourage clients to use a computer to research health information. (Source: *Foundations of Nursing*, 2nd ed., L. E. White, 2005, Clifton Park, NY: Delmar/Cengage Learning.)

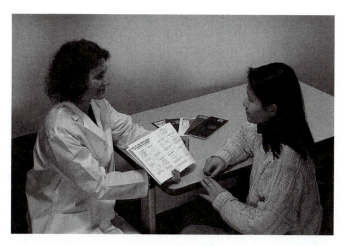

Figure 8–2 Printed resources can assist with client teaching.

In *Communication: The Key to the Therapeutic Relationship,* Schuster (2000) lists four factors that interfere with learning. These factors are emotional state, physiological issues, defense mechanisms, and cultural and value complexities.

Emotional State

Assess the client's emotional state before beginning a teaching session. If the client is anxious about his condition, his anxiety will interfere with his openness to being taught. Perhaps the client is grieving over the loss of a limb or limitations of the disease that will change his lifestyle. These emotions affect the client's ability and desire to comprehend what you are teaching. First address the client's emotional state with therapeutic communication techniques, and then teach small segments of information at separate intervals. This decreases his need to concentrate for longer periods of time. The client desires to learn what is taught but is unable to concentrate for long periods.

Box 8–1 Factors that Interfere with Learning

Emotional state

Physiological issues

Defense mechanisms

Cultural and value complexities

Physiological Issues

Delay the teaching to a different time of day if a client is hungry, tired, nauseated, or in pain. Some clients may hesitate to tell the nurse how they are feeling. Others may ask the nurse to return later, when they are feeling better, so they can concentrate on the information. It is important to assess the client's physiological state to determine the best teaching moment.

Defense Mechanisms

A client who needs to make a lifestyle change because of a disease may not be ready to make changes and puts up barriers or makes excuses not to change. An example is a client with an elevated cholesterol level. The client is not ready to make the needed diet, exercise, or medication changes. He makes excuses for why the new diet will not work or denies the need to exercise because a friend with the same problem lived for many years without exercising. The nurse develops a relationship of trust and educates the client about the disease until he sees the need for and desires to make the change. The nurse assists the client by discussing possible ways his present lifestyle could change to accommodate the needed diet and exercise changes.

Cultural and Value Complexities

A client's culture or value system may present barriers to teaching. For example, a client with heart disease who likes high-fat foods may find it difficult to adjust to the decreased fat content in the diet. The nurse considers the client's culture and assists him with menu modifications to accommodate his physical condition.

CRITICAL THINKING ACTIVITY

1. Write an example of one interfering factor you have seen in providing client teaching.

CLIENT TEACHING

Hood and Leddy (2005) define the **teaching-learning** process as "an interpersonal process in which both the teacher and the learner acquire new information, experience new relatedness, and behave in new ways as a result of the relationship" (p. 489). Nurses often think of the teaching-learning process as conveying information to the learner and forget the fact that we as nurses learn significant information from the clients. Information learned during nurse-client interaction includes how to phrase teaching statements, what type of teaching methods work best, and what to include in the teaching plan. Nurses are changed with each interaction with others and, therefore, have the opportunity to perceive the world differently and change personal behavior.

An informal teaching process is teaching when walking with a client or changing a dressing. The formal teaching process includes writing teaching objectives/goals, planning teaching content, implementing the teaching plan, and evaluating the teaching process. The nursing process and the teaching process use the same steps: assessment, diagnosis, outcome identification and planning, implementation, and evaluation, as shown in Table 8–1.

Table 8–1 Comparison of Nursing Process and Teaching Process

	Nursing Process	Teaching Process
Assessment	Assess client physical, psychosocial, spiritual, and cultural needs	Assess client knowledge base
Diagnosis	Identify actual and potential problems	Identify client teaching-learning needs
Outcome Identification and Planning	Set goals to achieve or maintain optimum health	Set goals to achieve teaching-learning needs
Implementation	Complete nursing interventions to meet client's needs	Develop teaching plan to meet client's learning needs
Evaluation	Evaluate attainment of client goals/outcomes	Evaluate attainment of educational goals and learning objectives

Assessment

First, the nurse assesses the client's knowledge base and understanding by asking questions. What does the client know about the disease condition? What does he know about treating the condition? What does he know about the prescribed medications? Is a diet change required? Does the client need special equipment? Does the client know how to operate the equipment? Once the client's knowledge base is determined, decide what further information is needed for the client to attain optimum health. A client's educational level or lack of degree does not always indicate his intelligence, comprehension, or knowledge level.

Diagnosis

Nursing diagnosis is the second step of the nursing process. This step reviews collected data and determines actual and potential problems. Likewise in the teaching process, nursing diagnosis is equivalent to identifying a client's teaching-learning needs. The most common nursing diagnosis when addressing teaching learning needs is knowledge deficit. Knowledge deficit covers a wide range of problems such as diagnoses, medications, diet, diagnostic procedures, and individualized treatment plans.

Box 8–2 Questions to Ask to Determine the Client's Teaching Needs

What does the client know about the disease condition?

What does the client know about treating the condition?

What does the client know about the prescribed medications?

Is a diet change required?

Does the client need special equipment?

Does the client know how to operate the equipment?

Outcome Identification and Planning

After diagnosis, the next step is planning. Plan what to teach the client, writing down client objectives or learning goals. It is important for the nurse to obtain input from the client as to what he desires to learn.

When developing the formal teaching plan, make the teaching plan simple and preferably teach only one concept, such as information about the disease, or medications, or changing a dressing. The client may learn and retain more information if the teaching sessions are short and one segment of information is taught at a time rather than multiple concepts.

To change a client's behavior we must teach to three domains: cognitive domain (knowledge), affective domain (emotions), and psychomotor domain (application or behavior change) (Anderson & Krathwohl, 2001). When preparing a teaching plan, write an outcome for each of the domains. An easy way to write an outcome for each domain is to remember the words *know* (knowledge), *feel/desire* (emotions), and *do* (application/action). Know addresses the knowledge level and translates to the nursing process as a nursing diagnosis of "knowledge deficit. . . ." Feel/desire activates the emotions. And, do, results in application and action. If teaching about medications, an outcome could be:

1. The client will state (know) the actions, administration times, side effects, and special considerations when taking the medications.
2. The client will state a desire (feel/desire) to learn the described information about medications.
3. The client will explain (do) the medication actions, administration times, side effects, and special considerations.

Box 8–3 Example of a Goal and Outcomes for a Teaching Plan

Educational goal

The client will live a healthy lifestyle to avoid cardiac complications.

Action-oriented outcomes

List	factors that contribute to heart disease
List	foods low in fat
List	foods low in sodium
Develop	a low-fat, low-sodium diet
Describe	an exercise program to reduce cardiac complications (Spicer, 2003)
Discuss	present lifestyle factors that may lead to heart disease

Write one educational goal and then list other related learning outcomes. The educational goal is written in broad terms, and then learning outcomes are written in specific, action-oriented terms so the client can attain the main goal. Write outcomes in realistic, specific, measurable terms so they can be evaluated easily. When writing learning outcomes, attach action verbs to the knowledge or skill statement desired of the client. Defining goals and outcomes is effective in breaking down content when teaching complex material (Spicer, 2003). Refer to Box 8–3 to examine an educational goal and learning outcomes when teaching a client a cardiac lifestyle change.

Goals are written so that each health care provider interprets them the same and works to achieve them with the client. When outcomes are written in specific, realistic, and measurable terms, it is easier to determine if the goal has been met.

Implementation

The fourth step in the teaching process corresponds to implementation in the nursing process. The nurse prepares content material to meet the cognitive goal. An example is a nurse discussing information with a client about medication actions, times of administration, side effects, and special considerations in taking the medication. This information is written down so that the client can refer to the material as needed. Prepared instruction sheets are great tools for client teaching. Nurses and clients both benefit. When nurses access the instruction sheets easily, they can use them in client teaching. The client receives all the needed information, and important items are not omitted.

If teaching is done in a structured setting, the teaching session includes three sections: introduction, body, and conclusion (Cornett, 2003). During the introduction the nurse introduces himself to the client, explains the purpose of the teaching session, and lists the expected outcomes. The client is included in setting goals for the teaching-learning session. In the body of the teaching session, the information is presented with as much client involvement as possible. Handouts, videos, computer instruction, or other teaching materials are offered. In the conclusion, the client is asked to do or perform the expected outcomes. The nurse gives positive feedback when the client restates information correctly or does a return demonstration satisfactorily (Cornett).

Evaluation

When evaluating the teaching-learning session and client knowledge, check if each teaching outcome is completed. If the outcomes are written in specific, measurable terms, the evaluation of the teaching goal is completed rather easily. Evaluate whether the teaching methods and content were appropriate. Could more effective methods have been used? Does the content need to be presented in a different order? Include client feedback on the teaching-learning session. The evaluation process will guide the revision of the next teaching-learning session. What needs to be retaught to the client? What new teaching does the client need?

APPLICATION

An example of a teaching plan using the concepts presented in this chapter appears in Box 8–4. Review that example and then, using it as a model, use Box 8–5 to create a teaching plan from your own clinical experience with a client.

Box 8–4 Teaching Plan Example

Teaching Plan Example

Scenario: Lorenzo was admitted to the medical unit with a deep vein thrombosis in his right leg. He has responded well to the heparin drip and has transitioned to Coumadin. He is now ready to be dismissed on Coumadin. The physician has asked the student nurse to teach Lorenzo about the action, side effects, needed laboratory appointments, and dietary precautions for Coumadin. Because this is the first time the student has taught a client about a medication, he asks his professor for assistance. The professor offers a teaching-plan sample to the student, who then proceeds to write the following teaching plan.

Assessment

Knowledge base of client:

Lorenzo has an associate degree from a local community college.

Past experiences with health, illness, health care, and lifestyle:

Lorenzo works on the assembly line at a major car manufacturing plant. He states he generally is healthy and has only had the flu twice in his life. He has regular dental checkups and yearly physical exams. This is his first clot.

Interfering factors: emotional, physical, defense mechanisms, cultural and value complexities:

Several friends visit Lorenzo in the hospital. He is fairly active and enjoys working on cars in the evening and weekends. He states that he is concerned how taking Coumadin will affect his lifestyle. He wants to know if he can work on cars and drink beer while watching ball games with his friends.

Questions to ask the client to determine knowledge base:

1. Describe what you do at work.
2. What do you know about how clots form?
3. What are the complications of having a clot?
4. Do you know any methods to prevent clot formation?
5. What do you know about Coumadin?

Diagnosis

Identify teaching-learning need:

Knowledge Deficit related to taking Coumadin

Outcome Identification/Planning

Bloom's goal-writing method

Client's learning goals:

Lorenzo will describe the action, list the side effects, explain the importance of regular laboratory appointments, and state dietary changes relating to Coumadin.

Write a goal to each domain: cognitive, affective, and psychomotor:

Cognitive: State the action, list the side effects, explain the importance of regular laboratory appointments, and state dietary changes relating to Coumadin.

Affective: Express a desire to make the lifestyle adjustments of taking Coumadin.

Psychomotor: Take Coumadin at the correct times, observing for side effects, with regular lab appointments, and following dietary specifications.

Spicer's educational goal and learning objectives method

Educational goal:

Lorenzo will learn to take Coumadin safely.

Learning outcomes:

Action verb	Desired knowledge/skill
List	the action of Coumadin
List	the side effects of Coumadin
Describe	the rationale for regular laboratory appointments
State	the normal INR level
List	dietary specifications while on Coumadin

Box 8–4 (continued)

Implementation

In outline form, complete the teaching information for each section: introduction, body, and conclusion. List the teaching method that you will use for each concept. List supplies and equipment needed to teach the content adequately using the chosen method.

Introduction

Information to teach:

Introduction of self:

Hello. I am _____ and I am a student nurse.

Purpose of teaching session:

Your physician has asked that I explain how you can safely and effectively take Coumadin.

Expected outcomes:

At the end of our discussion you will state the action of Coumadin, list some side effects, state the importance of maintaining regular laboratory appointments, and list specific dietary considerations.

Review client goals for the teaching-learning session:

Is there anything else you would like to know about taking Coumadin?

Teaching method:

Discussion

Client involvement:

Give the client time to think of other information he would like to know about taking Coumadin.

Supplies/equipment needed:

Goals of the teaching session written for the client.
List of the main points about taking Coumadin.

Body

Information to teach:

Outline of teaching information:

The clot may have formed in your leg because of standing in one spot for an
    extended period. Flexing your leg several times and exercising your legs as much
    as possible while working on the assembly line would improve circulation.

Box 8–4 (continued)

Coumadin is an anticoagulant. That means it prevents blood from clotting.

Every medication has some side effects. Coumadin causes you to bleed and bruise easily. Notify your doctor if you notice blood when you brush your teeth, urinate, defecate, or if you have a nose bleed. Your Coumadin dose may need re-evaluating.

It is important for you to have a lab test called an INR drawn on a regular basis. It is drawn more frequently at first and then on a regular basis once the Coumadin dose is regulated.

The normal desired INR for an individual on Coumadin with a history of clots is 2–3. The Coumadin dose is regulated according to the level of the INR.

When taking Coumadin, avoid foods high in vitamin K. These foods are the dark green vegetables like spinach, cabbage, brussels sprouts, and broccoli. Alcohol also has an anticoagulant effect so excessive amounts of alcohol is avoided. If you eat broccoli twice a week and have one beer a week, then continue as you presently are eating. Just do not eat broccoli three times in one day. Maintain a somewhat routine diet of green leafy vegetables and moderate alcohol consumption.

Teaching method:

Discussion with client followed by questions and answers.
Review brochure on Coumadin.

Client involvement:

Question and answer with client.
Review brochure with client.
Discuss regular eating habits with client.

Supplies/equipment needed:

Brochure on Coumadin

Conclusion

Information to teach:

What is the client to do or perform?

1. State the action of Coumadin.

2. List the side effects of Coumadin.

3. State the importance of maintaining regular laboratory appointments.

4. List specific dietary considerations.

Box 8–4 (continued)

Nurse's positive feedback to the client:

Give Lorenzo positive feedback on information he has learned.
Correct any information that he has misunderstood.
Ask if he has any questions.

Teaching method:

Question and answer

Client involvement:

Have the client complete each teaching outcome.

Supplies/equipment needed:

List of learning outcomes to review with client

Evaluation

Were the learning objectives achieved?
What would have improved this teaching-learning session?
What was effective?
What was not as effective as desired?
What could have been included?
What could have been deleted?
Could more effective teaching methods been used?
Did the content sequence need rearranging?
What did the client think of the teaching-learning session?
How did I facilitate or enhance communication in the teaching-learning session?
Did anything interfere or block communication in the teaching-learning session?

Information to Reteach:

What needs to be retaught for clarification.
What new teaching does the client need?

Box 8–4 (continued)

Now refer to Box 8–5 and create your own teaching plan.

Box 8–5 Create Your Own Teaching Plan

Assessment

Knowledge base of client:

Past experiences with health, illness, health care, and lifestyle:

Interfering factors: emotional, physical, defense mechanisms, cultural and value complexities:

Questions to ask the client to determine knowledge base:

1.

2.

3.

4.

5.

Diagnosis

Identify teaching-learning need

Outcome Identification/Planning

Bloom's goal-writing method

Client's learning goals:

Write a goal for each domain: cognitive, affective, and psychomotor:

Cognitive:

Affective:

Psychomotor:

Spicer's educational goal and learning objectives method

Educational goal:

Learning outcomes:

Action verb   Desired knowledge/skill

Implementation

In outline form, complete the teaching information for each section: introduction, body, and conclusion. List the method that you will use for each teaching item. List supplies and equipment needed to teach the content adequately using the chosen method.

Introduction

Information to teach:

Introduction of self:

Box 8–5 (continued)

Purpose of teaching session:

Expected outcomes:

Review client goals for teaching-learning session:

Teaching method:

Client involvement:

Supplies/equipment needed:

Body

Information to teach:

Outline of teaching information:

Teaching method:

Box 8–5 (continued)

Client involvement:

Supplies/equipment needed:

Conclusion

Information to teach:

What is the client to do or perform?

Nurse's positive feedback to the client:

Teaching method:

Client involvement:

Supplies/equipment needed:

Box 8–5 (continued)

Evaluation

Were the learning outcomes obtained?
What would have improved this teaching-learning session?
What was effective?
What was not as effective as desired?
What could have been included?
What could have been deleted?
Could more effective methods been used?
Did the content sequence need rearranging?
What did the client think of the teaching-learning session?

Information to Reteach:

What needs to be retaught for clarification.

What new teaching does the client need?

Box 8–5 (continued)

SUMMARY

Teaching is a vital part of health care. The chapter reviewed adult learning principles, factors that interfere with learning, and specific techniques to improve client teaching-learning sessions. An example of a teaching plan was presented and an opportunity was provided to create a teaching plan for an assigned client.

As an LPN you have played a vital role in the client teaching process. You participated in the client teaching role by gathering data, identifying client teaching needs, and reporting the information to the RN. You also may have taught some basic information to the client.

Now, as you become an RN, you can expect to play a larger role in client teaching. As an RN you will be expected to complete thorough assessments, finding any factors that interfere with or enhance client teaching and to develop the most appropriate method of client education. The RN usually oversees and coordinates the client's teaching care plans and reviews and coordinates discharge-teaching. Not only does the RN do client teaching, he also completes client family teaching, staff education, and participates in unit continuing education. RNs are also involved in client teaching positions such as staff education, diabetic teaching, and organ procurement.

You have tools to impart needed information to your clients in a new role. Now is your opportunity to improve nursing care by putting these principles into nursing practice.

THEORY TO PRACTICE

Charles, who is 30 years old, is admitted with a blood sugar of 210. His vital signs are T 99, P 80, R 20, BP 130/92, SpO_2 93. He has slight abdominal cramping. He states he has urinated more frequently in the last month. He states, "I am always hungry and I can't get enough water." After lab tests, Charles is diagnosed with diabetes mellitus.

You are Charles' nurse and are to assist in teaching him about diabetes. You explain the insulin injection technique to Charles as you give him his morning insulin dose. Charles listens attentively to the instructions and asks questions as you teach. After the injection, Charles says, "A friend of mine has diabetes and he said his father and grandfather also had diabetes. Will my children have diabetes?"

1. How do you respond to Charles?
2. After leaving the room, you reflect on the week's class discussion on client teaching. Was the teaching with Charles formal or informal?
3. What principles of adult learning apply in Charles' case?
4. Did you have a goal and outcomes in mind when you showed Charles how to administer his injection?
5. How did you develop a climate of trust?
6. What principles of client teaching did you follow?
7. Did you follow the teaching principles presented in the text and classroom setting or did the teaching just happen?
8. What prepared you for that teaching moment?
9. Were there any interfering factors in the teaching interaction?
10. How has working through these questions prepared you for your next teaching experience?
11. After reading the article by Levensky, Forcehimes, O'Donohue, and Beitz (2007) titled *Motivational Interviewing* listed in the end-of-chapter Suggested Resources, has the article changed your thoughts about client teaching?

CHAPTER REFLECTIONS

1. After reading this chapter, how will you change your client teaching experiences?

2. Obviously not all the teaching you do will require a teaching plan as described in this chapter, but if you use a teaching plan, how will it affect your client teaching?

3. How did working through the teaching plan and teaching a client change your approach, attitude, or ideas about client teaching?

Journaling Your Journey

Reflect on client teaching that you have done. Evaluate your teaching, preparation for teaching, client readiness to learn, content of presentation, style and delivery of presentation, client behavior or attitude change because of teaching, and attainment of teaching goal/outcomes. What has worked for you in client education up to this point in your career and what do you hope to improve or enhance as you transition into your RN role?

ೞ   ೞ   ೞ

My Story…

I decided to continue my education to become an RN so that I could be a traveling nurse. I will admit I always thought the only difference between an RN and an LPN was a title and wages. I worked hard as an LPN and was placed in many traditional RN roles. Now that I have earned my RN, I realize there are many differences. I was an LPN for ten years before going back to school and my attitude about returning to college was that I just needed to do the work and get through it. Well, was I in for a surprise.

As an LPN I learned things systematically. As an RN I learned the critical thinking skills needed to evaluate my patients. As an RN, I am equipped to teach my patients about their disease processes and explain the rationale for ordered medications and treatments. Now as an RN, I have come to understand these restrictions and am thankful I made the decision to go back to school. As a single mother who worked full time, it was tough to go back to school. But often things worth having in life require a great deal of hard work. You just have to make the decision to do it and remember there is always a light at the end of the tunnel.

Cindy Deemer, RN

REFERENCES

Anderson, L., & Krathwohl, D. (2001). *A taxonomy for learning, teaching and assessing: A revision of Bloom's taxonomy of educational objectives.* New York: Longman.

Cornett, S. (2003). *Principles for patient teaching* [On-line]. Available: devweb3.vip.ohio-state.edu/ Materials/PDFDocs/principles-teach.pdf

Hood, L., & Leddy, S. (2005). *Leddy and Pepper's conceptual bases of professional nursing* (6th ed.). Philadelphia: Lippincott Williams & Wilkins.

Knowles, M. (1980). *The modern practice of adult education: From pedagogy to andragogy.* Chicago: Follett.

Lawler, P. (1991). *The keys to adult learning: Theory and practical strategies.* Philadelphia: Research for Better Schools.

Marcum, J., Ridenour, M., Shaff, G., Hammons, M., & Taylor, M. (2002). A study of professional nurses' perceptions of patient education. *Journal of Continuing Education in Nursing, 33*(3), 112–118.

Schuster, P. (2000). *Communication: The key to the therapeutic relationship.* Philadelphia: F.A. Davis.

Spicer, M. (2003). *How to design and use a patient teaching module* [On-line]. Available: www .PubMed.com

SUGGESTED RESOURCES

Barber-Parker, E. (2002). Integrating patient teaching into bedside care: A participant-observation study of hospital nurses. *Patient Education Counsel, 48*(2), 107–113.

Levensky, E., Forcehimes, A., O'Donohue, W., and Beitz, K. (2007). *Motivational Interviewing.* American Journal of Nursing, 107(10), 50–58.

Russell, S. (2006). An overview of adult learning processes. Retrieved 6/16/2009 from www .medscape.com/viewarticle/547417_print

Chapter 9
The Nurse as Leader

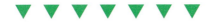

LEARNING OBJECTIVES

By the end of this chapter, you should be able to:

1. Define leadership.
2. Define manager.
3. Explain different leadership theories.
4. Explain different leadership styles.
5. Explain different management theories.
6. Define basic concepts of nurses in leadership roles.
7. Define the differences between LPN and RN leadership roles and responsibilities.

KEY TERMS

Accountability

Autocratic/Authoritarian leader

Delegation

Democratic leader

Facilitation

Human relations-oriented manager

Interdependence

Laissez-faire leadership

Leader

Leadership style

Manager

Mutuality

Scientific manager

Transformational leadership

SCENARIO

Tony is not looking forward to the charge nurse role as a new RN. He has always hated "telling people what to do." He prefers to just take care of his clients. He wonders how one attains the skills to be in charge. He feels he does not have the qualities to be in charge because he has never been an assertive person. The one time Tony was in charge as an LPN, he had a hard time making assignments and delegating tasks. He cannot picture himself in the charge nurse role. He wonders what else is involved with being a manager. His classmate, Chance, cannot wait to be in charge. He feels it is his turn to get to tell people what to do. These are two very different leadership and management views.

THINK ABOUT IT

1. Do you think being a leader means "telling people what to do"?
2. Do you feel that Tony and Chance have an appropriate perception of the leadership role?
3. What qualities do you appreciate in a nurse leader?
4. What qualities do you appreciate in a nurse manager?
5. Is there a difference between a leader and a manager?

INTRODUCTION

Leadership growth is comparable to a flower's petals continually opening in slow motion. As each petal unfolds, the leader gains knowledge, matures, expands, takes risks, is challenged in new ways, and constantly strives to be better. Just as most flower petals do not go back into a tight bud, so the leader cannot take back his mistakes but must continue to unfold and find new ways to handle the unremitting challenges. The bud may develop into a beautiful bloom and the leader into an effective facilitator. Sometimes frost or insects make dark spots on some of the petals. Rough times in leadership leave dark spots or scars in the leader's mind and heart. As the flower's petals continually unfold to full bloom, the nursing leader faces new challenges that strengthen the leadership skills and develop confidence.

The role of the leader has blossomed, changed, and evolved over the years, and the complex concept of leadership is still evolving and conforming to societal changes. Gregory-Dawes (2000) stated in "Changing Times, Changing Roles" that because of business influences on health care, "Managerial responsibilities were expected to change from that of sole decision makers to supportive, coaching, and nurturing roles" (p. 177).

In this chapter leadership and management are defined and the role of the RN as leader and manager is explored. The leadership and management role of delegation is discussed and accountability is defined. The impact of the nursing shortage on nursing leadership, and nursing in general, are reviewed. Different leadership styles are explained and leadership and management theories are briefly discussed.

LEADERSHIP THEORIES

Leadership styles and behaviors have been studied for years, and several theories have developed from this process. Leadership theories reflect the changing attitudes of each generation toward leadership styles and behaviors. Leadership theories include the traditional views of leadership, transformational leadership theory, leadership tasks theory, and new science leadership theory.

Traditional Views of Leadership

Christmas (2009) says "true leadership requires equal parts vision and humility, with the ability to confront hard truths and to coach and mentor" as defined in the book *Good to great, why some companies make the leap . . . and others don't* (Collins, 2001). Christmas (2009) articulates that leadership skills are required at every level and that RNs display the leadership role when making daily decisions about client care. Epstein (1982) defined leadership as a process of "influencing individuals or groups to take an active part in the process of achieving agreed-upon goals" (p. 2). The traditional concept of a leader is an individual with a vision and a plan to implement who interacts with and motivates others to reach the same vision or goal.

For a leader to lead there must be followers. The relationship between leader and followers is crucial to the success of the leader. The leader has a plan and a goal, but the relationship with the followers determines whether the leader reaches that goal. The followers must desire the same goal to follow the leader, and the leader must motivate and guide the followers.

Transformational Leadership Theory

Today, many believe that the term follower could be more accurately defined as collaborator. The leader works *with* his team, while requiring that the team work for him. Kerfoot (2007) reflects on the value of engagement with the whole health care team and believes "with engagement, staff will become loyal, highly productive, and excited about their work" (p. 47). Longevity and work dedication will come from individuals who are more excited about their work and lead to higher quality client care. Taking the time to recognize and appreciate the staff's strengths makes those individuals feel valuable, which leads to mutual respect. Kerfoot also says "the science of leadership/management can be seen as a game of chess where the pieces can move in all directions all over the board based on the uniqueness of each player" (p. 48). This more current definition of leadership involves empowerment and mutual goal setting and is known as **transformational leadership**. The term *collaborators* rather than *followers*, indicates mutuality in goal setting and goal attainment. Kearney-Nunnery (2008), states that "the transformational leader operates out of a deeply held personal value system, is visionary, has strong convictions, and interacts significantly with followers to see that the vision is realized" (p. 195). To refine this definition for more current concepts, the leader draws strength from personal values, has a vision, and interacts with collaborators. Personal beliefs, values, and past experiences set the tone for the leader's leadership style.

It is vital for the transformational leader to assess and evaluate all collaborators consistently. Are all individuals a part of the team? Do some of the individuals have different goals than stated or than others in the group? Do some individuals have their own agenda? A leader listens attentively to the verbal and nonverbal communication of the team members. When listening, the leader clarifies what is said to fully comprehend the message being sent. Frequent communication and assessment is imperative for the transformational leader to be successful.

Leadership Tasks Theory

John Gardner, the developer of the leadership tasks theory, listed nine tasks of a leader (1990). These leadership tasks are envisioning goals, affirming values, motivating, managing, achieving workable unity, explaining and teaching, serving as a symbol, representing the group, and renewing (Gardner, n.d.). See leadership tasks as shown in Figure 9–1.

The first task, envisioning goals, involves setting goals and motivating others to achieve those goals. This task is the heart and soul of a leader. The leader knows what he wants

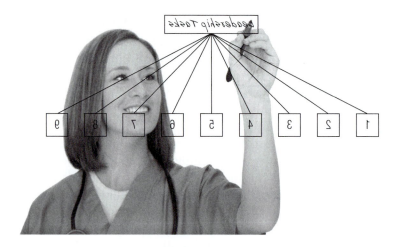

1. Envisions	4. Manages	7. Symbolizes
2. Affirms	5. Achieves	8. Represents
3. Motivates	6. Explains	9. Renews

Figure 9–1 Nine Leadership Tasks. (Source: Image copyright visi.stock, 2009. Used under license from Shutterstock.com)

to accomplish and how to get there. The goal must be so clear that he can communicate it to others and inspire them to achieve the goal. Some leaders' vision extends beyond their time and influences many generations. Florence Nightingale is an example of such a leader:

> One of the purest examples of the leader as agenda setter was Florence Nightingale. Her public image was and is that of the lady of mercy, but under her gentle manner, she was a rugged spirit, a fighter, a tough-minded system changer. She never made public appearances or speeches, and except for her two years in the Crimea, held no public position. Her strength was her formidable authority on the evils to be remedied, she knew what to do about them, and she used public opinion to prod top officials to adopt her agenda. (Gardner, 1990, pp. 15–16)

Every community has beliefs, ideas, and customs it values. A leader sanctions and believes in the values and norms of the community. In the leadership role, the leader represents and affirms the community's values.

Gardner (1990) states that leaders "unlock or channel existing motives" (p. 14). Leaders are able to harness the desires and will of people and make them move toward the established goals of the leader or group. Ideally, the leader does not force people to action but motivates them to action.

Managing includes five steps for the leader: planning and priority setting, organizing and institution building, keeping the system functioning, agenda setting and decision making, and exercising political judgment (see Box 9–1). Once the leader has set the goals, someone must plan the steps, set the path, and shift priorities to accomplish the goals. A leader does not center the focus on himself but establishes the goals, motivates, and instills direction in others, thus building an "institution" of the people. Then if something happens to the leader the institution carries on the action. During the Great Depression, President Franklin Roosevelt encouraged, inspired, and motivated the American people to press on for success. After his death, many future generations were influenced by his vision. To keep the system functioning, the leader provides resources, supplies staff,

Box 9–1 Five Steps for the Leader While Managing

Planning and priority setting

Organizing and institution building

Keeping the system functioning

Agenda setting and decision making

Exercising political judgment

directs, guides, develops procedures, delegates, coordinates, and keeps the system productive. Some leaders have a goal and visualize the fulfillment of the goal, but they lack the ability to plan the step-by-step process to reach the goal. The leader who is not a detailed person drafts others to assist him in determining the step-by-step activities to achieve the goal. The leader exercises political judgment by preventing conflicts from interfering with the accomplishment of the goal.

The leader strives to achieve a workable unity. Conflict does not have to be viewed as a negative but can be seen as a stimulant or a challenge. The leader determines whether an issue is a conflict or a lack of cooperation from the group. Part of the leader's time is spent in establishing and maintaining unity in the group.

Great leaders are willing to explain, explain, and reexplain. People want to know the rationale behind being asked to do certain things and why things are being done in a specific manner. Clear, candid, concise explanations assist the leader in developing unity. The people want and need to be informed.

The leader represents the members of the group both within the group and outside of the group. What he does and says represents the group. The leader does not represent his personal desires or thoughts but speaks and thinks as the group when he acts on its behalf in an outside context.

The leader has a global focus. Sometimes a leader guides the people down a tried and true, unchanging path. However, he must constantly be aware of the new thoughts and technology and keep abreast of new and better ways to accomplish new goals.

According to leadership tasks theory, a leader does not have to be in an appointed position to lead others. Nurses can apply this theory to their own lives by remembering that they do not have to be appointed to a leadership position to lead. By applying any of these principles, they are acting as leaders and make the nursing profession better and improve client care.

New Science Leadership Theory

The concepts of the new science leadership theory are coherent with the transformational leadership theory and leadership tasks theory. Wheatley (1994) presented the new science leadership theory, emphasizing that the leader must value and establish relationships with an acceptance of the values of all members. He views chaos as productive and inevitable in an ever-changing, evolving world. An environment where members are valued produces flexibility and an openness to change. It encourages the exchange of ideas and creativity. This leadership style is the essence of collaboration. Brandt, Holt, and Sullivan, in "How to Make Conflict Work for You" (2001), state, "Where collaboration reigns, strife wanes" (p. 32). A collaborative leadership style takes longer to develop and achieve but fosters individual growth, empowerment, and self-esteem.

Box 9–2 Leadership Theories

> Traditional Views
> Transformational Leadership Theory
> Leadership Tasks Theory
> New Science Leadership Theory

CRITICAL THINKING ACTIVITIES

1. Write your definition of a leader.
2. Review your personal definition of a leader. Which leadership theory does it best fit?
3. In your opinion, which leadership theory has the best fit with the nursing profession?
4. Conflict does not have to be viewed as a negative but can be seen as a stimulant or a challenge. Think of a conflict in your life. How could this conflict be approached as a stimulant or challenge? If the conflict is viewed as a stimulant or challenge, how will that change you?
5. Do you agree with Brandt, Holt, and Sullivan's statement, "Where collaboration reigns, strife wanes?" Give the rationale for your answer.

LEADERSHIP STYLES

Leadership is a learned process. Leadership can be learned from examples of previous leaders within the home, social environment, work setting, or textbooks, discussions of leadership. **Leadership style** is an individual fulfilling his responsibilities through the fulfillment of needs, distribution of power, decision-making ability of the group, and attainment of goals. A person's leadership style evolves from personal values, past experiences, and previous work environments. These previous influences form one's concept of the way a leader should lead.

There are three basic leadership styles: *autocratic, laissez-faire,* and *democratic.* The **autocratic or authoritarian leader** dominates, controls, gives orders, and expects the orders to be followed. There is little doubt to who is in charge. The leader is task oriented. Decisions are made from the top downward, generally without consulting the workers. The needs of individual group members are not considered. Often this type of leader lacks effective communication skills. When referring to the work environment, the words he most frequently uses are *I, my,* and *mine.* The autocratic leader has difficulty adapting to new concepts, ideas, or options. Autocratic leadership style squelches creativity and makes workers feel stymied and controlled. It diminishes individual initiative.

The democratic style of leadership is also known as the *collaborative* or *participative* style. The **democratic leader** makes the final decision after gathering the input and ideas of the group. The leader recognizes that the staff often has the best ideas to attain the goals. More time is consumed in obtaining each individual's ideas, but each person can buy in to the project or goal and feels that he is a part of the team. The words most often used by this leader are *we* and *our*. If there is conflict in the group, the democratic approach is not the most effective style of leadership. It takes time to create a collaborative, trusting atmosphere in which the staff trusts the leader. The democratic, collaborative environment encourages others within the group to develop their leadership abilities. Group and individual efforts are generously acknowledged and applauded. The leader is an effective communicator and has the healthy self-esteem necessary to admit and own errors as they occur.

The laissez-faire style of leadership is at the opposite end of the continuum from the autocratic leadership style. In the **laissez-faire leadership**, it is difficult to identify the leader because he is passive and provides little direction to the group. The leader relies on the strengths of each individual to meet loosely defined goals. The group has total autonomy and may lack direction. Laissez-faire leadership works if the individuals have worked together for a long period of time, know the group goals, and are well motivated. Otherwise, individuals become complacent and dissatisfied.

Sometimes leaders use different leadership styles in varied circumstances. For instance, in critical situations an authoritarian approach is more appropriate. In noncritical situations, a democratic approach is more appropriate.

One philosophy of nursing leadership is explained in the following quotation:

> The "command and control" style that has been a strong component of the leadership/management culture of nursing for much of our history just doesn't work anymore. Leadership is effective only if it can create a positive, supportive environment that frees people to do their best creative work. No longer do we believe that all of the knowledge of how things should be done is invested solely in the leader or manager. (Kerfoot, 1998, p. 180)

Successful leaders utilize the talents and skills of those they lead. Table 9–1 recaps the three basic leadership styles.

CRITICAL THINKING ACTIVITIES

1. Do you agree or disagree with the definition of leadership style? What would you change in the definition? What would you add to the definition? Discuss the leadership style definition with your peers.

2. What leadership style do you prefer? Discuss your rationale. What life influences have led to your preference?

3. In your opinion, do the business and technology professions need a different type of leadership style than the nursing profession? Give the rationale for your answer.

Table 9–1 Comparison of leadership styles

	Fulfillment of needs	Distribution of power	Decision-making ability of the group	Attainment of goals	Communication skills	Flexibility
Autocratic	Group member needs are not considered. Individual initiative is diminished. Creativity is squelched.	Leader gives orders.	Decisions are made from top downward without consulting the group.	Leader is task oriented.	Most frequently used words are *I, my,* and *mine.* Leader is often a poor, ineffective communicator.	Creativity is squelched. Leader has difficulty adapting to new concepts, ideas, or options.
Democratic	Group and individual efforts are generously acknowledged and applauded. Leader admits and owns errors as they occur.	Encourages others within the group to develop their leadership abilities. Each person buys in to the project and goal and feels part of the team. Staff trusts the leader.	Leader makes final decision after gathering the input and ideas of the group.	Leader recognizes that staff often has the best ideas.	Most frequently used words are *we* and *our.* Leader is an effective communicator.	Time is taken to obtain each individual's ideas.
Laissez-faire	Individuals may become complacent and dissatisfied.	Difficult to determine the leader Leader is passive and provides little direction to the group.	Leader relies on the strengths of each individual to meet loosely defined goals. Group has total autonomy and may lack direction.	Attained only if group knows goals and are well motivated	Group oriented	Extremely flexible Produces the most individual creativity.

MANAGEMENT THEORIES

We will briefly discuss two management theories: *scientific management* and *human relations–oriented management*. The scientific management theory is task oriented. A **scientific manager** focuses on the results: number of clients provided with care, number of procedures each nurse performs, adequate equipment to do the job, and documentation of work accomplished by each staff member.

The **human relations–oriented manager** would be concerned about employee morale and makes every effort to keep employees motivated to do their best. The human relations–oriented manager cares about employees' hopes, dreams, and concerns. He makes every effort to work out conflict in a smooth and efficient manner. If employees are content, the manager believes they will do their best work. The human relations–oriented manager cares about quality client care and an efficiently functioning unit but believes that contented employees make the unit more efficient and productive.

CRITICAL THINKING ACTIVITIES

1. Write your own definition of a manager.
2. Review your definition of a manager. Which management theory does it best fit?
3. In your opinion, which management theory is best suited for the nursing profession? Give the rationale for your answer.

DIFFERENCES BETWEEN LEADERSHIP AND MANAGEMENT

A **leader** seeks input and collaborates with all members of the team, guiding them toward mutually agreed-upon goals. A **manager** values individuals' needs while planning the tasks to accomplish the team's goals. The leader is a facilitator and a guide. The leader does not disdain chaos as an enemy but sees it as an opportunity to grow, change, and remain flexible to meet the needs of the ever-changing environment. The manager component of leadership is more task or planning oriented than the leader component but must not eliminate the value and needs of the team members in accomplishing the plan.

THE RN AS LEADER

According to Morgan (2000), "approximately one third of all nurses in management positions in the United States have associate degrees as their highest nursing-related educational preparation" (p. 181). Generally, management prefers that nurses in leadership have at least a baccalaureate degree and encourages nurses in leadership positions to attain higher degrees.

In the past, the leader or manager had a title to accompany the position. The business and technology concepts of cost containment, quality outcomes, and customer service have

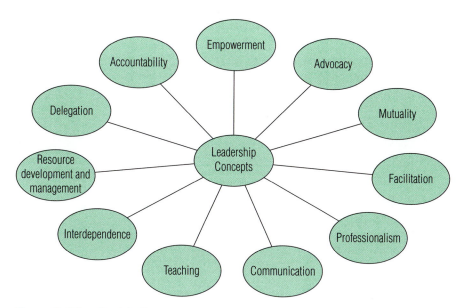

Figure 9–2 Leadership Concepts.

entered the health care arena. With these business and technology influences and the nursing shortage, health care management has had to revamp unit staffing and the utilization of equipment and supplies. According to Gregory-Dawes (2000), "Leaders without titles surfaced and showed their abilities to improve outcomes" (p. 177). In the health care setting, staff nurses started taking on leadership roles, and management was open to these changes in an attempt to cut costs as it provided quality client care.

Leadership concepts include empowerment, advocacy, mutuality, facilitation, professionalism, communication, teaching, interdependence, resource development and management, delegation, and accountability (see Figure 9–2). These leadership concepts become reality when a nurse transitions into leadership roles.

Empowerment

Currently power is shared in leadership. Staff nurses share leadership roles. At some hospitals, one staff nurse is in charge of a unit one day, and the next day another nurse shares that responsibility. In this way, leaders are developed and nurses who have leadership abilities have an opportunity to exercise their leadership skills.

Knowledge is power. Nurse leaders continually seek out opportunities to increase their knowledge base. They also share this knowledge with other nurses and clients to empower them.

Nurses empower clients by encouraging them to discuss their condition openly. Often, clients are hesitant to approach the health care provider or discuss treatment plans.

The nurse explains the disease process so the client has a knowledge-based understanding of his condition. Then the nurse guides the client in appropriate discussion, questions, and treatment approaches with the provider. As the nurse's knowledge increases about disease pathophysiology and treatment options, it becomes easier to instruct clients more thoroughly.

Advocacy

Nurses spend quality time with clients and often during this time clients share their treatment desires and wishes. The nurse becomes an advocate for the client by relating these desires to the health care provider or facilitating opportunities for the client to communicate his desires.

A nurse is an advocate for those who do not have access to care. A nurse advocate takes action when clients are shortchanged because of policies whose taproots are embedded in cost containment.

LPNs function as advocates. Very often these situations are accomplished by reporting to and collaborating with an RN or other members of the health care team. You will have increased responsibility, and oversee situations in which you or others will be the client advocate, as you transition to the RN role.

Mutuality

Mutuality is the joint sharing of power, resources, and knowledge. Staff nurses must have mutual trust in one another for this to work well. As the leaders on the unit promote and exhibit mutuality, other staff will grow into this camaraderie style of leadership. As an RN, there are resources to build knowledge and become a leader who promotes mutuality.

Mutuality also extends from nurse to client. With the development of technology, clients are much more knowledgeable about their disease conditions. Therefore there is a mutual sharing of knowledge and acceptance between nurse and client. In mutuality, nurses see the client as having the control and ability to manage the treatment regimen. The client views the nurse as a facilitator in the treatment process. The nurse seeks increased knowledge about the disease process, searches for resources to meet the client needs, and assists the client to gain maximum outcomes.

Facilitation

The nurse acts as a facilitator not only for the client but also for colleagues. **Facilitation** means to assist, ease the way, or make a smooth transition for a process or another person. The RN orients new employees to the unit. He eases the transition to the new working environment by teaching the philosophy of the unit, acting as a role model, and orienting the new nurse to the routines of the floor.

The RN facilitates the workload of other nurses. He makes suggestions to improve client care, decrease workloads, and make more appropriate use of resources. The goal is to make the unit run smoothly and efficiently for both nurses and clients.

Professionalism

The nurse leader draws from an underlying knowledge of personal values and needs. He knows the reason he went into nursing and what drives him to return to work each day. He knows the value of the client and desires to deliver quality care. When times get rough, he reviews the reason he chose nursing as a profession. When the morale on the unit starts to sag, he reminds other nurses of the opportunities of the nursing profession and motivates them to do their best.

The LPN is a valued member of the nursing team. Generally, the LPN's role is defined as task oriented, meaning that the LPN concentrates on completing assigned nursing tasks. The RN's professional role includes decision making and problem solving. The LPN makes basic decisions and collaborates with the RN in making more detailed decisions. The RN has more autonomy than the LPN in decision making and is accountable for decisions made. It is vital that the nurse continually update his knowledge base, as RNs are responsible for making serious decisions. The Professional RN relies on evidence-based research findings to practice, and keeps abreast of new issues in the nursing profession.

Communication

Nursing education prepares the nurse for a more effective communication style. Therapeutic communication is listening and effectively smoothing the way for a client to express verbal and nonverbal feelings and thoughts. It involves trust, empathy, listening, and respect as demonstrated in figure 9–6. This style of communication encourages the nurse to truly listen to the client, offer every opportunity for the client to verbalize concerns, and clarify communication between nurse and client. Therapeutic communication takes practice and constantly needs refining. Hopefully, the nurse becomes so comfortable with therapeutic communication techniques that he incorporates them into everyday life and utilizes them with co-workers, family members, and friends. Nurses eliminate much conflict by listening and clarifying communication with co-workers.

Gossip has no place in the conversation of the nurse leader. The leader avoids discussing co-workers with other nurses at all costs. Gossip is one vice that can quickly break cohesiveness on the unit. Good communicators avoid gossip by clarifying meanings with others or speaking candidly *to* the appropriate person rather than *about* the person.

Teaching

Leading is teaching. Nursing leaders teach graduates, new staff, and clients. For nurses, many co-worker and client interactions throughout the day are teaching opportunities. Teaching is explaining information to all involved parties. It is important for a leader to explain to co-workers the rationale behind decisions, schedules, and assignments. The staff wants and needs communication from the leader. Kerfoot (2008) states that mutuality and engagement is the core to a winning organization.

Transitioning into the RN role, one becomes a leader and is responsible for teaching clients, clients' families, and colleagues. As an RN, in charge of a unit teaching takes on an even bigger role.

Interdependence

Interdependence is reliance, mutual sharing, mutual assistance, and confidence that the other person will provide support when needed. No one nurse can care for all the clients and make the unit run smoothly. Nurse leaders recognize and promote co-worker interdependence. Kerfoot (2008) states creativity and individuality does not exist in authoritarian environments. Nonhierarchical organizations develop workplaces where relationships are mutual and have interdependence rather than independence. Interdependence promotes a creative, cohesive environment and does not smoother an individual's courage and strength.

The LPN-RN educational experience includes working in groups on projects or reports. These group interactions prepare the student for the interdependent role of an RN leader.

Resource Development and Management

Kerfoot (2008) believes that it is not uncommon for nurses to become formal leaders without formal leadership education or experience. Leaders provide information and opportunity for growth and the opportunity to obtain information externally for further knowledge and strength. Information is an important resource for development and success. Organizations are on the cutting edge of development only as leaders can continually seek new information. Swearingen (2009) concludes that "leadership development is a dynamic, ever-changing process directed at improving leaders and their organizations" (p. 111). A leader shares potential opportunities and encourages participation in continuing education activities. It is important for leaders and staff nurses to participate regularly in seminars and conferences and to keep up to date with the current literature.

As a leader it is important to conscientiously manage client care resources. Nurses watch for ways to decrease costs to the client and the facility. These measures do not decrease the quality of care or jeopardize client outcomes. LPNs are aware of costs to client. The RN role is responsible for finding the most cost-effective ways to provide continuing education for all staff members and quality client care.

Delegation

Delegation is assigning responsibilities to competent and qualified individuals for satisfactory completion. It is impossible for one person to accomplish all the daily tasks without the assistance of the health care team. Therefore, it is vital to learn the skill and diplomacy of delegation. Not only do nurse leaders delegate, but delegation takes place at all levels of the health care team. As you transition from LPN to RN, your ability to delegate becomes even more valuable to your success as a nurse leader.

The nurse leader is knowledgeable about the nurse practice act and the scope of practice for those to whom he is delegating. Prior to delegating, he considers the strengths and weaknesses of each individual. He does not hesitate to delegate responsibilities to qualified employees within their scope of practice. The nurse leader is legally responsible for the outcomes of the delegated tasks. He distributes work assignments to all employees fairly and treats all employees with respect. The leader does not delegate jobs that he himself would not be willing to perform. He communicates his expectations for the job so that the job is completed appropriately. The nurse leader makes sure the employee has the needed resources to complete the job adequately. He trusts that the employee will do his best in completing the task and relies on him to complete it. Together, the leader and the employee review the outcomes of the delegated work. The leader gladly recognizes and celebrates the employee's accomplishments.

Accountability

The terms *responsibility* and *accountability* are often used interchangeably because they have similar meanings. Responsibilities are the actual tasks that have been assigned. **Accountability** is being responsible and liable for one's personal actions and for the inaction of oneself and those under supervision. A person can delegate a task but cannot delegate accountability for task completion.

The nurse is accountable for the consequences of all his actions. He provides the best care possible to the assigned client and is held accountable for that care. Accountability to clients includes providing ample care to clients to meet their needs. It also includes obtaining resources to meet the client's needs that the nurse is unable to meet, such as physical therapy, diabetic teaching, or social services. Nurses are responsible for educating the community so that individuals make appropriate health decisions. Educating the community provides individuals with an opportunity to have a healthier lifestyle and decreased health care costs.

Nurses have a responsibility to participate in political efforts to assure adequate health care to everyone. This includes educating the community on political issues that affect their health and health care. The nurse functions as the client advocate in political situations and direct nursing care. Nurses are accountable for the provision of quality health care.

Accountability involves practicing safely within the job description of the agency according to the Nurse Practice Act and the nurses' scope of practice. If the job description is inappropriate, measures should be taken to correct its inadequacies. Accountability includes giving an employer an adequate quantity and quality of assigned work.

The nurse is accountable not only to the nursing profession but also to himself and his family. It is important to frequently assess whether the personal wellness needs of self and family are being met.

LPNs are accountable for the quality of care provided to clients. In transitioning into the RN role, the LPN's accountability increases. The RN is accountable for larger numbers of clients and for the staff providing care to the clients. The RN's ability to communicate and make wise decisions is vital as he becomes accountable for the decision made and communicated.

CRITICAL THINKING ACTIVITY

1. Give an example of an RN you have observed exercising each of these leadership concepts. State how each concept is exercised differently by an RN as opposed to an LPN.
   - Empowerment
   - Advocacy
   - Mutuality
   - Facilitation
   - Professionalism
   - Communication
   - Teaching
   - Interdependence
   - Resource development and management
   - Delegation
   - Accountability

THE RN AS MANAGER

Traditional management theories focused on tasks. The contemporary view is that a manager focuses on planning, monitoring results, decision making, decision analysis, resource control, and development. Kearney-Nunnery (2008) states that "a manager focuses on directing the group to meet the desired outcomes for the organization through thoughtful and careful planning, direction, monitoring, recognition, development, and representation" (p. 216). This definition includes the human relationship component of a manager.

Some literature implies that the manager is an appointed position. An RN can be in an appointed position, but staff nurses also have managerial skills. To be a successful manager one must be results oriented; however, to be only task or results oriented negates the human interaction needed for a collaborative working environment. Kerfoot (2008) summarizes leadership/management concepts by stating that a leader serves those under his guidance "first in order that they may serve their customers better because they are skilled and fulfilled human beings" (p. 134).

Mintzberg (1975) states that there are four managerial roles: *interpersonal, informational, decisional,* and *entrepreneurial.* The interpersonal role deals with developing productive relationships, conflict management, and employee growth. The informational role involves being a representative for staff and administration, relaying information appropriately, and monitoring the progress of the staff and unit. In the decisional role, the manager evaluates employees, monitors budget issues, and resolves conflicts. In the entrepreneurial role, the manager keeps abreast of new concepts and ideas to make the unit effective and profitable.

THEORY TO PRACTICE

Spend 16 hours observing a nurse leader/manager at work. Take notes on her actions, communication, interactions, and guidance/mentoring. Then, take a few minutes to talk to some of the staff to assess their job satisfaction and understanding of client satisfaction on their unit. Compare and contrast that information to the things you have just read about in this chapter. As you reflect on those notes, what do you believe is working for that leader/staff/unit/clients and what is not working?

SUMMARY

In transitioning from the LPN role to the RN role, take time to review the qualities and responsibilities of a mature nurse leader. Nursing presents the RN leader with many challenges and constant change. Through these challenges and changes, the RN chooses the appropriate leadership style and learns the best way to facilitate and guide, collaborate, and communicate with the health care team to provide the best possible care to each individual. Model nurse leaders have gleaned knowledge from their surroundings and bloomed into respected and admirable leaders who make a difference in the nursing profession.

CHAPTER REFLECTIONS

1. How have your perceptions of the leader role changed?
2. What positive qualities can you identify in yourself that will help you to assume the leader role as an RN?
3. Can you identify a role model who you feel is a good nurse leader? What qualities does the individual possess that makes that person a good nurse leader in your eyes? How could you incorporate these positive qualities into your own practice?
4. How have your perceptions of the manager role changed?
5. What positive qualities can you identify in yourself that will help you to assume the manger role as an RN?

Journaling Your Journey

1. Look at your life experiences and describe times when you functioned as a leader and/or manager.

2. Evaluate these times exploring what went well and what was most challenging, what were your strengths and areas you could have improved in those roles?

3. Anticipating your transition from LPN to RN and understanding that very often new RNs are placed in charge nurse and leadership type positions within 3 to 6 months after graduation, how might you prepare for this new responsibility? What can you do to enhance your leadership skills and the success of your future nursing teams?

 Cฦ Cฦ Cฦ

My Story...

Through my education experience, I gained greater respect for the nursing staff as a whole. I realized it takes all health care personnel to complete the process of patient care. LPNs, RNs, CNAs, QMAs, receptionists, and ancillary staff are all required to work together to care for the patient as a whole and accomplish their daily needs. I thought the nurse was ultimately responsible for all patient care. The nurse is the one who is ultimately responsible, but it takes the team to accomplish the tasks.

The biggest benefit of becoming an RN is the opportunity for advancement into different aspects of nursing. RNs can work in ambulatory care, long-term care, acute care, management, and home health care. RNs can also be consultants. These positions are not always open to LPNs. Nursing is a very dynamic profession that carries a lot of responsibility. If a nurse is burned out in one area of nursing, there are multiple avenues that can be explored.

I think being an LPN before becoming an RN helped me in my education process. There are multiple aspects of my LPN education that were clear, but made so much clearer once I had additional education and classes in the RN program. My learning experience was enhanced by more complicated RN clinicals. My experience as an LPN with assessments and patient care made my education process easier than some of my classmates who did not have the same educational background. I recommend obtaining an LPN license first and working as an LPN while obtaining an RN license. I feel my LPN education enhanced my RN learning experience.

Lori Covey, RN

REFERENCES

Brandt, M., Holt, J., & Sullivan, M. (2001). How to make conflict work for you. *Nursing Management,* *32*(11), 32–35.

Christmas, K. (2009). 2009: The year of positive leadership. *Nursing Economics, 27*(2), 128–129, 133.

Ellis, J., & Hartley, C. (2008). *Nursing in today's world: Trends, issues, and management* (9th ed.). Philadelphia: Lippincott Williams & Wilkins.

Epstein, C. (1982). *The nurse leader: Philosophy and practice.* Reston, VA: Reston.

Gardner, J. (1990). *On leadership.* New York: Free Press.

Gardner, J. (n.d.). Tasks of leadership. Retrieved June 5, 2002, from www.leader-values.com

Gregory-Dawes, B. (2000). Changing times, changing roles. *AORN Journal, 72*(2), 177–178.

Kearney-Nunnery, R. (2008). *Advancing your career: Concepts of professional nursing,* (4th Ed.). Philadelphia: F.A. Davis.

Kerfoot, K. (1998). Leading change is leading creativity. *Dermatology Nursing, 10*(2), 142–144.

Kerfoot, K. (2007). Staff engagement: It starts with the leader. *Nursing Economics, 25*(1), 47–48.

Kerfoot, K. (2008). Bossing or serving?: How leaders execute effectively. *MedSurg Nursing, 17*(2), 133–134.

Mintzberg, H. (1975). The manager's job: Folklore and fact. *Harvard Business Review, 53,* 49–61.

Morgan, B. (2000). Testing leadership and management concepts: The relevancy factor. *Nurse Educator, 25*(4), 181–185.

Swearingen, S. (2009). A journey to leadership: Designing a nursing leadership development program. *The Journal of Continued Education in Nursing, 40*(3), 107–112.

Wheatley, M. (1994). *Leadership and the new science learning about organizations from an orderly universe.* San Francisco: Berrett-Koehler Publishers.

SUGGESTED RESOURCES

Asselin, M. (2001). Time to wear a third hat? *Nursing* Management, 32(3), 24–28.

Carroll, P. (2006). Nursing leadership and management: A practical guide. New York: Delmar Cengage Learning.

Grossman, S. & Valiga, T. (2009). *The new leadership challenge.* (3rd Ed). Philadelphia: F.A. Davis

Hickey, P. (2010). 7 Summits: A nurse's quest to conquer mountaineering and life. Boston: Jones and Bartlet Publishers.

Hood, L., & Leddy, S. (2005). *Leddy and Pepper's conceptual bases of professional nursing* (6th Ed.). Philadelphia: Lippincott Williams & Wilkins.

Swansburg, R., & Swansburg, R. (2002). Introduction to management and leadership for nurse managers (3rd Ed.). Sudbury, MA: Jones & Bartlett Publishers.

Tappen, R., Weiss, S., & Whitehead, D. (2006). *Essentials of nursing leadership and management* (4th Ed.). Philadelphia: F.A. Davis.

Chapter 10
Managing Client Care

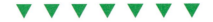

LEARNING OBJECTIVES

By the end of this chapter, you should be able to:

1. Identify ways to manage your time on the clinical unit effectively.
2. Relate methods to solve conflicts.
3. Identify methods to improve clinical decision making.
4. Identify ways to utilize resources appropriately.

KEY TERMS

Conflict

Conflict resolution

Resources

Time management

SCENARIO

Ling, a new RN, feels overwhelmed by her assignment on the medical-surgical floor. The floor has been very busy this shift. She is preparing to change the surgical dressing in Room 202. When she enters the room, she realizes that she forgot to bring tape and leaves to retrieve it. Once she uncovers the wound, she realizes that she did not bring enough dressings with her and must obtain more. While she is changing the dressing, the client contaminates the sterile field and Ling must get more supplies to complete the procedure. Ling feels frustrated that "everything I do today seems to go wrong." To make the situation worse, one of Ling's co-workers is reading a magazine while everyone else is so busy. Ling informs the co-worker, "It might be nice to have some help around here!"

THINK ABOUT IT

1. Can you recall a day when each procedure seemed to take you twice as long as it should? Reflecting on the situation, does it seem that the delays were the result of a lack of organization?

2. Do you usually have a plan in mind when you approach a particular activity?

3. Identify someone who you feel is good at performing her job in a high-quality and timely manner. What organizational skills does the person display? What organizational tools does the person use?

INTRODUCTION

The chapter discusses the tasks of effectively managing time, conflicts, decisions, and resources. Nursing is a career that involves human beings with a variety of needs and values. LPNs deal with each of the above-mentioned tasks. As you move into the role of an RN, your role will change with each of these tasks. As an RN, you may be in charge of mentoring a team of caregivers and be responsible for time management, conflict management, decision making, and managing resources. Each of these tasks, if handled competently, provide a more efficient and effective work environment.

MANAGING TIME ON THE CLINICAL UNIT

Each of us views time from our own personal perspective of values, ideals, beliefs, and experiences. Some people have a relaxed view of time and amble through life. Some are always trying to beat the clock and slide in under the wire. Others approach time in a more organized, matter-of-fact manner, calculating how each minute can be utilized to the fullest. How we view time depends on whether we see time as rigid and exacting or flexible and free.

CRITICAL THINKING ACTIVITY

1. How do you view time?
2. How does your view of time affect how you live and work?

As nurses, our daily schedules are generally packed as soon as we arrive on the job, especially now with the nursing shortage. Daily, we have more to do than we can comprehend accomplishing. Through the years, nursing has developed many methods to improve workload organization, such as daily planning sheets, client kardexes, chart dividers, functional health patterns, and computer-generated flowcharts. Yet time management is a constant challenge.

Reflecting on time management, do you take a minute to fluff a suffering client's pillow or document a dressing change and attempt to stay somewhat on schedule? Do you offer a sip of water to a thirsty client or grab a snack for break? Do you talk to a distressed client or rush off to a committee meeting? (See Figure 10–1.)

Time management is productively performing tasks in an organized, efficient manner. Writing down a schedule or list is part of time management. It gives direction and serves as a visual reference point throughout the day. Daily planning sheets help nurses organize

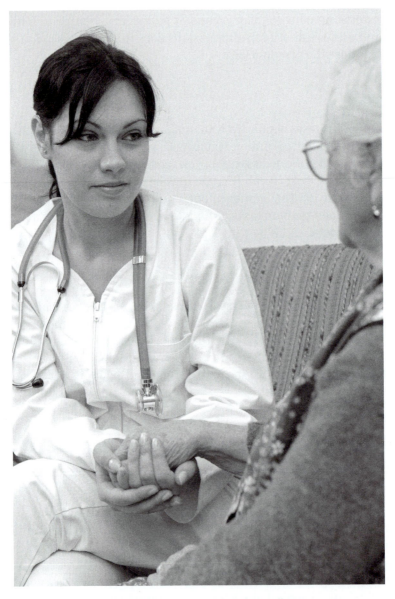

Figure 10–1 Time management includes taking time for a client.
(Source: Image copyright Kacso Sandor, 2009. Used under license from Shutterstock.com)

their days. At the beginning of a clinical day, place all routine items on the daily planning sheet (Figure 10–2). Include such things as vital signs, treatments, medication administration, bathing the client, charting, and shift report. Only by listing all activities can you truly see the complete day. Refer to the planning sheet frequently throughout the day. Crossing off completed items gives a sense of progress and prevents errors and omissions. By placing treatments in designated time sections on the planning sheets, nurses are able to determine priorities and plan needed activities appropriately. As your organizational skills improve, you can omit some routine activities from the sheet. However, it is important that we not become so focused on individual procedures that we lose the holistic view of our client's needs.

Client	0700	0800	0900	1000	1100	1200	1300	1400	1500

Figure 10–2 Daily Planning Sheet.

CRITICAL THINKING ACTIVITIES

1. Design your own daily planning sheet to help you be more organized. It could include a separate column or space for intravenous fluids, diet, intake and output, and so forth. Be creative. Share this with your peers.

2. Discuss the meaning of the statement, "it is important that we not become so focused on individual procedures that we lose the holistic view of our client's needs."

If you are struggling with organizational skills, it is a good idea to arrive a few minutes early to organize the day's planning sheets before the shift begins. Another tip to assist with organizational skills is to complete a time log. Use the daily planners discussed in Chapter 1 for three to seven days. Keep track of how you spend your time by listing everything you did in 15- or 30-minute segments. At the end of three days, analyze your schedule for items that could be deleted, combined, or revised. You may be surprised at how your time is spent.

Some jobs or activities cannot be accomplished in a few minutes. You may need to set aside a block of time to prepare a report, analyze data, or prepare a time schedule.

3. Complete the following time log for three days.

Time	Activities	Time	Activities	Time	Activities
7:00		7:00		7:00	
7:30		7:30		7:30	
8:00		8:00		8:00	
8:30		8:30		8:30	
9:00		9:00		9:00	
9:30		9:30		9:30	
10:00		10:00		10:00	
10:30		10:30		10:30	
11:00		11:00		11:00	
11:30		11:30		11:30	
12:00		12:00		12:00	
12:30		12:30		12:30	
1:00		1:00		1:00	
1:30		1:30		1:30	
2:00		2:00		2:00	
2:30		2:30		2:30	
3:00		3:00		3:00	
3:30		3:30		3:30	
4:00		4:00		4:00	
4:30		4:30		4:30	
5:00		5:00		5:00	
5:30		5:30		5:30	
6:00		6:00		6:00	
6:30		6:30		6:30	
7:00		7:00		7:00	

Time	Activities	Time	Activities	Time	Activities
7:30		7:30		7:30	
8:00		8:00		8:00	
8:30		8:30		8:30	
9:00		9:00		9:00	
9:30		9:30		9:30	

4. After completing the time log, ask yourself these questions:
   - How have I wasted time?
   - Where have I duplicated activities?
   - What activities could have been combined?
   - Did I plan each day's activities? Did I follow my plan?
   - Did I complete priority items first each day?
   - What activities took longer than I thought they would? Why?
   - How could I revise my time log or my schedule to use my time more efficiently?
5. Refer to the article by Debra Spidal (2009) entitled *Time Management* under Suggested Resources at the end of the chapter.

Nurses should continually analyze their work for duplication and repetition of duties. Tasks are often routinely performed without evaluating whether the task could be done differently to save time, whether it could be appropriately delegated, or whether the task needs to be done at all. Consider obtaining supplies for the next few planned treatments rather than obtaining supplies for one treatment at a time. Obtaining all the needed supplies will save time and eliminate unnecessary trips to the supply room. Review activities to see if you can complete more than one task at a time. Document a procedure immediately when it is completed. Plan ahead, and allow a buffer zone to complete tasks in case an emergency occurs. Using these time-saving tips assists in utilizing time more effectively. Monitor your schedule periodically to see how effectively you are using your time.

Personal ambition, drive, job requirements, and future goals often get in the way of our ability to say no when asked to serve on a committee or work an extended or second shift. Some nurses have such a need to be needed or wanted that saying no is very difficult for them. It is all right to say no. If your personal schedule is packed, or if the goals and plans of the committee do not interest you, learn to say no politely. Each of us needs time to replenish our souls to be productive and enjoy work. As you attempt to utilize your time more effectively, remember to save time for relaxation and personal endeavors. Include time to take walks in the park, meet a friend for lunch, see a funny movie, or attend a worship service. Take time for whatever it is that you find the most relaxing, fun, and rejuvenating.

CRITICAL THINKING ACTIVITIES

1. Complete the time assessment tool. Do the results surprise you?

2. Using suggestions presented in the text and your own creativity, review your clinical experience this week and identify ways you could use your time more effectively. Write observations of your time management.

MANAGING CONFLICT

Conflict is a complex situation in which two parties have opposing views that may interfere with one of the two parties' reaching the desired goal. Conflict is multidimensional, stemming from varying values, beliefs, attitudes, and cultures. Conflict is often avoided. Most people do not desire or seek conflict. Rarely is conflict seen as a welcome occasion to grow, an opportunity to expand horizons, or a chance to produce a change. However, conflict handled productively can produce growth and constructive change. A challenge is to change how one views conflict. Effective conflict management is an essential learned skill. It is imperative that nurses learn to handle conflict constructively to provide quality client care (see Figure 10–3). If a nurse has to work in an environment of constant conflict, she cannot effectively concentrate

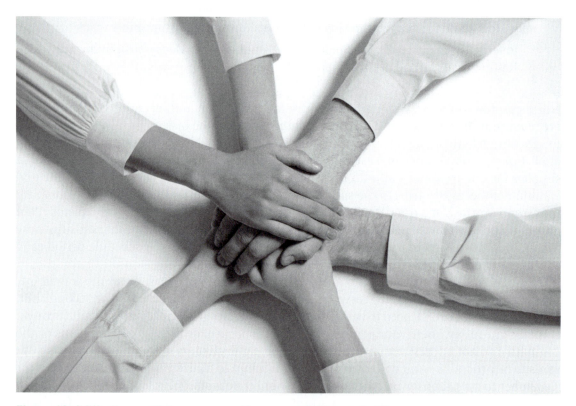

Figure 10–3 Effective conflict management is an essential learned skill.
(Source: Image copyright Dmitriy Shironosov, 2009. Used under license from Shutterstock.com)

on client needs and care. Bartol, Parrish, and McSweeney (2001) state, "Ineffective intervention can lower employee morale, decrease productivity, increase absenteeism and turnover, foster resistance to change, and interfere with employee development" (p. 35). Therefore, it is essential that we learn to handle conflict in a mature, positive manner.

Identifying Personal Attitudes toward Conflict

Identifying your attitude toward conflict and your usual method of handling conflict is the first step toward effectively handling conflict. Bartol and McSweeney's Conflict Management Scale, which is based on the ideas of Hall (1973), measures attitude toward managing conflict (Bartol, 1976). This tool is reproduced in Figure 10–4 (pp. 197–202) and can be useful in determining your approach to conflict.

CRITICAL THINKING ACTIVITY

1. Complete the Bartol and McSweeney Conflict Management Scale. According to this assessment tool, what is your style for handling conflict?

BARTOL/McSWEENEY CONFLICT MANAGEMENT SCALE

DIRECTIONS: Please darken in the space to the right of each statement that most closely indicates the extent to which you agree or disagree that the statement reflects your style of managing interpersonal conflict. Please respond to all items.

1 = Strongly agree   2 = Agree   3 = Disagree   4 = Strongly disagree

	1	2	3	4
1. It is important to recognize tension in relationships and confront the difficulty if problems are to be solved.	❏ 1	❏ 2	❏ 3	❏ 4
2. I give in for the sake of the common good, knowing I will get another chance later.	❏ 1	❏ 2	❏ 3	❏ 4
3. When conflict is honestly admitted and accurately interpreted, relationships can be strengthened.	❏ 1	❏ 2	❏ 3	❏ 4
4. I stick to the rules to avoid disagreements because I can't be bothered with arguments.	❏ 1	❏ 2	❏ 3	❏ 4
5. Compromise can be reached if extreme positions are eliminated by negotiation.	❏ 1	❏ 2	❏ 3	❏ 4
6. Attempts to resolve conflicts are fruitless in the long run; it is best to keep your distance.	❏ 1	❏ 2	❏ 3	❏ 4
7. I keep out of the way when I see disagreements among my co-workers; one needs to learn to sidestep conflict.	❏ 1	❏ 2	❏ 3	❏ 4
8. There is no room for hesitancy or doubt in conflict resolution or others may see you as wishy-washy.	❏ 1	❏ 2	❏ 3	❏ 4

Figure 10–4 Bartol/McSweeney Conflict Management Scale. (Source: Printed with permission of Dr. Bartol and Dr. McSweeney.)

1 = Strongly agree   2 = Agree   3 = Disagree   4 = Strongly disagree

9. It is better to sacrifice your goals than to threaten a relationship.	❏ 1	❏ 2	❏ 3	❏ 4
10. All is fair when you believe your goal is the correct one.	❏ 1	❏ 2	❏ 3	❏ 4
11. Progress through compromise is the best way to resolve conflict.	❏ 1	❏ 2	❏ 3	❏ 4
12. Arguing is futile, silence can be eloquent and helps you avoid trouble.	❏ 1	❏ 2	❏ 3	❏ 4
13. I overlook others' shortcomings for the sake of maintaining relationships and keeping peace.	❏ 1	❏ 2	❏ 3	❏ 4
14. I let things ride rather than risk causing irreparable damage to a relationship.	❏ 1	❏ 2	❏ 3	❏ 4
15. I worry when I have a disagreement with another because I don't want to create divisions.	❏ 1	❏ 2	❏ 3	❏ 4
16. I try to encourage brainstorming when differences arise. Many ideas are explored and often I am pleasantly surprised at the results.	❏ 1	❏ 2	❏ 3	❏ 4
17. It is better to remain aloof and disengaged than to get involved in useless discussion when there is disagreement.	❏ 1	❏ 2	❏ 3	❏ 4
18. People should face the fact that there is only one correct way to do things.	❏ 1	❏ 2	❏ 3	❏ 4
19. I will give in a little in the beginning if it affords me an opportunity to get something else later.	❏ 1	❏ 2	❏ 3	❏ 4
20. I am careful not to step on another's toes; no idea is worth destroying a relationship.	❏ 1	❏ 2	❏ 3	❏ 4
21. I talk about differences openly in an effort to resolve possible underlying conflict before taking any actions.	❏ 1	❏ 2	❏ 3	❏ 4
22. I feel insecure when someone disagrees with me because I am afraid that means I am disliked.	❏ 1	❏ 2	❏ 3	❏ 4
23. I try to encourage the expression of what underlies conflict; it helps all parties to be aware of the problems.	❏ 1	❏ 2	❏ 3	❏ 4
24. The only sensible thing to do when there is conflict is to simply withdraw and wait for things to blow over.	❏ 1	❏ 2	❏ 3	❏ 4
25. Conflict may be a sign of incomplete understanding, or hidden personal feelings. The underlying causes can only be discovered through honest discussion.	❏ 1	❏ 2	❏ 3	❏ 4
26. Exploration and discussion of differing viewpoints lays the groundwork for creative resolution of conflict.	❏ 1	❏ 2	❏ 3	❏ 4
27. Avoiding arguments is important to me because I've learned discussion of different opinions gets you nowhere.	❏ 1	❏ 2	❏ 3	❏ 4
28. A problem-solving approach based on respect for other people and their goals should characterize our approach to conflict.	❏ 1	❏ 2	❏ 3	❏ 4
29. Conflicts should not be explored nor the underlying tensions identified; avoidance is the best course.	❏ 1	❏ 2	❏ 3	❏ 4

Figure 10–4 (continued)

1 = Strongly agree   2 = Agree   3 = Disagree   4 = Strongly disagree

30. Whenever there is conflict it is the best team that wins, and that is how it should be. ❏ 1   ❏ 2   ❏ 3   ❏ 4

31. When there is disagreement, I call attention to that fact and suggest that we explore the needs and opinions of everyone involved. ❏ 1   ❏ 2   ❏ 3   ❏ 4

32. When there is conflict, I am curious about how others are thinking and feeling, and concerned with getting everything out into the open that needs to be. ❏ 1   ❏ 2   ❏ 3   ❏ 4

33. Indifference is the best shield in conflict; in that way you can sidestep the problem. ❏ 1   ❏ 2   ❏ 3   ❏ 4

34. I give in to others on lesser points and try to win what is more important to me. ❏ 1   ❏ 2   ❏ 3   ❏ 4

35. When there is a disagreement with others, I suggest we discuss our differences. Closer relationships and creative solutions are often the result. ❏ 1   ❏ 2   ❏ 3   ❏ 4

36. I would forget my goals rather than risk displeasing a friend. ❏ 1   ❏ 2   ❏ 3   ❏ 4

37. When there is conflict, I try to open it up so that every aspect of people's feelings and the issue at hand gets thoroughly considered. ❏ 1   ❏ 2   ❏ 3   ❏ 4

38. When there is conflict, I am interested in knowing what others are thinking and feeling; getting everything out into the open that needs to be. ❏ 1   ❏ 2   ❏ 3   ❏ 4

39. When there is a disagreement the minority should give into the majority so progress can be made. Everyone gets their chance. ❏ 1   ❏ 2   ❏ 3   ❏ 4

40. The underlying reasons for conflict can only be discovered through candid and objective discussion. ❏ 1   ❏ 2   ❏ 3   ❏ 4

41. Sometimes it is necessary to give into others if progress is to be made. You will get another chance later. ❏ 1   ❏ 2   ❏ 3   ❏ 4

42. You can't win all the time; good sportsmanship requires compromise. ❏ 1   ❏ 2   ❏ 3   ❏ 4

43. Personal relationships are more important than achieving personal goals. ❏ 1   ❏ 2   ❏ 3   ❏ 4

44. It is unrealistic to think you can always win; you should expect to compromise on some points. ❏ 1   ❏ 2   ❏ 3   ❏ 4

45. I owe it to myself to accomplish what I set out to do, regardless of whose feelings get hurt. ❏ 1   ❏ 2   ❏ 3   ❏ 4

46. Impersonal tolerance is the most enlightened approach to handling conflict and the best way to avoid trouble. ❏ 1   ❏ 2   ❏ 3   ❏ 4

47. It is better to go along with others than to provoke antagonism. ❏ 1   ❏ 2   ❏ 3   ❏ 4

48. Conflicts are a necessary evil, but I have learned to dodge them and avoid involvement. ❏ 1   ❏ 2   ❏ 3   ❏ 4

49. One must guard against causing irreparable damage to a relationship just to achieve some goal. ❏ 1   ❏ 2   ❏ 3   ❏ 4

Figure 10–4 (continued)

1 = Strongly agree   2 = Agree   3 = Disagree   4 = Strongly disagree

		1	2	3	4
50.	Maintaining good interpersonal relationships is more important than achieving personal goals.	❏ 1	❏ 2	❏ 3	❏ 4
51.	The only sensible thing to do when there is conflict is to wait it out.	❏ 1	❏ 2	❏ 3	❏ 4
52.	I would lay my personal goals aside before I would jeopardize a relationship.	❏ 1	❏ 2	❏ 3	❏ 4
53.	Keeping your distance is the best policy when you see a conflict developing.	❏ 1	❏ 2	❏ 3	❏ 4
54.	Conflict requires self-sacrifice and placing the importance of continued relationship above one's own goals.	❏ 1	❏ 2	❏ 3	❏ 4
55.	I owe it to myself to prevail in conflicts with others whose goals are different.	❏ 1	❏ 2	❏ 3	❏ 4
56.	In disagreements with others, I owe it to myself to avoid any pressure to compromise.	❏ 1	❏ 2	❏ 3	❏ 4
57.	Power, and even force may be used when your goal is important to you.	❏ 1	❏ 2	❏ 3	❏ 4
58.	Survival of the fittest applied to human relations is a basic test of one's ability to deal effectively with conflict.	❏ 1	❏ 2	❏ 3	❏ 4
59.	You never get anywhere if you give in to others when there is a disagreement about goals.	❏ 1	❏ 2	❏ 3	❏ 4
60.	I avoid calling attention to disagreements with the hope they will just disappear.	❏ 1	❏ 2	❏ 3	❏ 4
61.	Conflicts should be explored and the underlying tensions identified if problem solving is to be successful.	❏ 1	❏ 2	❏ 3	❏ 4
62.	Exploration and discussion of conflict leads to creative resolution of conflict.	❏ 1	❏ 2	❏ 3	❏ 4
63.	I find conflict disturbing so I give in readily to others and try to keep everyone happy.	❏ 1	❏ 2	❏ 3	❏ 4
64.	It is a fact of life, some people are right and some are wrong; I aim to win regardless.	❏ 1	❏ 2	❏ 3	❏ 4
65.	I am willing to bargain and negotiate to preserve the common good.	❏ 1	❏ 2	❏ 3	❏ 4
66.	I prefer to walk away when I see an argument is starting.	❏ 1	❏ 2	❏ 3	❏ 4
67.	Arguments should be avoided because they only drive people apart.	❏ 1	❏ 2	❏ 3	❏ 4
68.	I won't reveal any hesitancy or doubt when I become involved in a disagreement, because it may be seen as a sign of weakness.	❏ 1	❏ 2	❏ 3	❏ 4
69.	When there is a disagreement I prefer to wait it out rather than become involved in useless discussion.	❏ 1	❏ 2	❏ 3	❏ 4
70.	Persuasion, power, and even force are all acceptable ways to resolve a conflict.	❏ 1	❏ 2	❏ 3	❏ 4
71.	I enjoy using my skills and persuasive ability to maneuver toward my goals when there is conflict.	❏ 1	❏ 2	❏ 3	❏ 4

Figure 10–4 (continued)

SAMPLE OF COMPLETED HAND SCORE SHEET—CONFLICT MANAGEMENT

ID# _____

Place the numeral (1, 2, 3, or 4) corresponding to your choice next to the number of the item on the score sheet. Then, total the numerals you chose in each column and write the total in the space provided. Last, divide the total by the number of items in each column. For example, divide the total in the collaborative column by 16 and by 11 in the compromise, etc. The lowest score represents your preferred conflict management style. The next lowest score, your second choice, etc. The five scores will show your pattern of managing conflict.

Collaborative	Compromise	Accommodative	Forcing	Avoidant
_1_ 1	_2_ 2	_3_ 9	_4_ 8	_1_ 4
_3_ 3	_2_ 5	_3_ 13	_4_ 10	_2_ 6
_3_ 16	_3_ 11	_4_ 14	_4_ 18	_1_ 7
_4_ 21	_2_ 19	_2_ 15	_3_ 30	_2_ 12
_3_ 23	_2_ 34	_2_ 20	_4_ 45	_2_ 17
_2_ 25	_2_ 39	_3_ 22	_4_ 55	_3_ 24
_2_ 26	_2_ 41	_4_ 36	_3_ 56	_2_ 27
_2_ 28	_1_ 42	_2_ 43	_4_ 57	_3_ 29
_3_ 31	_1_ 44	_3_ 47	_3_ 58	_1_ 33
_2_ 32	_2_ 65	_3_ 49	_3_ 59	_2_ 46
_4_ 35	_3_ 71	_2_ 50	_4_ 64	_1_ 48
_3_ 37		_3_ 52	_3_ 68	_3_ 51
_3_ 38		_3_ 54	_4_ 70	_1_ 53
_4_ 40		_3_ 63		_1_ 60
_1_ 61				_1_ 66
_3_ 62				_2_ 67
				_1_ 69

	Collaborative	Compromise	Accommodative	Forcing	Avoidant
Total Columns	_43_ Total	_22_ Total	_40_ Total	_47_ Total	_29_ Total
Divide by	16	11	14	13	17
Final Score	_2.69_	_2.00_	_2.86_	_3.62_	_1.71_

1. Preferred Choice - Avoidant
Pattern of back-up choices
2. Compromise   3. Collaborative   4. Accomodative
Least Preferred - Forcing

Figure 10–4 (continued)

HAND SCORE SHEET—CONFLICT MANAGEMENT

ID# _____

Place the numeral (1, 2, 3, or 4) corresponding to your choice next to the number of the item on the score sheet. Then, total the numerals you chose in each column and write the total in the space provided. Last, divide the total by the number of items in each column. For example, divide the total in the collaborative column by 16 and by 11 in the compromise, etc. The lowest score represents your preferred conflict management style. The next lowest score, your second choice, etc. The five scores will show your pattern of managing conflict.

Collaborative	Compromise	Accommodative	Forcing	Avoidant
___ 1	___ 2	___ 9	___ 8	___ 4
___ 3	___ 5	___ 13	___ 10	___ 6
___ 16	___ 11	___ 14	___ 18	___ 7
___ 21	___ 19	___ 15	___ 30	___ 12
___ 23	___ 34	___ 20	___ 45	___ 17
___ 25	___ 39	___ 22	___ 55	___ 24
___ 26	___ 41	___ 36	___ 56	___ 27
___ 28	___ 42	___ 43	___ 57	___ 29
___ 31	___ 44	___ 47	___ 58	___ 33
___ 32	___ 65	___ 49	___ 59	___ 46
___ 35	___ 71	___ 50	___ 64	___ 48
___ 37		___ 52	___ 68	___ 51
___ 38		___ 54	___ 70	___ 53
___ 40		___ 63		___ 60
___ 61				___ 66
___ 62				___ 67
				___ 69

	Collaborative	Compromise	Accommodative	Forcing	Avoidant
Total Columns	___ Total	___ Total	___ Total	___ Total	___ Total
Divide by	16	11	14	13	17
Final Score	_____	_____	_____	_____	_____

Figure 10–4 (continued)

According to Hall's ideas on conflict, there are five methods or styles of handling conflict in relationships and in attaining goals. The five styles of handling conflict are *collaborative, compromise, accommodative, forcing,* and *avoidance* (See Figure 10–5).

The collaborative style values relationships and goals. A person with a collaborative style approaches a situation in a manner that seeks to creatively solve the problem with the belief that the process of working through the problem together strengthens the relationships.

In the compromise style, an individual approaches the problem believing she can use persuasive influence to sway or convince the group to choose a certain option and put aside personal desires for the good of the group. Relationships are maintained by considering the interests of the group. All group members are encouraged to express personal opinions and views. The basic belief is that everyone will win sometimes.

The accommodative style views relationships as most important. An accommodative person willingly releases her goals for the sake of the relationship. She avoids conflict at all costs.

The forcing style centers on the goal and forsakes the relationship. An individual with a forcing style uses confidence, firmness, power, and force to obtain the goal. Others' desires are forced aside.

In the avoidance style, the individual ignores personal goals and does not value relationships. This person expects to lose in conflicts, so she avoids all issues that approach conflict and becomes detached in such situations. She sees energy spent on resolving conflict as wasted, especially because the individual will not win anyway.

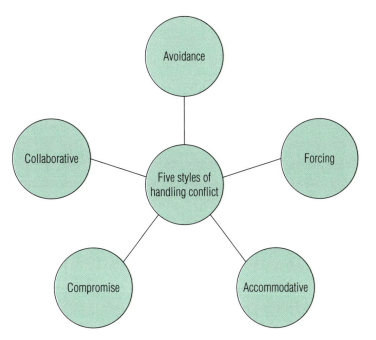

Figure 10–5 Five Styles of Handling Conflict

An individual's view of conflict directly influences the approach to conflict resolution. Changing an individual's view of conflict frees the individual to approach the situation more objectively and confidently. It gives freedom to move more creatively and productively toward a collaborative approach where goals and relationships can be preserved and maintained.

Sources of Conflict

In the health field, various cultures, genders, socioeconomic groups, and educational levels merge. Each individual in these groups approaches a situation a little differently leading to a potential conflict. Sources of conflict are personal conflicts, role definition, resources, group conflict, and workload.

Personal Conflicts

Each person makes decisions based on personal values and beliefs. Thus each person approaches problems differently. As these individual problem solving approaches converge, conflict may arise.

Role Definition

In times of nursing shortages and economic downturns, management requests individuals to assume multiple roles. Sometimes these roles overlap or are not well defined, and confusion arises as to who is to perform what role. This leads to role conflict.

Resources

As people scramble for limited supplies, pay raises, equipment, and personnel, conflict can occur because each person or department wants a share. This is especially likely to occur when resources are at a premium.

Group Conflicts

Each individual belongs to a variety of group types, such as gender, occupation, culture, and role. Two groups may disagree and have conflict with each other. Nurses may disagree with an administrative decision. Conflicts over wages and job assignments occur. Consider nurses who have worked at a facility for several years at one pay level and newly hired nurses with less experience start at a higher or equal pay level. The issue causes conflict between the groups.

Workload

Workloads may increase in times of nursing shortages. Some individuals may not mind the overload if it means more pay, while others desire more personal time more than the extra money. Increased workloads also make employees tired, and tensions increase when personal resources are exhausted.

RESOLVING CONFLICT

Resolving conflict is not like a boxing match in which one person or group is knocked out and the other one wins with a few bruises. Conflict resolution is not about winning or losing. Instead, **conflict resolution** is two individuals or groups working effectively together to come to an agreement both can accept. In this way, no one is a winner who must stay on top and watch for the next battle. No one is a loser who wastes energy plotting the next round in a disagreement. Nor is there a tie leading to a stalemate with no resolution to the issue.

When conflict arises there are strategies to resolve the situation effectively. Consider the following ideas on effective conflict resolution:

1. Concentrate on issues, not on individual personalities.
2. Claim responsibility for personal involvement where appropriate.
3. Communicate openly and assertively without aggression.
4. Listen attentively to the other's statements and concerns.
5. Creatively look for commonalities and solutions.
6. Examine the consequences of each solution. (Zerwekh & Claborn, 2009)

Gottlieb and Healey (1990) present a practical process in solving conflict that includes identifying the source of conflict, generating possible solutions, examining suggested solutions, choosing the best solution, implementing the chosen solution, evaluating the effectiveness of the solution for the conflict, and deciding if the conflict has been resolved or if the conflict-solving process needs repeating (See Figure 10–6).

Identifying the Source

Sometimes the source of conflict is obvious, and other times it is hidden in other agendas. Emotional involvement can color a person's objectivity, hiding the solution to the real problem of conflict. If the problem is not obvious, objectively discuss the situation to bring the problem into focus. It is important for all parties involved to attentively listen to one another's concerns until the source of conflict is identified. At times a third party can assist in objectively identifying the problem.

Generating Possible Solutions

During the solution generation phase it is important to state your personal desires for the solution to the conflict. It is also important to brainstorm during this phase. All potential

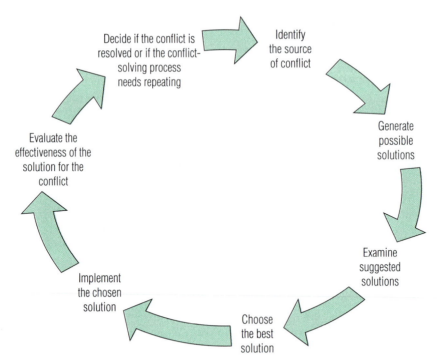

Figure 10–6 Conflict-solving process.

solutions that come to mind are presented even if they appear unconventional. Such suggestions lead to a creative, satisfying solution that might otherwise have been overlooked.

Examining Suggested Solutions

Once all solutions are presented, open-mindedly and impartially review them and evaluate which solution or solutions might work. Evaluate the suggested solutions without considering who made the suggestions. Sometimes a suggestion is rejected because of personal status or personal feelings about the person who made the suggestion. Be aware of personal feelings about others when examining possible solutions. Discuss these feelings as appropriate, but stay focused on the issues, not personalities. Flexibility is important during the problem-solving process.

Choosing the Best Solution

After carefully considering the ramifications of all suggested options, chose the best solution to appropriately resolve the conflict. Sometimes by combining several suggestions a more creative and satisfying solution is obtained.

Implementing the Chosen Solution and Evaluating Its Effectiveness

Once the solution has been implemented, choose a date to evaluate the results. Allot an appropriate amount of time for the implemented solution to be effective. Aborting the process before allowing adequate implementation time may be unfair to the solution and to the parties involved.

Deciding if the Conflict Has Been Resolved

Repeat the conflict resolution process if the solution does not work and the conflict is not resolved. Perhaps the real issue was not identified in the first attempt. Spend time discussing the conflict further to truly identify the issue. Conflict resolution takes time and energy. If each step of the conflict resolution process is followed and given adequate time for solution emergence, creative solutions are identified and the end product is an effective, quality solution to a puzzling conflict. Conflict is a growth process.

CRITICAL THINKING ACTIVITIES

1. Analyze the advantages and disadvantages of Zerwekh and Claborn's strategies to resolve conflict (2009).

Conflict Style	Advantages	Disadvantages
• Concentrate on issues, not on individual personalities.	_____ _____ _____	_____ _____ _____
• Claim responsibility for personal involvement where appropriate.	_____ _____	_____ _____
• Communicate openly and assertively without aggression.	_____ _____ _____	_____ _____ _____
• Listen attentively to the other's statements and concerns.	_____ _____ _____	_____ _____ _____
• Creatively look for commonalities and solutions.	_____ _____	_____ _____
• Examine the consequences of each solution.	_____ _____	_____ _____

2. How have your thoughts about conflict been challenged or changed after reading this section?

MANAGING DECISIONS

Chapter 7 discusses clinical judgment, problem solving, decision making, and the nursing process. Nurses make quick, accurate decisions regarding client care. A nurse determines a client's future when making clinical decisions regarding care. It is a sobering thought that "patients' lives hang in the balance of skilled nursing judgment" (Tanner, 2000, p. 338).

Faculty members assist students to apply theory to practice so future clinical judgments are sound. Faculty members encourage students to think critically and creatively in classroom discussions, clinical experiences, and nursing-related blog posts. Various methods used to encourage critical thinking are case studies/scenarios, computer-simulated clinical experiences, and journaling. Classroom discussions and written case studies or scenarios do not replace the clinical experience of working with a client needing immediate, appropriate, therapeutic nursing action. "Written scenarios may not capture the unpredictable, dynamic, moment-to-moment reasoning of nursing practice" (Fowler, 1997, p. 350). According to a research study by Fowler, "experiential knowledge is a component of clinical reasoning" (p. 361). Knowledge gained and applied in a clinical situation assists students in making decisions and determining decisive, appropriate nursing actions.

"Clinical decision making is a problem-solving activity that focuses on defining patient problems and selecting appropriate treatment interventions" (Higuchi & Donald, 2002, p. 145). Higuchi and Donald describe six thinking processes that nurses use in clinical decision making: *description, selection, inference, hypothesizing, synthesis,* and *verification.*

Description is the listing of facts as they relate to the client, for example, the data collected in a client assessment such as vital signs, breath sounds, and heart sounds. Nurses also describe nursing actions taken to meet client needs.

Selection is choosing relevant data or information about the client to report or chart. The nurse must know the data to collect and sorts out the relevant, important data to share in report. Selection as a thinking skill requires knowledge from theory and critical decision-making abilities. Skill in making decisions is gained and improved by following the decision-making process described in Chapter 7.

Inference includes three thinking functions: categorizing, discovering relationships among the separate parts, and hypothesizing. A nurse with sound clinical judgment is able to place appropriate data in different categories or sections so the data is documented and communicated in an effective way. An example of categorizing would be placing data relating to the heart in one category and data relating to the renal system in another category. The nurse needs knowledge to know what data to collect and needs nursing judgment to review the data as a unit. To discover the relationship between these separate parts, the nurse reviews the data in the cardiac system and the data in the renal system and then discovers how the renal function is affecting the heart and how the heart is affecting the renal function. The conclusion the nurse draws from the data she reviews is her hypothesis or assumption; for example, she could hypothesize that the kidneys are not producing enough urine because the heart cannot adequately pump the blood through the body to the renal system.

Synthesis is combining the separate parts of a whole and determining a nursing action; for example, after obtaining and reviewing cardiac, renal, and respiratory system data, the nurse determines that the client with congestive heart failure needs oxygen. "The ability to intuitively grasp a situation as a whole is one of the characteristics of nursing expertise" (Higuchi & Donald, 2002, p. 151).

Verification is assessing the validity of data and asserting appropriate results. Nurses verify data by documenting it and asserting the nursing action taken as appropriate. In our congestive heart failure example, verification is the nurse documenting assessment data after starting oxygen that confirms appropriate nursing action occurred to improve client status.

Every day, nurses use description, selection, inference, hypothesizing, synthesis, and verification in the clinical setting. Use the following critical thinking activity to evaluate your clinical thinking skills.

CRITICAL THINKING ACTIVITY

1. Review your clinical experiences over the past few weeks and describe examples of each of the thinking processes you used in making clinical decisions.
   - Description
   - Selection
   - Inference (include examples of categorizing, discovering relationships among the separate parts, and hypothesizing)
   - Synthesis
   - Verification

MANAGING RESOURCES

Resources are usable commodities available to meet a need. These resources include personnel, equipment, supplies, and finances. All of these must be managed and utilized effectively to provide quality client care. Resources are distributed sparingly in an economic downturn.

Wise use of personnel is especially important to improve job satisfaction, prevent burnout, and provide sufficient nurse-client ratios. Providing an encouraging, supportive, nonthreatening environment for nursing personnel is one of the best ways to care for the resource of personnel.

Facility resources include a convenient layout to prevent wasted time and energy. It is important to have and maintain state-of-the-art equipment, quality client care, accurate diagnoses, and time-saving devices. Continuing education provides staff with updated education. Nurses can do their jobs more efficiently with assistance from members of the ancillary team such as housekeeping, pastoral care, and volunteer services. Ideally, if available resources are used wisely, overhead is decreased, needed resources are purchased, and nursing salaries increased.

CRITICAL THINKING ACTIVITY

1. What are some ways you could use your facility's resources more productively?

THEORY TO PRACTICE

Time management

Shadow an RN to observe organizational skills and time management.

- Describe the positive organizational skills you observed.
- What did you learn about clinical organization skills and time management?

Conflict

- Did any role conflicts arise? Describe.
- How did the nurse handle the role conflict?
- Evaluate the conflict situation.
- What could have been done to prevent the conflict?
- Once the conflict began, according to Zerwekh and Claborn, what steps could have been taken to resolve the conflict?
- Were any of Zerwekh and Claborn's steps taken to resolve the conflict?
- What did you learn from observing this conflict?

Managing Decisions

- What quick decisions did the nurse make today?
- Evaluate the decisions and the outcomes of the decisions?

Managing Resources

- Describe and evaluate the management of
- personnel
- equipment
- supplies
- finances

SUMMARY

Job satisfaction improves when individuals learn to manage time, conflict, decisions, and resources. Wise use of time provides quality client care, excellent job performance, and valuable self-care. Work becomes more enjoyable when an individual realizes that conflict occurs and that it does not have to be viewed as a battleground but, rather, as an opportunity for change and growth. Self-confidence in the workplace improves as an individual learns to make effective, sound decisions. These sound decisions allow an individual to provide safe and competent client care. Increased self-confidence, while caring for clients, is comforting to them and eases their anxieties, leading to a more pleasant healing process. Wise use of resources provides an adequate quantity of supplies and improves fiscal security. Knowing and understanding these concepts related to management of client care will prove valuable as LPNs move ahead in their nursing career.

CHAPTER REFLECTIONS

Looking back on the opening scenario in this chapter, answer the following questions:

1. What were the dynamics in the scenario that frustrated Ling?
2. What could Ling do to manage her time more appropriately?
3. What is the source of the conflict between the co-workers?
4. What effective approach could Ling have taken with her co-worker to obtain assistance?

Journaling Your Journey

1. Define conflict in your words.
2. Describe a personal experience with conflict and explain how you responded.
3. Describe a professional experience with conflict and explain how you responded.
4. How could you change your approach to conflict and conflict resolution?

✌ ✌ ✌

My Story...

To be honest, I felt I was doing the same job as an RN and being paid a lot less for the same amount of hard work. So I decided to return to school and get my RN degree. At this point, I was no longer finding the coursework as difficult, I had established a good knowledge base, and I was working as a nurse. I felt a lot of the course content was repetition from my LPN schooling. I did not think the school had all that much to teach me; I thought I would do my time and then be an RN. I did not think that much would change. I would just be making more money for doing the same job. I was in for a few surprises.

Once I became an RN, I very quickly realized that not only did RNs earn more money and have more autonomy, but they also had a lot more responsibility. What I had not realized until

I was put into a leadership role myself was that I had always had a mentor or colleague nearby to guide me through any difficult situation. Suddenly, as an RN, I was that lead individual. I was thrust into a leadership role and expected to guide other nurses and co-workers.

RNs do the patient assessments, make instant decisions, and delegate tasks to others. There was more to learn as an RN because the scope of practice is different from the LPN. As an RN I needed a deeper knowledge base to enhance my critical thinking skills. I was dependent on the RNs if I needed help or guidance, I now had be able to take independent actions and be responsible for the unit as well as the patients. I had aspired to make more money and have more autonomy and respect. Now I needed to earn it and be able to put everything into action.

I realize that with more education comes more responsibility, and although LPNs and RNs strive to help others, there are differences in the two roles. The RNs had more job opportunities and more autonomy in their scope of practice. My responsibilities are now broader, encompassing patient care planning, managing and delegating, and having the responsibility of mentoring, managing, and guiding others.

Jennifer Foley MSN, RN

REFERENCES

Bartol, G. (1976). *The styles of conflict management used in co-worker relationships by nurse practitioners employed in hospitals.* Unpublished doctoral dissertation, Teachers College, Columbia University.

Bartol, G., Parrish, R., & McSweeney, M. (2001). Effective conflict management begins with knowing your style. *Journal for Nurses in Staff Development, 17*(1), 34–40.

Fowler, L. (1997). Clinical reasoning strategies used during care planning. *Clinical Nursing Research, 6*(4), 349–362.

Gottlieb, M., & Healy, W. (1998). *Making deals: The business of negotiating (*2nd ed.). New York: New York Institute of Finance.

Hall, J. (1973). *Conflict management survey.* Conroe, TX: Telemetric International.

Higuchi, K., & Donald, J. (2002). Thinking processes used by nurses in clinical decision-making. *Journal of Nursing Education, 41*(4), 145–155.

Tanner, C. (2000). Critical thinking: Beyond nursing process. *Journal of Nursing Education, 39*(8), 338 [On-line]. Available: http://80-proquest.umi.com

Zerwekh, J., & Claborn, J. (2009). *Nursing today: Transition and trends* (6th ed.). St. Louis: Saunders.

SUGGESTED RESOURCES

Asselin, M. (2001). Time to wear a third hat? *Nursing Management, 32*(3), 24–29.

Brandt, M., Holt, J., & Sullivan, M. (2001). How to make conflict work for you. *Nursing Management, 32*(11), 32–35.

Carroll, P. (2006). *Nursing leadership and management: A practical guide.* New York: Delmar Cengage Learning.

Childress, K. (2006). A dozen time-saving ideas you can use today. *Podiatry Management, 25*(4), 155–158.

Cox, S. (2006). Better time management: A matter of perspective. *Nursing2006, 36*(3), 43.

Kelly, J. (2006). An overview of conflict. *Dimensions of Critical Care Nursing, 25*(1), 22–28.

Riesz, N. (2008). Tips to help you maximize your time. *Clinical Leadership and Management Review, 22*(4), E1–E6.

Spidal, D. (2009). *Time Management.* Retrieved June 30, 2009 from www.asindexing.org/site/keycont.shtml

Tappen, R., Weiss, S., & Whitehead, D. (2006). *Essentials of nursing leadership and management* (4th ed.). Philadelphia: F.A. Davis.

Tomey, A. (2008). *Guide to nursing management and leadership* (8th ed.). St. Louis, MO: Mosby.

Valentine, P. (2001). A gender perspective on conflict management strategies of nurses. *Journal of Nursing Scholarship, 33*(1), 69–74.

Walczak, M., & Absolon, P. (2001). Essentials for effective communication in oncology nursing: Assertiveness, conflict management, delegation, and motivation. *Journal for Nurses in Staff Development, 17*(3), 159–162.

Chapter 11
Nursing Theory as a
Basis to Practice Nursing

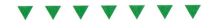

LEARNING OBJECTIVES

By the end of this chapter you should be able to:

1. Define nursing theory.
2. Identify major concepts in nursing.
3. Identify scientific theories that influence nursing theory.
4. Explain how nursing theory is a basis for nursing practice.
5. Examine the relationship of nursing theory, nursing research, and nursing practice.

KEY TERMS

Concepts
Metaparadigm
Nursing concept
Nursing theorists
Nursing theory
Paradigms
Phenomena
Philosophy
Science
Theory
Validity
Variables

SCENARIO

Kory is studying for a test and is wondering why theory is such a big deal in nursing. He feels that theory is of no use to the nurse working on the floor. After all, he has been an LPN for five years and has never had to use theory to give what he considers good care to his clients. Kory thinks that theory is "just something nurses with big degrees talk about using in practice." He has never heard anyone say that the facility is providing care in a particular manner because of a nursing theory or research studies.

THINK ABOUT IT

1. What is nursing theory?
2. Are you familiar with any nursing theorists? If so, which ones?
3. Is your school of nursing curriculum based on a nursing theory? If so, which one? Discuss the rationale for choosing this theory (see Journaling your Journey at the end of this chapter).

INTRODUCTION

In this chapter we discuss nursing theory and the major nursing concepts. We explore the definition of nursing theory and how it defines nursing as a respected science, art, and profession. We examine how scientific theories influence nursing theory and how nursing theory and research influence and relate to nursing practice. Finally, we look at the RN's role in nursing theory and research with regard to nursing practice. What does nursing theory mean to you as you transition into your new role as an RN?

MAJOR CONCEPTS IN NURSING

Have you had an idea that would either make your nursing practice better or improve client care or outcomes? This type of idea can and does inspire nursing theory. An individual has an idea and then sets out to prove it in a systematic fashion. The development of a nursing theory leads to an increase in knowledge, research, and education for the practice of nursing and, therefore, an opportunity to provide better quality client care. Nursing theory is not a new concept. Florence Nightingale, the first nursing theorist, developed her environmental theory during the Crimean War more than 140 years ago (See Figure 11–1). In her 1859 *Notes on Nursing*, Nightingale identified factors that affected health and wellness and documented her beliefs with observations, statistics, and deductive reasoning (Kearney-Nunnery, 2008).

Nursing theory gives us a philosophy and is the framework that guides nursing actions. This theoretical approach to nursing helps provide supportive, researched data to improve nursing practice by describing, predicting, and controlling **phenomena** (Tomey & Alligood, 2002). A phenomenon is any fact or event that we can detect through the use of our senses.

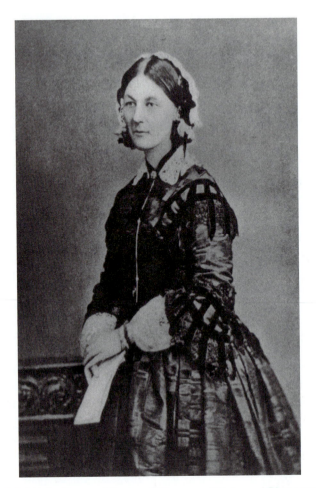

Figure 11–1 Florence Nightingale. Source: Library of Congress Prints and Photographs Division Washington, D.C. 20540 USA

An example of a phenomenon is a nurse taking client's blood pressure and detecting variations when he is in different positions, such as sitting, standing, or lying down. A nurse can control the position or phenomenon. **Nursing theory** consists of ideas that attempt to explain a relationship between two or more **concepts** (views or ideas about something). The concepts in the blood pressure illustration are the variations in the blood pressure with the different, controlled positions. Concepts are considered to be the subject matter or building blocks of nursing theory. These concepts or ideas are the labels given the phenomenon in question. They are ideas or mental images that originate in the mind of an individual or group of individuals from a particular experience that they had in their nursing career. For example, when you turn an immobile client every two hours, you have the concept or idea that turning prevents the client from skin breakdown.

Concepts are either *abstract* or *concrete*. Abstract concepts do not refer to a specific time or place and are sometimes defined as a mental image or picture. Concrete concepts relate to a

Table 11–1 Abstract and Concrete Concepts Using Nightingale's Environment Theory

Abstract Concepts	Concrete Concepts
Environment	Ventilation
	Light
	Cleanliness
	Warmth
	Noise level
	Diet

particular time, place, or thing (Tomey & Alligood, 2002). A **nursing concept** is a concrete or abstract idea about nursing. Table 11–1 gives examples of abstract and concrete concepts as they apply to Nightingale's environmental theory.

Concepts are referred to as **variables** when they are measured in research studies to develop a theory. The terms measurable concept and variable mean the same thing and are used interchangeably. A client's blood pressure is a measurable concept or variable. A client's blood pressure is measured and compared to his blood pressure in different situations or in relation to different variables.

CRITICAL THINKING ACTIVITIES

1. Share an idea you think would improve your nursing practice.
2. Share examples of concepts that are measurable.

When a relationship is assumed to exist between a set of variables, a theoretical statement is developed and then systematically tested. When the relationship between a set of variables is scientifically proven, and it is proven that the theoretical statement is applicable to nursing practice, it is recognized as a nursing theory.

Nursing theory exists to scientifically define and support the realm of nursing as a profession with its own body of knowledge. Perhaps the most abstract or general level of nursing knowledge is referred to as the **metaparadigm** of nursing. *Metaparadigm* is defined as the main phenomena of interest to a particular discipline. The main phenomena to nursing centers around the concepts *person, environment, health,* and *nursing.* These concepts are the universal tools that nursing theorists and nursing organizations use to write their individual philosophies of nursing. In addition, each person has a personal definition of what the concepts of the nursing metaparadigm mean to his practice of nursing. For example, you may feel that health is the absence of illness. As you continue to practice in the field of nursing, your experiences will change your definition of what these concepts mean.

CRITICAL THINKING ACTIVITY

1. Write your personal definitions of the following concepts.
   - Person:
   - Environment:
   - Health:
   - Nursing:

Philosophy (a broad or global view of the world) specifies the definitions of the concepts or ideas of the metaparadigm. It is in the process of defining the universal concepts of the nursing metaparadigm that the development of a nursing philosophy occurs. Theories are then derived from these definitions. A researcher uses these concept definitions as a starting point to develop a theory. For example, the definitions of person, environment, health, and nursing that you just wrote are the groundwork of your nursing theory.

Researchers have developed their individual philosophies into conceptual models or frameworks that are referred to as **paradigms.** *Paradigm* is a term that explains the existing network of science, philosophy, and theory accepted by the field of nursing. These conceptual models (established examples) serve as a guide to systematically test a proposed theory and to verify the theory's appropriateness for application to nursing practice. Frameworks are sometimes borrowed from other scientific fields, such as sociology or psychology, and applied to the field of nursing.

A **theory** is an abstract statement that explains the relationship of concepts. In essence, a theory is a set of organized information that explains facts, ideas, principles, or laws. With regard to nursing, theory is the organized body of information about phenomena that is unique to nursing. Nursing theories provide nursing with a set of guidelines that give nurses a real purpose, meaning, and value; a framework that will support what we do, how we do it, and when we do it. Nursing theories support measures to improve quality care by collecting scientific data. Figure 11–2 outlines the steps in theory development.

SCIENTIFIC THEORIES INFLUENCING NURSING THEORY

Science, philosophy, and theory are parts of any scientific discipline. As a science, nursing is a relatively new field; in fact, there is little reference to the field of nursing as a science before the 1950s. Compared to other scientific fields as they relate to theory, nursing is in its infancy.

To develop its knowledge base as a science, nursing borrowed from established scientific fields such as psychology and sociology. An example of the use of knowledge from other fields to build nursing as a science is Abraham Maslow's Theory of Human Motivation and Hierarchy of Human Needs. Maslow's theoretical model contributed to nursing practice by determining the order of importance in which nurses address the needs of clients. Maslow proposed that human motivation is explained by five levels of human needs. The first level

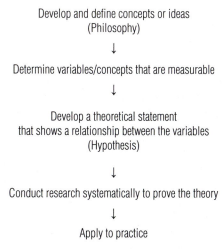

Figure 11–2 Steps in theory development.

represents very basic needs such as food and water. The second level is the need for safety and security. The third level is the need for love and belonging. The fourth level is self-esteem, and the fifth is self-actualization (Frisch & Frisch, 2010). Maslow's theory for understanding human behavior is one example of how nursing theory developed as a discipline using psychological and other scientific theories as a foundation. However, because nursing deals with the complexity of clients, nursing needs to develop its own body of science and scientific knowledge. **Science** is defined as the observation, identification, description, experimental investigation, and theoretical explanation of natural phenomena (Tomey & Alligood, 2002). Science gives meaning to who nurses are and what they do; that is, it defines the paradigm of nursing.

Nurses in the early era of nursing did not provide poor or unsafe care; they did what they thought was best based on values and the prevalent thinking of their time. The continued development of a scientific base for nursing practice is a high priority for the discipline. These are exciting times for the nursing profession as the foundation of knowledge continues to grow and expand. It is important to recognize the nursing leaders who have worked so hard over the last centuries to help develop this body of knowledge for nursing.

In the 1960s and 1970s nursing theorists began investigating development of certain issues and theories pertaining to nursing, which focused on the academic needs of nursing students. They developed appropriate curricula for each of the different levels of nursing. Then, in the mid-1970s, there was a change of focus and a new goal to make nursing more than a vocation but, rather, a profession (Tomey & Alligood, 2002). In the 1980s the universally accepted concepts of the nursing metaparadigm (person, environment, health, and nursing) were developed and lead to a more organized and consistent body of knowledge for nursing. Nursing theory was accepted in nursing and in nursing education programs (Tomey & Alligood). The acceptance of nursing theory allowed nursing leaders to begin publishing and presenting their newfound knowledge in journals, newspapers, books, and oral presentations. In the 1990s nursing professionals debated if nursing is a basic science, an applied science, or a practical science. Nursing's central concepts were defined in nursing literature. Scholars were trying to demonstrate the connection between nursing as an art and nursing as a science.

The "scientists" for the field of nursing are referred to as **nursing theorists.** Many of them devoted a large part of their careers to theory development and are commended and respected for their great efforts. Theorists worked in a systematic manner. They made the stages of theory development explicit so that others can review, replicate, and test a theory to give it **validity** (i.e., prove the theory's accuracy). The major theorists worked hard to define nursing as a profession with their own body of knowledge. Each of these theorists developed her theory based on her definitions of the metaparadigm of nursing. Refer to Table 11–2 for a list of a few of the nursing theorists who worked to further the development of the field of nursing. There are many others who contributed to the growth and development of nursing over the years. It is important for us as nurses to study these theorists and their theories to gain a better understanding of where nursing has been, where it is now, and where it is going. No one theory encompasses all of the ideas or concepts of nursing, and there may never be one, due to the complexity of dealing with human beings. Nursing theorists continue to develop new theories to improve the practice of nursing and quality of care.

NURSING THEORY AS A BASIS FOR PRACTICE

Nurses at all levels of education play a very important role in nursing theory and research. Practical nurses participate in research by communicating problems to administration, assisting with data collection, and utilizing evidence-based practice (EBP). The associate degree nurse assists with problem identification, collects data, and utilizes evidence-based practice to improve quality of client care. The baccalaureate nurse also helps identify problems, collects data, analyzes research literature, and implements evidence-based practice to improve quality of client care. The RN with a master's degree collaborates in research projects, and the nurse with a doctorate degree conducts independent, funded research projects as shown in Table 11-3 (Burns & Grove, 2005). As a registered nurse, you have an important role in research and nursing theory. If nurses collaborate and explore new ideas, the nursing profession grows as a science with a respected and specialized body of knowledge. Clements and Frederick (2009) stress the importance of EBP when they say "multiple studies demonstrate that clients who receive care, based on evidence, have a more positive outcome and less adverse incidents." (p. 185).

CRITICAL THINKING ACTIVITY

1. Review your nursing practice and think of a situation that could be researched to promote a change in client care. Describe this situation.

Table 11-2 Nursing theorists' contribution to nursing

Theorist	Theory	Description of Theory	Application to Nursing
Florence Nightingale	Environmental Theory	A belief that a person's surroundings such as clean air, water, and lighting can play a part in their healing process and their quality of care.	Made nurses more aware of the environment in which the clients receive care.
Virginia Henderson	Definition of Nursing	Nurses should help a client regain as much independence as quickly as possible with a holistic approach.	Helps us treat each client as an individual, including them in the plan of care and assisting them with a quick and healthy recovery.
Jean Watson	Philosophy and Science of Caring	Supports the idea of humanistic and holistic care; focus is on "caring," promoting health, and preventing illness.	Focuses on the importance of the "caring" relationship and communication in an individual's health.
Patricia Benner	From Novice to Expert: Excellence and Power in Clinical Nursing Practice	Nurses move through stages of expertise and skill as they practice nursing; defines a set of competencies from novice to expert nurse.	Has made nursing aware of effects of clinical skills on client care and client outcomes. Benner's goal was to make the community more aware of nursing as a responsible and caring practice.
Dorothea Orem	Self-Care Deficit Theory of Nursing	Nurses assist clients to their highest level of self-care.	Has made nurses aware of individualized client care, their participation in plan of care and return to their highest possible level of self-care.
Martha Rogers	Unitary Human Beings	Human beings are the focus of nursing. Humans and their environments are made up of energy fields and are continually working together to maintain harmony.	Supports and encourages scientific research and professional development of nursing; encourages letting go of tradition and constantly building on continued education. Rogers continued to expand her knowledge base and theory ideas to keep current with technological advances.
Imogene King	Systems Framework and Theory of Goal Attainment	Involves three systems: personal, interpersonal, and social; these systems form the connection between the client and the nurse. These components make up the process of nursing.	Encourages nurses to collaborate with each client to determine individualized goals and their plan of care.

Table 11-2 (continued)

Theorist	Theory	Description of theory	Application to nursing
Betty Neuman	Systems Model	A wholistic approach to client care; addresses the homeostasis of the client and the environmental effects with a focus on primary prevention.	Nurses use this theory in the clinical area, classrooms, and in continued research to prevent illness and encourage health through a wholistic systems approach to assessment and client-centered care; includes the client at the center of care; encourages continued research and growth with nursing knowledge and theories.
Hildegard Peplau	Psychodynamic Nursing	Client-nurse relationships use interpersonal skills and knowledge gained through previous research from other disciplines; you must understand your own behavior before you can help someone else understand his behavior.	Used in the mental health field to develop therapeutic interpersonal communication skills in meeting the needs of each client.
Madeline Leininger	Culture Care: Diversity and Universality Theory	Culturally specific care is provided in a "caring" manner.	Encourages nurses to gain an awareness of the uniqueness of each culture to meet the individualized needs of each client.
Rosemarie Rizzo Parse	Human Becoming	Views nursing as a human science that can function independently; attention is focused on individual definitions of health and quality of life and assists in making the client and the nurse partners in the plan of care.	Allows nursing the opportunity to grow into a profession with its own body of knowledge and a special approach to each individual client.
Nola Pender	Health Promotion Model	Health promotion for all ages is the priority in nursing care.	Refocuses nurses on health promotion and disease prevention.

Table 11–3 Nursing roles in nursing theory

Nursing Role	Relationship to Nursing Theory
Licensed Practical/ Vocational Nurse	The LPN/VN reports to the charge nurse that clients who have the support of family seem to recover more quickly and are dismissed sooner.
Associate Degree Nurse	The ASN notices that her surgical clients have better outcomes and are discharged sooner when family has been allowed unlimited visitation. She keeps a record of this.
Baccalaureate Nurse	The BSN does a literature review and finds that the literature verifies the assumption that the emotional support surgical clients receive from their families contributes to better outcomes and shorter hospital stays. She applies this acquired knowledge to her nursing practice by encouraging family interactions with clients.
Master's Level Nurse	The MSN collaborates in a research project that seeks to prove that emotional support provided to surgical clients by their families contributes to better outcomes and shorter hospital stays.
Doctorate Level Nurse	The Ph.D. RN conducts research funded by a health-related organization to determine if family support promotes better outcomes and/or reduces hospital stays for surgical clients.

RELATIONSHIP OF THEORY TO PRACTICE

Theory, practice, and research are related and intertwined. They all work together to demonstrate nursing as a science using nursing's body of knowledge to guide nursing practice. The application of nursing theory to nursing practice depends on the skills of observation, questioning, comparing, and contrasting what is observed (Johnson & Webber, 2001). It is nursing theory that guides the practice of nursing in an effective manner. Research tests the theories and questions that arise in nursing practice. Nursing practice applies theory and research in client care. Nursing practice provides the study questions for research that is relevant to the field of nursing. Theory, practice, and research are interdependent as shown in Figure 11–3 (Kearney-Nunnery, 2008).

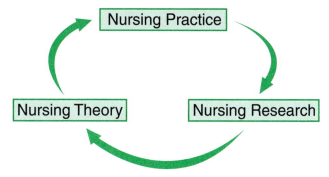

Figure 11–3 Theory, practice, and research are interdependent. (Source: From *Nursing Fundamentals, Caring & Clinical Decision Making*, 2nd ed., R. Daniels, 2010, Clifton Park, NY: Delmar/Cengage Learning.)

SUMMARY

Nursing is a profession supported by scientific knowledge. As we practice nursing, we gain knowledge from our experiences that we can use to enlarge our scientific knowledge base. In other words, the art of nursing, or the care we provide, lends itself to the science of nursing. As nurses, we practice using principles provided by our metaparadigm and nursing theory. This principle-based practice provides us with the tools for critical thinking, client care, education, administration, research, and collaboration (Kearney-Nunnery, 2008).

As you continue to grow personally and professionally, remember the professional role you play in the field of nursing. Ideas that you gain from your care of one client could easily benefit many more clients. Nursing theory begins with a simple idea or concept that someone or a group of individuals begins to question and develop into a researchable concept or idea. These new concepts or ideas may develop into the next research project or theory. It is this collaboration among health care providers that leads to research resulting in improved quality care.

CHAPTER REFLECTIONS

1. How does nursing theory affect nursing as a profession?
2. Share an idea or theory of yours that could improve client care.
3. How could you apply nursing theory to your own nursing practice?

THEORY TO PRACTICE

1. Using the four components of the nursing metaparadigm (health, environment, nursing, and person), define your philosophy of nursing.

2. How does your own theory and ideas compare to the other theorist in this chapter?

3. How does your own theory compare to your peers? Share ideas and rationale.

4. Linda Ryan's (2005) article, "The Journey to Integrate Watson's Caring Theory with Clinical Practice" (see references), is an example of integrating theory into practice. Ryan believes through this experience that a common bond developed among members of the health care team and that quality of care improved. Research different facilities, organizations, and businesses that adopted one specific theory to guide their practice? Who did they chose? How did the process work? How does it impact the care they give?

Journaling Your Journey

1. What does nursing mean to you?

2. Describe your nursing practice—on what do you focus the most attention and time? Why?

3. Identify different approaches to nursing care. Describe the similarities and differences.

ↁↁ ↁↁ ↁↁ

My Story...

I loved being an LPN. I did not return to school for my RN because I felt pressured by co-workers, wanted to make more money, or got sick of hearing "Oh, you're *just* an LPN." I did it for myself, because I knew that if I got my RN I would have more responsibilities and then in turn, could help more people and work in more critical areas.

I did not become an RN to make more money even though there are some high-dollar nursing jobs out there. I did not do it for more prestige, or to be a charge nurse, or to one day be a chief nurse executive. I did it because I knew I could help more people. When a patient or co-worker asks me, "How long have you been a nurse?" I don't say "Well, I was an LPN for 2 years and an RN for 8 years". The *title* really doesn't matter as much to me. I have been a *nurse* for ten years. I have been caring for people, helping families let go of their loved ones, and celebrating with families when new life arrives.

"As an RN you will have a lot more responsibility. You will be a shift charge nurse, experience many code blues, resolve staff conflicts, and attend to client, family, and staffing needs and issues. All of these are accomplished through strong critical thinking skills and the ability to apply the nursing process to any given clinical situation."

Stacy Fladhammer, RN

REFERENCES

Burns, N., & Grove, S. (2005). *The practice of nursing research: Conduct, critique, and utilization* (5th ed.). Philadelphia: W.B. Saunders Company.

Clements, P., & Frederick, A. (2009). Toto rides again: Evaluating the evidence. *Journal of Forensic Nursing* 5(3), 185–188.

Frisch. N., & Frisch, L. (2006). *Psychiatric mental health nursing* (4th ed.). Clifton Park, NY: Thomson Delmar Learning.

Johnson, B., & Webber, P. (2001). *An introduction to theory and reasoning in nursing.* Philadelphia: Lippincott.

Kearney-Nunnery R. (2008). *Advancing your career: Concepts of professional nursing* (4th ed.). Philadelphia: F.A. Davis Company.

Ryan, L. (2005). The journey to integrate Watson's caring theory with clinical practice. *International Journal of Human Caring, 9*(3), 26-30.

Tomey, A., & Alligood, M. (2002). *Nursing theorists and their work* (5th ed.). St. Louis, MO: Mosby.

SUGGESTED RESOURCES

Malinowski, A., & Stamler, L. (2001). Comfort: Exploration of the concept in nursing. *Journal of Advanced Nursing, (39)*6, 599–606.

Schwartz-Barcott, D., Patterson, B., Lusardi, P., & Farmer, B. (2002). From practice to theory: Tightening the link via three fieldwork strategies. *Journal of Advanced Nursing, (39)*3, 281–289.

Smith, C., Pace, K., Kochinda, C., Klein Beck, S., Koehler, J., & Popkess-Vawter, S. (2002). Caregiving effectiveness model evolution to a midrange theory of home care: A process for critique and replication. *Advances in Nursing Science, (25)*1, 50–64.

Chapter 12
Ethical and Legal Considerations

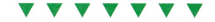

LEARNING OBJECTIVES

By the end of this chapter, you should be able to:

1. List the organizations that regulate nursing practice.
2. Explain legal issues that affect nursing practice.
3. Define personal values.
4. Explain the relationship between ethical principles and nursing practice.
5. Explain an ethical decision-making process.

KEY TERMS

Assault
Autonomy
Battery
Beneficence
Bioethics
Clinical ethics
Code of ethics
Confidentiality
Delegation
Deontology
Ethical rights
Ethics
HIPAA
Justice
Licensure
Malpractice
Mandatory licensure
Morals
Negligence

Nonbeneficence
Option rights
Protected health information
Rights
Standard of care
Utilitarianism
Values
Veracity
Welfare rights

SCENARIO

Paula, a new RN on a medical-surgical floor, often follows Deb, a nurse who has worked on the floor for many years. Several times clients have complained that they have asked for pain medication and not received it. When Paula reviewed the medication records on these clients, she noted that Deb had charted that each client received pain medication at each prn interval that it was ordered. Paula notices that sometimes when Deb gives her report she is somewhat distant and not connected to shift report. Paula is not certain what is happening, and she also feels that she is new and could be crossing her boundaries if she says anything about her concerns.

THINK ABOUT IT

1. Have you ever experienced an ethical situation that placed you in an awkward position?
2. Do you think that it is your professional responsibility to report all ethical concerns?
3. Do you think Deb is guilty of stealing client pain medications, or can you come up with alternative explanations?

INTRODUCTION

As nurses, we make many decisions daily about client care. The decisions become more difficult when a variety of personal values and beliefs are involved. Conflict may occur between the health care provider's values and the client's values and requests. At that point, moral and ethical decision making becomes a very important and valuable tool for a nurse. Ethical decisions may involve legal issues. The RN functions as a leader and is a vital member of the team involved in making ethical and legal decisions.

The moral, ethical, and legal boundaries of nursing are maintained by successful organizations that are well informed and plan sufficient time for nurses to build a good working relationship with clients, families, and other health care professionals. Good relationships help provide the highest quality care possible. Nursing is usually a profession that focuses its efforts and energies on the good of others. The success of the professional relationship is often credited to open communication built on trust and honesty (Day, 2007).

In this chapter we will review key ethical and legal principles that are important to understand in transitioning into the RN role. We will discuss the development of personal values and their influence on ethical issues and the ethical decision-making process. We will explore how nursing practice is guided by legislative acts and client rights. An ethical decision-making process is presented to guide nurses in making ethical decisions. Finally, we will discuss how values, ethics, legal issues, and ethical decision making influence nurses and the nursing care they provide.

VALUES AND ETHICS

Why do we make the decisions we make? How do we decide the appropriate actions in various situations? Personal **values** are beliefs that guide our thoughts and actions and drive our decisions. We develop these values from our family, friends, culture, environment, and life experiences. In a sense, our values are our philosophy of life.

Our values determine our ethics or code of conduct. We form professional values and ethics from personal and educational experiences (see Figure 12–1). Professional values and ethics determine our thoughts and response in ethical dilemmas that we face with clients and their families each day in nursing.

Nurses, who understand their personal values, find it easier to separate ethical opinions and nursing knowledge. A good understanding of personal values, and a strong knowledge base, helps nurses show respect to clients and their families while making more independent and informed decisions (Sizemore, 2006).

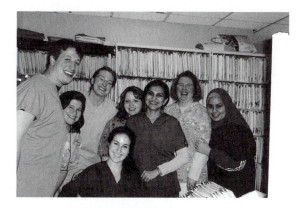

Figure 12–1 Nursing staff enjoys each other and formed their values and ethics from a varied personal and educational background. (Source: *Heath Assessment and Physical Examination* 4th ed., by M. Estes, 2010, Clifton Park, NY: Delmar/Cengage Learning.)

Morals, Ethics, and Bioethics

Morals, ethics, and *bioethics* are key terms to understanding the principles of ethics. **Morals** are the rules of right and wrong that serve as the standard for decision making and behavior. An example of a moral is "Good people do not cheat." Therefore, respectable citizens do not cheat.

Lawrence Kohlberg (1977) studied the development of morals in individuals. Kohlberg was not concerned with the morality of a decision but concentrated on the reasons people make decisions. He described three levels and six stages of moral development from childhood to adulthood. Table 12–1 contrasts Piaget's development of cognitive stages, Erickson's psychosocial stages, and Kohlberg's moral judgment stages. The first level is called the preconventional, or premoral level. In this level, an individual makes decisions based on fear of the consequences of actions rather than respect for the authority figure. The second level is the conventional level. The individual makes decisions based on a desire to conform to the norms of the family, group, community, or nation. The third level is the postconventional, or principled, level. The individual is not concerned with conforming to the group but makes decisions based on an internalized set of rules (Kozier, Erb, Berman, & Snyder, 2008).

Ethics define how people should act because of the moral standard. An ethicist is concerned about the morality of a decision and would analyze the moral standard to see if it is correct in all circumstances. Ethics involve the analysis of actions. For example, an ethicist would analyze whether cheating is appropriate in some circumstances. **Bioethics** (also known as **clinical ethics**) applies ethical theories and principles to health care situations.

Code of Ethics

A **code of ethics** is the standard that members of a profession follow when performing the duties of the profession. The nursing code of ethics is the standard that nurses are expected to follow when providing nursing care. The American Nurses Association (ANA) and the International Council of Nurses (ICN) established the nursing professions' standards and expectations. See appendices D, E, and F to review these published standards. These standards are respected by the majority of nursing professionals and are used as a guideline for expected practice behaviors as demonstrated in Figures 12–2 and 12–3. The National Student Nurses Association (NSNA) Code of Conduct sets the expectations for professional, academic, and clinical conduct and introduces students to the ideals and principles of the nursing profession. The organizational standards and expectations become an important socialization component in the holistic and professional development of the new and growing RN. The standards are in appendices E and F and on the NSNA web page at: www.nsna.org. As members of the community see members of the nursing profession following the standard, or code of ethics, community members will view the members of the profession as reliable, trustworthy, and accountable.

Table 12–1 A Contrast of Piaget's Cognitive Stages, Erickson's Psychosocial Stages, and Kohlberg's Moral Judgment Stages

Stage/Age	Piaget's Cognitive Stages	Erikson's Psychosocial Stages	Kohlberg's Moral Judgment Stages
1. Infancy Birth to 1 year	**Sensorimotor** (birth to 2 years): Begins to acquire language Task: Object permanence	**Trust vs. Mistrust** Task: Trust Socializing agent: Mothering person Central process: Mutuality Ego quality: Hope	
2. Toddler 1 to 3 years	**Sensorimotor** continues **Preoperational** (2 to 7 years) Begins: Use of representational thought Task: Use language and mental images to think and communicate	**Autonomy vs. Shame and Doubt** Task: Autonomy Socializing agent: Parents Central process: Imitation Ego quality: Self-control and willpower	**Preconventional Level:** **1. Morality stage:** Avoid punishment by not breaking rules of authority figures
3. Preschool 3 to 6 years	**Preoperational** continues	**Initiative vs. Guilt** Task: Initiative and moral responsibility Socializing agents: Parents Central process: Identification Ego quality: Direction, purpose, and conscience	**2. Individualism, Instrumental Purpose, and Exchange Stage:** "Right" is relative, follow rules when in own interest
4. School Age 6 to 12 years	**Preoperational** continues **Concrete Operations** (7 to 12 years) begins: Engage in inductive reasoning and concrete problem solving Task: Learn concepts of conservation and reversibility	**Industry vs. Inferiority** Task: Industry, self-assurance, self-esteem Socializing agents: Teachers and peers Central process: Education Ego quality: Competence	**Conventional Level** **3. Mutual Expectations, Relationships, and Conformity to Moral Norms Stage:** Need to be "good" in own and others eyes, believe in rules and regulations
5. Adolescence 12 to 18 years	**Formal Operations** (12 years to adulthood): Engage in abstract reasoning and analytical problem solving Task: Develop a workable philosophy of life	**Identity vs. Role Confusion** Task: Self-identity and concept Socializing agents: Society of peers Central process: Role experimentation and peer pressure Ego quality: Fidelity and devotion to others, personal and sociocultural values	**4. Social System and Conscience Stage:** Uphold laws because they are fixed social duties

Table 12–1 (continued)

Stage/Age	Piaget's Cognitive Stages	Erikson's Psychosocial Stages	Kohlberg's Moral Judgment Stages
6. Young Adult 18 to 30 years	**Formal Operations** continues	**Intimacy vs. Isolation** Task: Intimacy Socializing agent: Close friends, partners, lovers, spouse Central process: Mutuality among peers Ego quality: Intimate affiliation and love	**Postconventional Level:** 5. **Social Contract or Utility and Individual Rights Stage:** Uphold laws in the interest of the greatest good for the greatest number; uphold laws that protect universal rights
7. Early Middle Age 30 to 50 years		**Generativity vs. Stagnation** Task: Generativity Socializing agent: Spouse, partner, children, sociocultural norms Central process: Creativity and person-environment fit Ego quality: Productivity, perseverance, charity, and consideration	
8. Late Middle Age 50 to 70 years		**Generativity vs. Stagnation** continues	6. **Universal Ethical Principles Stage:** Support universal moral principles regardless of the price for doing so
9. Late Adult 70 years to death		**Ego Integrity vs. Despair** (65 years to death) Task: Ego integrity Socializing agent: Significant others Central process: Introspection Ego quality: Wisdom	

(Source: *Health Assessment and Physical Examination* 4th ed., by M. Estes. Cengage Learning/Delmar. 2010.)

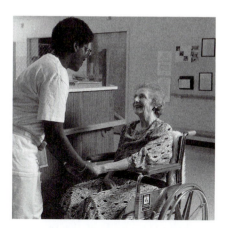

Figure 12–2 "The nurse, in all professional relationships, practices with compassion and respect for the inherent dignity, worth, and uniqueness of every individual, unrestricted by considerations of social or economic status, personal attributes, or the nature of health problems." (American Nurses Association, *Code of Ethics for Nurses with Interpretive Statements*, © 2001 American Nurses Publishing, American Nurses Association, Washington, DC.) (Source: *Heath Assessment and Physical Examination* 4th ed., by M. Estes, 2010, Clifton Park, NY: Delmar/Cengage Learning.)

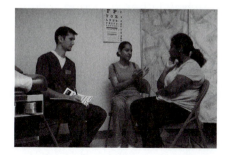

Figure 12–3 "In providing care, the nurse promotes an environment in which the human rights, values, customs and spiritual beliefs of the individual, family and community are respected." (International Council of Nurses, (2000). *The International Council of Nurses Code of Ethics,* Geneva, Switzerland.) (Source: *Heath Assessment and Physical Examination* 4th ed., by M. Estes, 2010, Clifton Park, NY: Delmar/Cengage Learning.)

CRITICAL THINKING ACTIVITY

1. List your expected standards and behaviors for nurses.

2. Share your belief system and thoughts about the Code for Conduct/Code of Ethics?

3. Review the different Codes of Conduct in Appendices D through G. Identify similarities and differences between each. Do you think this is a complete Code of Ethics for nurses and student nurses? If not, what is missing?

4. How do you believe these Codes of Conduct impact the profession of nursing?

Ethical Theories

Why do I make the decisions I make? What guides my actions? What determines how I respond to my neighbor? An ethical theory is a framework for personal beliefs that guide one's values, decisions, and actions and determines responses in life. Therefore, it is important for us to study ethical theories to determine how an individual makes decisions and responds in life.

One ethical theory is **utilitarianism** (or situational ethics). It was first proposed by David Hume (1711–1776) and further developed by Jeremy Bentham (1748–1826) and John Stuart Mill (1806–1873). The two supporting concepts of utilitarianism are:

1. "Achieve the greatest good for the greatest number." In other words, "utilitarian values give greater moral weight to the needs of the many than to the needs of the few, even if the few are much worse off." (Hein, 2001, p. 245)
2. "The end justify the means."

According to this theory, an individual does not have rights but is considered as one with the whole population. The right action is the action by which the greatest number of people benefit. The situation determines whether an action is done with honor or is morally right or wrong.

An example of utilitarianism is spending more federal money on people with curable diseases than on the smaller number of people with incurable diseases. In the movie *Pearl Harbor,* casualties were so numerous that the hospital personnel could not care for all the injured. A nurse was asked to assess all incoming clients to determine which ones could be assisted and which ones were too badly injured to benefit from assistance. This is an example of triage, an accepted concept in health care.

A second ethical theory is Immanuel Kant's (1724–1804), theory of **deontology**. This theory states that the right or wrong of an action is dependent upon the morality of the action. The action is moral if it is based on good will. To do one's duty is right or good, not to do one's duty is wrong. This theory is further divided into two ideologies: *act deontology* and *rule deontology.*

Act deontology gathers all the facts about a situation and determines the appropriate action. The generalized decision then becomes the right action or judgment for all similar situations. These rules regarding actions or judgments then apply to all similar situations, even if the external circumstances surrounding the situation change.

Rule deontology states that principles or rules determine our actions. These principles or rules do not change with the situation. A rule could be "Never cheat another person" or "Always be kind to elderly people." The rule applies in all situations. Rule deontologists are not concerned with consequences or the situations in which the rule is applied, only that the rule is followed. A nursing example of rule deontology is the rule in most facilities that states, "Clients must be turned every two hours." If the rule is followed, clients are turned every two

Box 12–1 Ethical Principles Affecting Nursing

Justice	—	treat all people fairly
Autonomy	—	ability to make and act on personal decisions
Beneficence	—	duty to do good to others
Nonbeneficence	—	not to intentionally or unintentionally harm others
Veracity	—	principle of truthfulness

hours regardless of the client's desires or condition. What if the client is terminally ill and in severe pain? What if the client refuses to be turned? Is the rule still followed?

Ethical Principles

Ethical principles are based on the right of each person to be treated with respect (Chitty, 2007). Ethical principles are justice, autonomy, beneficence, and veracity.

Justice

The principle of **justice** states that all people are treated fairly (Kearney-Nunnery, 2008). In nursing, this would indicate that all clients would receive quality care regardless of diagnosis, care needs, or financial concerns. This becomes a concern in the allocation of funds. Does the 89-year-old client with a terminal disease and multiple complications or the 20-year-old with a broken leg receive the funded care? Some say the 20-year-old is given the care because the elderly man is going to die regardless of treatment. From this perspective, clients with terminal or extensive needs will not get the funds because others with lesser needs are given more reasonable or equitable care. The principle of justice makes us question the ethics of a situation but does not provide the answers.

Autonomy

Autonomy is based on self-determination and independence. Autonomy provides each person the option to make personal decisions and act on those decisions. Thus, each person has the right to determine her personal health care (Chitty, 2007; Kearney-Nunnery, 2008). Health care workers following the principle of autonomy respect each individual person to make sound decisions. Strictly taken, autonomy offers the individual the right to make a health care decision, even if the nursing staff does not agree. An example is an 18-year-old client who is a Jehovah's Witness and is refusing a needed blood transfusion. In this case, the client has the right to refuse the blood transfusion even if the nurses caring for her disagree with her decision. However, if the same client had tuberculosis or a highly contagious disease that could harm others, she could be isolated for the good of society. Thus a client's autonomy can sometimes be overruled.

A nurse is not allowed to withhold information from a client to prevent her from making a decision with which she disagrees. She must inform the client of all health care options and provide care even if the client's health care decision differs from the nurse's beliefs.

Beneficence/Nonbeneficence

A nurse's duty is to do good or promote the well-being of clients (**beneficence**) and not to intentionally or unintentionally harm the client (**nonbeneficence**) (Rosenthal, 2001). Good care requires not only technical skill but also having a holistic view of the client that includes the client's values, beliefs, feelings, and desires. The nurse providing good care considers the family's and significant support person's input. A problem arises if the nurse does not agree with what the client thinks is good care. Who then can make the best ethical decision about the client's care? The nurse can discuss the situation with colleagues and physicians involved in the case. If she still has concerns after discussing the situation with others involved in the case, the situation is referred to an ethical committee within the facility.

Nonbeneficence also has another aspect that requires the nurse to protect from harm those who cannot care for themselves, such as the mentally challenged, cognitively impaired elderly, or children. The nurse guards the best interests of these clients and seeks quality, equitable care. For example, the nurse reports possible abuse or neglect cases.

Veracity

Veracity is the principle of truthfulness. Nurses have a responsibility to be truthful with clients. Trust is the basis of an open, sincere, meaningful relationship, and the basis of trust is truthfulness. Health care workers have a responsibility to share truthful information with their clients. It is difficult to share bad news with clients. We rationalize that the client is better off not knowing everything, or that she would not understand the information. These are not legitimate reasons to withhold truthful information from a client. Even if a client withholds truthful information from the health care worker, such as facts about her sex life, a socially unacceptable disease, or mental illness, the nurse does not have the right to withhold information from the client.

The Client's Rights

The principles previously discussed are based on **rights**. Ellis and Hartley (2007) define a right as "something that is owed to an individual on a legal, moral, or ethical basis" (p. 342). A right is something a person lays claim to or an entitlement that seems due a person. Rights are also described as a person's privileges, special considerations, or freedoms. There are three rights: *welfare rights*, *ethical rights*, and *option rights* (Aiken, 2004).

Welfare rights (legal rights) are a legal access or right to something that will give an individual an advantage or gain. In the United States everyone has a right to employment regardless of race, religion, or gender. Laws protect these rights. If an individual's rights are violated, she may appeal to a legal system for justice.

Ethical rights (moral rights) are based on a moral or ethical principle. Law does not support these rights. However, over time the belief in these principles gives them the conceptual backing of a legal right. An example of this is health care in the United States. Many people believe that everyone has the right to receive health care, but at the present time, obtaining appropriate health care is not a legal right.

Option rights are based on the dignity and freedom of choice for all individuals. As U.S. citizens, we have the freedom to choose where we live, the type of clothes we wear, and where we travel. This is because our country believes in the right of each individual to make choices and to have the free will to follow those choices as long as they do not infringe on the rights of others.

Summary of Ethical Principles

Concerns arise from ethical principles and the interpretation of individual rights. When a conflict of rights arises, how should the conflict be resolved? Obligations to clients may seem to conflict with obligations to the physician or to the institution. This is not really a moral dilemma although the decision may be an agonizing one. An important distinction is made between doing what is morally right and what is least difficult practically (Hood & Leddy, 2005). Do we take the action that is morally right, or the action that is least difficult? Which can be more agonizing? Doing what is morally right? Or taking the road of least resistance and then living with a seared conscience regarding the results of the actions? Ethical decision making is discussed in the next section.

CRITICAL THINKING ACTIVITIES

1. List some of your personal values.
2. Review the American Nurses Association Code of Ethics (Appendix E) and discuss with peers. Write some ideas to discuss.
3. Ethical Principle Scenario:

   Deana, a 76-year-old woman, has Parkinson's disease. She had an athletic build and has been very active her entire life. Slowly, the effects of Parkinson's have overtaken her body. Because her family is unable to care for her any longer in the home, she is admitted to a nursing home. She is unable to walk and is lifted from a wheelchair to the bed. The results of a swallow study indicate that she is unable to swallow any type of food. She is losing weight and a small pressure sore is developing on her coccyx. She had aspiration pneumonia twice in the last three months. The nursing home director requested permission from the family for placement of a feeding tube. The family refuses to have any type of feeding tube inserted knowing that she will starve to death.

   Refer back to the preceding discussion of ethical concepts. Put yourself in the place of the client, the client's family, and the nursing home personnel in the scenario for this Critical Thinking Activity. What would be your viewpoint as the client, the client's family, and nursing home personnel based on the ethical principles of justice, autonomy, beneficence, nonbeneficence, veracity, and client's rights? Refer to the example that is given here in the justice section and then write your own thoughts for the other five principles. Discuss your thoughts with your peers.

Evaluate the scenario from the viewpoint of the client, the client's family, and nursing home personnel as their views may relate to the ethical principle of justice.

Ethical principle	Ethical principle as it relates to the client, the client's family, and nursing home personnel
Justice	Client:
	My body has deteriorated and I would like a natural, dignified death.
	Family:
	We have provided the best care we can. The family's funds have been depleted in providing nursing home care. We feel she has suffered enough and prolonging life will only cause more suffering.
	Nursing home personnel:
	The nursing home director has offered nutritional supplements to provide quality nutritional care. Some of the nursing home personnel do not think Deana is being treated fairly because the family is starving her to death.
Autonomy	Client:
	Family:
	Nursing home personnel:
Beneficence	Client:
	Family:
	Nursing home personnel:
Nonbeneficence	Client:
	Family:
	Nursing home personnel:
Veracity	Client:
	Family:
	Nursing home personnel:
Client's rights	Client:
	Family:
	Nursing home personnel:

ETHICAL DECISION MAKING

The nursing process is the basis for decision making in nursing. How do the steps of the nursing process relate to the ethical decision–making process?

Nurses face many ethical issues. To make an ethical decision, a nurse reviews ethical principles, evaluates personal values and beliefs, and researches related legal issues. Chitty (2007) presented an ethical decision–making process with the following six steps:

1. **Clarifying the ethical dilemma**—What is the ethical problem? Who owns the problem? Who will be affected by the problem and results of the problem? What ethical principles are related to the problem? Is there a conflict with personal and professional values or professional duties? What is the time frame for making the decision?

2. **Gathering data**—How did this situation occur? Have all parties been contacted and had input into the situation? Has a legal and ethical literature review been completed? Are there any political or economic issues to consider?

3. **Identifying options**—Brainstorm and list all possible solution options. List new and creative alternatives.

4. **Making a decision**—Consider the pros and cons of the outcome of each potential solution. Consider ethical ramifications of each solution. Will other dilemmas occur because of the potential decision? Will any institutional, community, or government policies be affected? Make a decision. Not making a decision is not being accountable or responsible.

5. **Choosing and implementing a course of action**—Outline a plan of action to carry out the decision. Make sure that personal values and morals are not compromised. Communicate appropriately with all involved parties. Act as a team when completing the course of action.

6. **Evaluating the decision**—Analyze all the unexpected outcomes produced by the ethical dilemma. It is not uncommon that an ethical decision made in a crisis may result in other unsettled issues. Review and address all issues that arise. Only after a decision is made and the results of the decision occur can it be determined if the best decision was made. Evaluate if the best decision was made. If an alternative decision had been made, what would be the results? Is there a way to determine the real results? Are there any legal implications that need addressing? Are new policies needed or do other policies need changing because of the chosen decision and actions?

The steps in the ethical decision–making process have many parallels to the nursing process (see Table 12–2).

Table 12–2 Comparison of the nursing process and the ethical decision-making process

Ethical Decision-Making Process	Nursing Process
Clarify the ethical dilemma.	Assess patient needs.
Gather data.	Decide on appropriate nursing diagnosis.
Identify options.	Determine outcome identification
Make a decision.	Plan nursing care.
Choose and implement a course of action.	Implement nursing action.
Evaluate the decision.	Evaluate outcomes.

CRITICAL THINKING ACTIVITY

1. Using the ethical decision–making process presented in this chapter, discuss with your peers the best approach in handling Paula's situation in the chapter's opening scenario. Write your decisions for each section in the following chart.

Ethical decision–making step	Student's thoughts
Clarify the ethical dilemma	
Gather data	
Identify options	
Make a decision	
Choose and implement a course of action	
Evaluate the decision	

REGULATION OF NURSING PRACTICE

Licensure is mandatory for a nurse to practice nursing. A license is a legal document issued by each state certifying that a person has met minimum standards to qualify as a practitioner. Each state is responsible to its citizens to provide qualified, competent health care personnel. Each state has a nurse practice act that defines the requirements for licensure as an RN.

All 50 states license nurses using the National Council Licensure Examination for Registered Nurses. A student must graduate from a state-approved school of nursing and send an application to be approved by the State Board of Nursing. The NCLEX-RN is a computerized test given to nursing graduates at a local testing site. The candidate for licensure must pass the exam to be licensed and registered in the state. A nurse licensed in one state may apply for

Box 12–2 Legal Issues Affecting Nurses

Torts	—	a civil wrong against another person
Negligence	—	an action that leads to harm of another person that a reasonable prudent person would not have done in the same or similar situation
Malpractice	—	professional negligence
Delegation	—	giving authority for one person to act in place of another
Assault and Battery	—	threat, attempt, or actual injury to another person
Informed consent	—	a knowledgeable, voluntary decision to consent to treatment
Confidentiality	—	safe handling of client information

licensure in another state. The license is permanent but must be renewed every other year by paying a fee to the state where licensure is desired.

All states require **mandatory licensure** of nurses, meaning that a nurse must have a license to practice legally in that state. All states license and register graduates of all nursing education programs.

LEGAL ISSUES

Nurses are accountable for their own actions. Even though states regulate nursing practice by licensure and the state's nurse practice act, nurses are vulnerable to several types of legal action. Some legal concepts for the nurse to understand are: torts, negligence, malpractice, delegation, assault and battery, informed consent, and confidentiality.

Torts

Torts may be an intentional or unintentional civil wrong against a person that results in physical, emotional, or economic harm. An intentional act is a willful act against another person's rights or property; however, a tort needs no proof of intent to cause harm. An example of a tort is a nurse accidentally using the wrong solution to irrigate a client's bladder.

Negligence

Negligence is committing an act that a reasonable, prudent person would not do in the same or similar situation or failing to act as a reasonable, prudent person would act in the same or similar situation. For an act to be negligent, it does not need proof of premeditation or intent to harm, but it does require that proof of specific damage or harm was done. An example of negligence is a person driving on a narrow road, seeing a bicycler, and not slowing down. The driver hits the bicycler and causes injury to her.

Malpractice

Malpractice is professional negligence. Malpractice occurs when a professional person does not act as another reasonable, prudent professional person would act in the same or similar situation because of a lack of "professional knowledge, experience, or skill that can be expected of others in the profession or from a failure to exercise reasonable care or judgment in the application of professional knowledge, experience, or skill" (Mosby Elsevier, 2006, p. 1145). This action is classified as an unintentional tort because there is no need to prove that the professional intended to cause harm or be negligent. Malpractice includes acts of commission and acts of omission. An act of commission is committing an improper act. An act of omission is not doing an expected act. Acts of commission and acts of omission are grounds for legal action. In legal action, evidence must be presented that the nurse did not meet the standard of care. The **standard of care** is the minimal requirement of competent care that does not harm a client. The nursing standard of care is an act a reasonable, prudent nurse does under the same or a similar situation.

There are several issues that need to occur for an act to be defined as malpractice: (1) a nurse assumes the duty of care or responsibility for the care of a client, (2) the nurse fails to meet the standard of care when caring for the client, (3) the client is injured because of the break in the standard of care, and (4) the injury is confirmed (Chitty, 2007). An example of negligence is a nurse gossiping with co-workers and failing to answer a client's call light. The failure to act resulted in the client's falling and breaking a hip when trying to go to the bathroom alone. Because of the nurse's actions or failure to act (negligence), the client was injured.

Not only is the nurse responsible for personal actions, but the facility is also legally responsible because of the legal *respondeat superior* (master-servant) rule. This rule states that the master is responsible for the actions of the servants. It implies that the nurse's employer or facility is responsible for the actions of the nurse.

Legal Implications of Nursing

A nurse takes several actions throughout the course of a day that make her vulnerable to legal action. A review of some of these legal issues follows.

Delegation

Delegation is giving the authority for one person to act in the place of another. Professional nurses have the authority to delegate nursing activities to other health care personnel. The state nursing practice acts do not give LPNs/LVNs the right to delegate (Chitty, 2007). The professional nurse must know the scope of practice for the members of the health care team and delegate accordingly. She is held accountable for the actions of the persons to whom she delegates. The health care personnel are responsible for safely performing the delegated activity. The main concern in delegation is the safety of the client, therefore, the professional nurse assesses the capabilities of the person to whom the activity is delegated to make sure it is completed safely. A nurse is responsible to refuse an action that is not within her scope of practice or expertise, regardless of who requests her to perform the act.

Assault and Battery

Assault is a threat or an attempt to make physical contact with a person who does not desire the contact. **Battery** is a completed assault whereby a person has had physical contact with another person without the consent or permission of that person. An example of a potential battery is giving a client an injection without proper consent, or performing surgery on an unconscious client without consent.

Informed Consent

In signing an informed consent, a client gives written consent for treatment as shown in Figure 12–4. An informed consent implies that a competent client was given accurate and full information to make a prudent, knowledgeable, voluntary decision to consent to treatment (Rosenthal, 2001). A competent client has the mental capacity to comprehend the information given about the procedure or treatment. A knowledgeable decision is based on the completeness of provided information. Voluntary consent implies freedom to make the choice without excessive pressure (Rosenthal, 2001). The client receives information about risks, benefits, side effects, and costs.

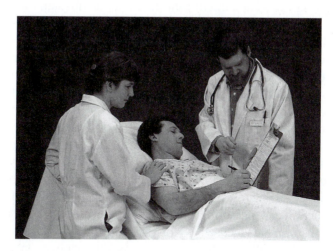

Figure 12-4 A client signs an informed consent after he receives information about risks, benefits, side effects, and costs. (Source: *Fundamentals of Nursing: Standards and Practice* 3rd ed., by S. Delaune and P. Ladner, 2006, Clifton Park, NY: Delmar/Cengage Learning.)

Confidentiality

Confidentiality is the safe handling of client information or the ability to keep a secret. Confidentiality is not a new concept, but, an old concept with new standards and disciplinary actions and consequences for those who choose not to comply with new regulations. Nurses have access to private information about clients. It is the nurse's responsibility to protect the client's private health care information. The nurse must make a conscientious effort to share needed information only with the appropriate people; such as the doctor, health care personnel, and family or friends as designated by the client, and to involve the client in this decision process.

In 1996 the Health Insurance Portability and Accountability Act (**HIPAA**) was enacted to ensure health care coverage for employees when they were changing jobs. The act soon grew into multiple regulations for the health care system. Technology boomed and offered an array of advances for the health care environment including electronic medical records. Confidentiality became an even greater concern in health care. The client's health information needed to be protected and not misused. Health care facilities were required to comply with the new HIPAA Privacy Regulations by April 14, 2003 ("HIPAA Privacy Policies").

HIPAA guidelines are mandatory for health care personnel. HIPAA protects the client from unauthorized personnel gaining access to private health information. HIPAA ensures that the right people use the client's information appropriately and discreetly for the right purposes.

According to the HIPAA Privacy Regulations, a health care facility gives the client a written copy of the Notice of Privacy Practices upon entrance for treatment. The Notice of Privacy Practices informs the client of the facility plans to access, use, and disclose the client's protected health information. The client is given an opportunity to ask questions and then to sign a statement indicating receipt of information. If the client does not sign the HIPAA statement of receipt, health care personnel document that the client did not sign the notice, including the reason for not signing. The facility keeps the receipt on record for at least six years.

HIPAA requires the facility to protect any information that could be used to trace a client's identity or lead to access of the client's medical information. This information is referred to as **protected health information (PHI)**. Information about the client's past, present, or future physical or psychological condition also falls under protected health information.

Information that can be disclosed without the client's consent is information shared between two doctors providing treatment to the client, between nurses directly providing care to the client, or between billing personnel to receive payment for the services provided. Before any protected health information is disclosed to a third party, the client must give written authorization for the disclosure except for reasons related to treatment, payment, or health care operations.

Health care personnel have a responsibility to protect client privacy. If HIPAA regulations are not followed, the health care personnel are liable to receive disciplinary actions. The Department of Health and Human Services' Office for Civil Rights (OCR) enforces civil disciplinary actions for violations of the HIPAA Privacy Regulations. The Department of Justice prosecutes criminal issues (HHS, 2009). The new standards and regulations developed through HIPAA empower clients and involve them directly in decisions regarding their medical records. The regulations force health care personnel to always be aware and to respect clients' rights.

Individuals no longer need to be hesitant to get lab tests done for fear that the test results could be accessed without their knowledge or consent. A person having tests done to detect the presence of cancer genes or HIV might have some serious concerns about confidentiality with insurance companies and employers. If the person applied for insurance but the potential insurance company obtained the test results, the company might have refused employment to the job applicant. This situation occurred in the 1970s when African Americans who tested positive for sickle-cell anemia were denied jobs by major airlines and were required to pay higher prices for health insurance coverage (Rosenthal, 2001). Situations of this type were the impetus for legislative confidentiality reform.

CRITICAL THINKING ACTIVITY

1. Access and read your state's Nurse Practice Act at the state's board of nursing web site. Identify five items that you learned or rethought as you read your state's Nurse Practice Act. Share these thoughts with your peers.

2. How does your current job description/role compare to your state nurse practice act?

POTENTIAL FUTURE ETHICAL CONCERNS

We have discussed ethical situations that nurses face such as tube feeding usage, reporting potential drug abuse by health care personnel, allocation of funds in client care, appropriate administration of blood, reporting neglect and abuse cases, and confidentiality of the client's private health care information. Some potential future ethical issues are gene research, cloning, organ transplants, euthanasia, and allocation of funds for the elderly versus younger, healthier people. As health care systems move in more of a profit-oriented direction, nurses may feel pulled between issues of nursing practice and economic shortcuts. These are only a few of the ethical situations that nurses will face in coming years. As you transition into the role of an RN, it is important that you examine the origin and development of your personal values and make the determination to provide quality care to your clients within those preset value parameters.

THEORY TO PRACTICE

Ethical dilemmas are not an uncommon occurrence although sometimes are seen as situations that only happen to other people. Most nurses experience some sort of ethical dilemma in their nursing careers. Take time to review your local community and national news. Search for a potential ethical or legal scenario occurring in a health care environment. Then:

1. Summarize that situation using some of the key terms from this chapter. Describe the situation as best you can from both the health care (professional) and your own (personal) views.

   - Are there any differences between those two views?
   - Is there a difference between nursing knowledge and ethical considerations in the situation?
   - Did you find it difficult to separate personal opinions from professional knowledge?

SUMMARY

Nurses face situations daily that could become legal or ethical issues. Personal values influence our thoughts, opinions, and actions. A nurse is responsible for her personal actions. Therefore, it is important that the nurse make wise decisions when caring for clients. By recalling ethical principles, legal nursing implications, and following the ethical decision–making process, an RN makes prudent decisions followed by prudent actions. In the RN role, nurses face many ethical and legal situations and are expected to function professionally as a leader and decision maker. Determine your own values, beliefs, ethics, and moral ideas or opinions so that when you find yourself in such situations you are better equipped and ready to face the situation. Clients deserve the best care possible.

CHAPTER REFLECTIONS

1. If you were Paula, would you approach Deb regarding the pain medication discrepancies?

2. Is approaching Deb the first step Paula should take? Why or why not?

3. What would be the ethical and legal implications to Deb if Paula went over Deb's head and was wrong?

4. How do your personal values and beliefs affect the way you approach this situation?

Journaling Your Journey

Describe an ethical, legal situation you have experienced in your life time. How did this make you feel? If experienced again, is there anything you might do differently? What would you do exactly the same way if repeated?

☙ ☙ ☙

My Story...

Transitioning to an RN role has opened many doors for me. Career options are endless in the field of nursing. In an age when many of us will be working for an extended amount of years, nursing offers choices for people of all ages. Financial security and job stability are only a small part of the benefits I have experienced. The emotional rewards from clients, families, and co-workers are invaluable. My nursing education has given me the confidence to face life challenges and make decisions both inside and outside of the nursing profession.

Julie Richardson, MSN, RN

REFERENCES

Aiken, T. (2004). *Legal, ethical, and political issues in nursing* (2nd ed.). Philadelphia: F.A. Davis Company.

Chitty, K. (2007). *Professional nursing: Concepts and challenge* (5th ed.). Philadelphia: W.B. Saunders Company.

Day, L. (2007). Courage as a virtue necessary to good nursing practice. *American Journal of Critical Care, 16*(6), 613–616.

Delaune, S., and Ladner, P. (2006). *Fundamentals of nursing: Standards and practice* (3rd ed.). Clifton Park, NY: Cengage Learning Delmar.

Ellis, J., & Hartley, C. (2007). *Nursing in today's world: Trends, issues, and management* (9th ed.). Philadelphia: Lippincott Williams & Wilkins.

Estes, M. (2010). *Health assessment and physical examination* (4th ed.). Clifton Park, NY: Cengage Learning Delmar.

Hein, E. (2001). *Nursing issues in the 21st century: Perspectives from the literature.* Philadelphia: Lippincott Williams & Wilkins.

Hood, L., & Leddy, S. (2005). *Leddy and Pepper's conceptual bases of professional nursing* (6th ed.). Philadelphia: Lippincott Williams & Wilkins.

Kearney-Nunnery R. (2008). *Advancing your career: Concepts of professional nursing* (4th ed.). Philadelphia: F.A. Davis Company.

Kohlberg, L. (1977). *Recent research in moral development.* New York: Holt, Rinehart, & Winston.

Kozier, B., Erb, G., Berman, A., & Snyder, S. (2008). *Fundamentals of nursing: Concepts, process, and practice* (8th ed.). Upper Saddle River, NJ: Prentice Hall.

Mosby Elsevier. (2006). *Mosby's dictionary of medicine, nursing and health professions* (7th ed.). St. Louis, MO: Mosby Elsevier.

Rosenthal, M. (2001). *Bioethics: What is the "right thing" in healthcare?* [On-line]. Available: www.sarahealth.com

Sizemore, R. (2006). Separating medical and ethical; Helping families determine the best interests of loved ones. *Dimensions of Critical Care Nursing, 25*(5), 216–220.

U.S. Department of Health and Human Services (HHS). (2009). Summary of the HIPAA Privacy Rule. Retrieved June 8, 2009 from www.hhs.gov/ocr/privacy/hipaa/understanding/summary/

SUGGESTED RESOURCES

Allen, S., Chapman, Y., Francis, K., and O'Connor, M. (2008). *Supporting nurses to make ethically sound decisions when nursing aged care residents at the end-of-life: Using the decide model.* Singapore Nursing Journal, 35(2), 4–11.

American Nurses Association (ANA), www.nursingworld.org/

Ludwick, R., & Silva, M. (2000). *Nursing around the world: Cultural values and ethical conflicts* [On-line]. Available: www.nursingworld.org

National Student Nurses' Association. [On-line]. Available: www.nsna.org

Seal, M. (2007). Patient advocacy and advance care planning in the acute hospital setting. *Australian Journal of Advanced Nursing, 24*(4), 29–36.

U.S. Department of Health and Human Services (HHS). www.hhs.gov (Search for HIPPA Privacy Act.)

Chapter 13
Intravenous Therapy Skills

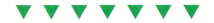

LEARNING OBJECTIVES

1. Explain the purpose of intravenous (IV) fluid and medication administration.
2. Explain the assessment of an IV site and IV equipment.
3. Demonstrate the preparation of an IV bag and tubing.
4. Calculate an IV flow rate.
5. Explain the different ways to administer medication intravenously.
6. Explain the procedure to discontinue an IV.

KEY TERMS

Incompatibility

Maintenance

Replacement

Restoration

Tonicity

Vesicants

SCENARIO

David, a new LPN graduate, is assigned a client who has IV fluids infusing in a central line. The health care provider ordered erythromycin lactobionate (E-mycin) 15mg/kg IV every 6 hours. David knows the facility does not let LPNs give IV medications through a central line, nor does the State Board of Nursing's Standards of the Nurse Practice Act give LPNs the right. However, all the RNs are so busy that he does not want to bother them by asking them to give the medication for him. If David gives the medication, is he following the Standards of Practice for the state in which he is practicing?

THINK ABOUT IT

1. What are the consequences of David giving the medication?
2. What are other options for David to handle the situation?
3. What are the State Board of Nursing's Standards of the Nurse Practice Act for the LPN in administering IVs in your state?

INTRODUCTION

Administering intravenous (IV) medications can be intimidating to nurses. Starting IVs and handling equipment are complicated procedures. The knowledge that medications and solutions immediately enter the vascular system is frightening. Other medication routes require several minutes to hours for the drug to reach the blood stream and become systemic. While many nurses find administering medications and solutions through central venous catheters even more daunting than through peripheral access devices, both introduce the pharmacological agents directly into the blood stream. The administration of any medication or solution through an IV route also has the potential of contaminating the blood stream with bacteria. Handling all connections between various parts of the infusion system requires aseptic technique to prevent hospital acquired infections.

Across the nation the LPN role in IV administration varies. Some states require the LPN nursing program curriculum to include IV administration. Other LPN curriculums only teach limited content about IV administration. Therefore, recognizing that LPNs have different backgrounds in IV administration, the chapter offers a review of IV skills to prepare the LPN/VN for the RN transition nursing program.

IV FLUIDS

Probably the most easily understood advantage of IV medication administration is rapid action of the medication. Likewise, the disadvantage is the adverse reaction is also immediate. Related to the disadvantage is the benefit of stopping the medication immediately if a reaction occurs. For many adverse reactions, there is an antidote that can be given to counteract the medication's affect. The IV route is used when oral and other medication routes are either unavailable or not appropriate for a particular medication.

Purposes of IV Infusions

Three purposes for infusing IV fluids are maintenance, restoration, and replacement. **Maintenance** infusions provide fluid volume and meet the client's needs for water, sugar (dextrose), and electrolytes.

Restoration infusion therapy involves supplying nutrients and fluid necessary to correct ongoing losses, such as draining intestinal fistulas. An example is total parenteral nutrition.

A nurse recording accurate intake and output enables health care providers to determine what type and amount of fluid is necessary to restore losses of fluid and electrolytes. Health care providers also monitor serum electrolyte levels to plan fluid and electrolyte restoration (Phillips, 2005).

Replacement infusion therapy provides water, electrolytes, and blood products for clients experiencing extreme disease or traumatic events. These amounts are generally infused over two days rather than 24 hours. To infuse the required amounts in a shorter period of time would overwhelm the vascular system and bring about pulmonary edema or congestive heart failure. Extremely ill clients often have renal insufficiency or acute renal failure making rapid fluid replacement difficult (Phillips, 2005).

Tonicity and Osmolarity

The word **tonicity** means the concentration of an IV fluid. The concentration or tonicity of an IV fluid causes fluid to move from one area to another by osmosis (Adams, Holland, & Bostwick, 2008). If an IV fluid is equal to the tonicity of plasma, it is isotonic (equal in tonicity). There are three different levels of tonicity available for infusion: hypotonic (less than the tonicity of plasma), isotonic, and hypertonic (more tonicity than plasma). Refer to Table 13–1 to review different tonicities of IV solutions, indications and incompatibilities, precautions, and contraindications.

ASSESSING THE IV SITE

Each agency has policies regarding who may start an IV. Agencies require that nurses have special education before performing the procedure. Check the client's fluid, electrolyte, and nutritional status to provide baseline data for comparison with the client's response to IV therapy. Check the health care provider's order for the type of therapy planned to determine the optimal needle size and type to use. Assess the client's understanding of the purpose for the IV. Teach the client about IV therapy and allow time for questions to clarify any concerns and to decrease anxiety. Assess the skin at the IV site so that the solution is not administered into an inflamed or edematous site, which could cause injury to the tissue. Assess the client's veins to determine the best IV site. Assess the patency of the IV to ensure that the solution will enter the vein and not the surrounding tissue.

GERIATRIC CONSIDERATIONS

When starting an IV on older clients, gently apply the tourniquet with minimal pressure because they often have fragile skin and veins. Use a 5- to 15-degree angle when inserting the needle because the older client's veins are more superficial. When taping the IV, use enough tape to secure the IV but do not use excess tape. Use the least abrasive tape available to reduce irritation to the skin. Take care when removing the tape as the skin may peel with the tape.

Table 13–1 Isotonic Infusions: Indications for Use and Precautions

Infusion	Osmolarity	Indications and Incompatibilities	Precautions, Comments, Contraindications
5% dextrose in water (D₅W) 50 g dextrose per liter pH 4.5 (3.5–6.5)	252.52 mOsm/L	**Indications:** Hydration: replaces water losses in dehydration Provides free water for the excretion of solutes Provides 20 kcal/100 ml (200 kcal/L) Diluent for medications **Incompatibilities:** Ampicillin sodium (after 2 hr) Diazepam Erythromycin lactobinate (after 6 hr) Fat emulsions Phenytoin sodium Procainamide Sodium bicarbonate Warfarin sodium Whole blood Vitamin B₁₂	D₅W is isotonic in the container. Once infused, the dextrose is rapidly metabolized and the infusion becomes hypotonic Do not administer to patients with increased intracranial pressure because it is hypotonic in the body and will increase edema D₂W does not contain electrolytes Because of excess ADH secretions, as a stress response to surgery, use cautiously in the early postoperative period to prevent water intoxication Hypokalemia can occur because, during the cellular use of glucose, potassium shifts from the ECF to the ICF Use cautiously in patients with signs of fluid overload and CHF Can cause dehydration from osmotic diuresis if infused too rapidly D₅W may alter insulin or oral hypoglycemic needs in diabetics Contraindicated in diabetic coma Contraindicated in patients allergic to corn and corn products
Normal saline (0.9% NaCl) Na 154 mEq/L Cl 154 mEq/L pH 5 (4.5–7.0)	308 mOsm/L	**Indications:** Replaces ECF losses by expanding the intravascular space when chloride loss is greater than sodium loss Corrects hyponatremia Corrects hypovolemia Replaces sodium losses	Accurately monitor I & O Can cause intravascular overload Can cause hypokalemia because saline promotes potassium excretion Can cause hypernatremia Can induce hyperchloremic acidosis due to loss of bicarbonate ions

Table 13–1 (continued)

Infusion	Osmolarity	Indications and Incompatibilities	Precautions, Comments, Contraindications
		Corrects mild metabolic acidosis	Normal saline can cause sodium retention during the intraoperative and early postoperative periods.
		Corrects metabolic alkalosis when fluid depletion exists because the chloride ions cause a decrease in bicarbonate ions	Does not provide free water
			Does not provide calories
		Only infusate compatible with blood; used to intiate and follow transfusions	Use with caution in patients with decreased renal function
			Use with caution in patients with altered circulatory function
		Diluent for medications	Use with caution in the elderly
		Used as an irrigant for intravascular devices	Contraindicated in the presence of edema with sodium retention
		Maintains patency of heparin locks	Causes excess sodium retention when used with glucocorticoids
		Incompatibilities:	
		Amphotericin B	
		Chlordiazepoxide hydrochloride	
		Diazepam	
		Fat emulsions	
		Lavarterenol	
		Mannitol	
		Methylprednisolone sodium succinate	
		Phenytoin sodium	
Dextrose in Saline Solutions		**Indications:**	To prevent circulatory overload, use with caution in the following:
		Rehydration by replenishment of salt and water	patients with CHF
0.2% dextrose in 0.9% NaCl	318.1 mOsm/L	Fluid replacement for burns	patients with pulmonary edema
2 g dextrose per liter (10.1 mOsm/L)		Supply calories	patients with edema with sodium retention
		Reduce nitrogen depletion	
Na 154 mEq/L		Used in place of plasma expanders (until they are available) to treat circulatory insufficiency and shock	patients undergoing corticosteroid therapy
Cl 154 mEq/L			patients with urinary obstruction
pH 4.5			Maintain strict I & O
(3.5–6.5)			Contraindicated in patients in diabetic coma

Table 13–1 (continued)

Infusion	Osmolarity	Indications and Incompatibilities	Precautions, Comments, Contraindications
2.5% dextrose in 0.45% NaCl 25 g dextrose per liter (126.26 mOsm/L) Na 69.3 mEq/L Cl 69.3 mEq/L pH 4.0 (3.5–6.5)	264.86 mOsm/L	Hypotonic saline with dextrose infusions (2.5% D in 0.45 NaCl and 5% D in 0.2% NaCl) are used to establish renal function prior to electrolyte administration D$_5$ in 0.2% NaCl is used as a maintenance infusion **Incompatibilities:**	Contraindicated in patients with allergies to corn and corn products May falsely elevate BUN laboratory reports Once renal function is assured, electrolytes must be supplemented to prevent hypokalemia
5% dextrose in 0.2% NaCl 50 g dextrose per liter (252.52 mOsm/L) Na 30.8 mEq/L Cl 30.8 mEq/L pH 4.0 (3.5–6.5)	314.12 mOsm/L	Amphotericin B Ampicillin sodium Diazepam Erythromycin lactobinate Mannitol Phenytoin Warfarin sodium Whole blood	
Ringer's solution Na 147 mEq/L K 4 mEq/L Ca 4 mEq/L Cl 155 mEq/L pH 5.5 (5.0–7.5)	301 mOsm/L	**Indications:** Restores fluid balance Restores electrolyte balance Replaces ECF loss resulting from dehydration, gastrointestinal losses, and fistula drainage Used instead of lactated Ringer's when patients have liver disease and are unable to metabolize lactate May be used as a blood replacement for a short period of time **Incompatibilities:** Ampicillin sodium Cefamandole Cyphradine	Provides no calories (when dextrose is added to Ringer's solution, the dextrose provides calories and spares protein loss) May exacerbate the following: Sodium retention CHF renal insufficiency Maintain strict 1 & O Added potassium is needed to correct severe hypokalemia Contraindicated in renal failure

Table 13–1 (continued)

Infusion	Osmolarity	Indications and Incompatibilities	Precautions, Comments, Contraindications
		Chlordiazepoxide Diazepam Erythromycin lactobinate Methicillin Phenytoin Potassium phosphate Sodium bicarbonate Whole blood	
Lactated Ringer's (Hartmann's solution) Na 130 mEq/L Cl 109 mEq/L K 4 mEq/L Ca 3 mEq/L Lactate 28 mEq/L pH 6.5 (6.0 – 7.5)	274 mOsm/L	**Indications:** Restores fluid volume deficit Used for rehydration in *most* types of dehydration Replaces fluid lost as a result of **bile loss, burns,** or **diarrhea** Treats mild metabolic acidosis Treats diabetic ketoacidosis Treats salicylate overdose **Incompatibilities:** Amphotericin B Ampicillin sodium Cefamandole Cephradine Chlordiazepoxide Diazepam Erythromycin lactobinate Methicillin Methylprednisolone sodium succinate Oxytetracycline Phenytoin sodium Potassium phosphate Sodium bicarbonate Thiopental Warfarin Whole blood	Resembles blood serum electrolyte content Provides 9 calories from lactate Lactate is metabolized to bicarbonate in the liver Does not provide free water for renal excretion Can precipitate hypernatremia because the amount of potassium is not sufficient for daily requirements Hyperkalemia can develop with use of potassium-sparing diuretics and potassium supplementation Contraindicated with severe metabolic acidosis and alkalosis Contraindicated in hypoxia Contraindicated with hepatic disease where the liver is unable to metabolize lactate May exacerbate the following: CHF edema sodium retention

Table 13–1 (continued)

Infusion	Osmolarity	Indications and Incompatibilities	Precautions, Comments, Contraindications
Multiple Electrolyte Solutions		**Indications:** Replace water and electrolytes caused by the following:	*Monitor electrolytes because, once the deficits have been replaced,* hyperkalemia can occur
Plasma-Lyte R® (Baxter) Isolyte E® (McGaw) Na 140 mEq/L Cl 103 mEq/L K 10 mEq/L Ca 5 mEq/L Mg 3 mEq/L Acetate 47 mEq/L Lactate 8 mEq/L pH 5.5 (4.0–6.5)	316 mOsm/L	severe diarrhea severe vomiting gastric suctioning	Monitor I & O Observe for signs of circulatory overloads
Plasma-Lyte 148® Na 140 mEq/L Cl 98 mEq/L K 5 mEq/L Ca 0 Mg 3 mEq/L Acetate 27 mEq/L Gluconate 23 mEq/L pH 5.5 (4.0–6.5)	296 mOsm/L		
Plasma-Lyte A®	296 mOsm/L	Plasma-Lyte® has the same constituents as Plasma-Lyte 148,® but has a pH of 7.4 (6.5–8.0) and is used in anesthesia	
Gastric replacement solutions			In addition to the constituents in the electrolyte replacement solutions, gastric replacement fluids have the addition of ammonium ions

Table 13–1 (continued)

Infusion	Osmolarity	Indications and Incompatibilities	Precautions, Comments, Contraindications
Alkalinizing Fluids **Sodium lactate 1/6 molar (M/6 sodium lactate)** Na 167 mEq/L pH 6.5 (6.0–7.3)	334 mOsm/L	**Indications:** Mild to moderate acidosis, not for the treatment of lactic acidosis Alkalinization of urine **Incompatibilities:** Oxytetracycline Sodium bicarbonate	Contraindicated in lactic acidosis Contraindicated with hypernatremia Contraindicated in hypoxic patients Can exacerbate respiratory or metabolic alkalosis Use with caution when administering to patients with conditions that increase lactate use, such as hepatic insufficiency Monitor glucose, electrolytes, and acid-base balance Strict I & O Daily weight Monitor for fluid retention Administer with caution to patients with altered (reduced) tissue perfusion
Sodium bicarbonate 1/6 molar (1.45% sodium bicarbonate) Na 166.70 mEq/L HCO$_3$ 166. 70 mEq/L pH 8.0 (7.0–8.5)	333 mOsm/L	**Indications:** Treats systemic acidosis Increases serum bicarbonate and buffers excess hydrogen Alkalinization of urine **Incompatabilities:** Numerous: consult pharmacist **Drug Interactions:** Numerous; consult pharmacist	Contraindicated in chloride depletion from gastrointestinal losses Contraindicated in hypocalcemia Use with caution in patients with renal insufficiency Use extreme caution in patients with edema due to sodium retention Monitor for signs of alkalosis (overdose) Take precautions to prevent extravasation
Acidifying Fluids **0.9% sodium chloride**	308 mOsm/L	**Indications:** Corrects metabolic alkalosis when fluid depletion exists because the chloride ions cause a decrease in bicarbonate ions	See comments under normal saline

Table 13–1 (continued)

Infusion	Osmolarity	Indications and Incompatibilities	Precautions, Comments, Contraindications
Ammonium chloride solution 0.9% NH_4 168 mEq/L Cl 168 mEq/L	336 mOsm/L	Systemic acidifier indicated for severe metabolic alkalosis resulting from vomiting, gastric suctioning, or chloride depletion from diuretic use Rids body of excess hydrogen ions in metabolic acidosis and supplies chloride Ammonium ion is converted to hydrogen ion and ammonium then excreted as urea in the urine **Incompatibilities:** Alkalides and their carbonates Dimenhydrinate Levorphanol tartrate Methadone Potent oxidizing agents Warfarin	Can produce dangerous dysrhythmias Accurate I & O Accurate respiratory assessment Seizure precautions Contraindicated in severe liver disease because the liver is unable to convert ammonium ions to urea; ammonia retention results in hepatic coma Contraindicated in primary respiratory alkalosis due to chance of development of systemic acidosis
Mannitol 5% in 0.45 NaCl (Osmitrol,® Resectisol®) pH 5.0 (4.5–7.0)	274 mOsm/L	**Indications:** Diuresis Treatment of oliguria Reduction of increased intracranial pressure Reduction of cerebrospinal fluid pressure Reduction of intraocular pressure **Incompatibilities:** Blood products Imipenem/cilastic sodium	Strict I & O Hourly vital signs Closely monitor BUN and electrolytes, especially sodium and potassium levels Contraindicated with anuria due to possibility of circulatory overload Can cause renal failure May induce dangerous dysrhythmias May exacerbate intracranial bleeding May cause congestive heart failure in patients with cardiopulmonary compromise May exacerbate electrolyte imbalances Monitor for rebound increase in intracranial, cerebrospinal, and intraocular pressures within 12 to 24 hours after administration

Table 13–1 (continued)

Infusion	Osmolarity	Indications and Incompatibilities	Precautions, Comments, Contraindications
Plasma Volume Expanders **Dextran 70 and 0.9% NaCl (6% Gentran® 70 and 0.9% NaCl)** Na 154 mEq/L Cl 154 mEq/L pH 5.0 (4.0–6.5)	308 mOsm/L	**Indications:** Restoration of circulatory dynamics Fluid replacement Treatment of perioperative shock Used prophylactically in surgical patients at risk for acute thrombosis and embolization Hemorrhage Trauma Moves water from body tissues to increase urinary output	**Caution:** Never add any medications to dextran infusions. **Contraindicated with:** Cardiac decompensation Coagulation defects Corticosteroid therapy Hypersensitivity to dextran Hypervolemia Pulmonary edema Renal failure Severe bleeding disorders
Dextran 40 and 0.9% NaCl (10% Gentran® and 0.9% NaCl) Na 154 mEq/L Cl 154 mEq/L pH 5.0 (3.5–7.0)	308 mOsm/L	**Incompatibilities:** Ascorbic acid Chlortetracycline Phytonadione Promethazine	Monitor for any signs of allergic reaction Never administer near site of trauma of infection Monitor I & O hourly Monitor pulse, blood pressure, and central venous pressure (CVP) hourly Monitor specific gravity
Dextran 40 and D₅W (10% Gentran® and D₅W) pH 4.0 (3.0–7.0)	255 mOsm/L	Protein hydrosylate	Monitor for fluid overload Monitor for signs of bleeding Monitor for exacerbation of bleeding Monitor site of infusion for venous thrombosis and phlebitis **Comments:** Solution must be clear—not cloudy Crystallization may occur; before administration, submerge bottle in warm water to dissolve crystals

Table 13–1 (continued)

Infusion	Osmolarity	Indications and Incompatibilities	Precautions, Comments, Contraindications
Hetastarch (HES) 6% in 0.9% NaCl Na 154 mEq/L Cl 154 mEq/L pH 5.5	308 mOsm/L	**Indications:** Similar to dextran but causes fewer allergic reactions Used in shock due to sepsis, acute hemorrhage, or burns Similar to human albumin in colloidal properties **Incompatibilities:** Amikacin Ampicillin Cefamandol Cefazolin Cefonicid Cefoperazone Cefotaxime Cefoxitin Cephalothin Gentamicin Phenytoin Ranitidine Theophylline Tobramycin	Contraindicated with severe bleeding disorders Contraindicated in congestive and renal failure Maintain strict I & O Monitor CVP and PCWP (hemodynamic monitoring) to assess for circulatory overload

Table 13–1 Hypotonic Infusions: Indications for Use and Precautions

Infusion	Osmolarity	Indications and Incompatibilities	Precautions, Comments, Contraindications
Dextrose in Water Solutions **2.5% dextrose in water 25 g dextrose per liter** pH 4.5 (3.6–6.5)	126 mOsm/L	**Indications:** Provides 85 kcal/L Diluent for medications Provides hydration to cells in hyperglycemic situations and in cellular dehydration associated with diuretic administration	Depletes intravascular compartment Monitor for signs of cardiovascular collapse from fluid volume depletion Contraindicated in patients with increased intracranial pressure Contraindicated in patients with decreased serum protein levels
5% dextrose in water (Reminder: D_5W is isotonic, but it becomes hypotonic when it is infused because the dextrose is metabolized rapidly.)	252.52 mOsm/L	Review Table 6-5: Isotonic Infusions **Incompatibilities:** Refer to isotonic dextrose in water above	Assess for hypokalemia after prolonged use without potassium supplementation Review under isotonic infusions. D_5W is isotonic in the container. Once it is infused, the dextrose is rapidly metabolized, and the infusion becomes hypotonic. Review Table 6-5: Isotonic Infusions
Sodium Chloride Solutions **0.45% (half normal) saline** pH 5.0 (4.5–7.0)	154 mOsm/L	**Indications:** Used when fluid losses exceed electrolyte depletion Preferable to 0.9% NaCl for electrolyte restoration of sodium and chlorides Provides free water for the renal elimination of solutes Lowers serum osmolality by moving body fluid from the blood vessels into the cells and interstitium Used in hyperosmolar diabetes when dextrose is contraindicated, but fluid without excess sodium is indicated	Contraindicated in hypernatremia Use with caution in situations of fluid retention Assess for cellular dehydration

Table 13–1 (continued)

Infusion	Osmolarity	Indications and Incompatibilities	Precautions, Comments, Contraindications
		Incompatibilities: Amphotericin B Levarterenol Mannitol	
Dextrose in Sodium Chloride Solutions No hypotonic infusions			
Multiple Electrolyte Solutions **Plasma-Lyte 56®** **or Normosol R® injection** Na 40 mEq/L Cl 40 mEq/L K 13 mEq/L Mg 3 mEq/L Acetate 16 mEq/L pH 5.5 (4.0–6.0)	112 mOsm/L	**Indications:** Maintenance solution; provides free water and electrolytes Provides water for retention of needed electrolytes and the excretion of excesses **Incompatibilities:** Refer to isotonic multiple electrolyte solutions	Monitor I & O Monitor electrolyte levels Use with caution in patients with impaired renal function Observe for signs of hyperkalemia Weigh daily to assess for water retention and intoxication
Sterile water for injection pH 5.5 (5.0–7.0)	0 mOsm/L	**Indications:** Use as a diluent	Never administer free water alone, as it causes cell rupture

Table 13–1 Hypertonic Infusions: Indications for Use and Precautions

Infusion	Osmolarity	Indications and Incompatibilities	Precautions, Comments, Contraindications
Dextrose in Water Solutions		**Indications:** Nonelectrolyte source of calories (protein-sparing) and water	Monitor for hyperglycemia and glycosuria Monitor for sepsis, with high glucose concentrations Accurate I & O
10% dextrose in water	505 mOsm/L	Provides 340 kcal/L	10% solution should be administered in a large arm vein. The site must be assessed frequently for pain, phlebitis, and thrombosis
20% dextrose in water	1,010 mOsm/L	Provides 680 kcal/L	
30% dextrose in water	1,510 mOsm/L	Provides 1,020 kcal/L	Solutions over 10% must be delivered via a central line into a large vessel for adequate dilution and the prevention of peripheral vein sclerosis
40% dextrose in water	2,020 mOsm/L	Provides 1,360 kca/L	
50% dextrose in water	2,520 mOsm/L	Provides 1,700 kcal/L	
60% dextrose in water	3,030 mOsm/L	Provides 2,040 kcal/L	
70% dextrose in water pH 4.5 for all strengths	3,530 mOsm/L	Provides 2, 380 kcal/L	
Sodium Chloride Solutions **2.225% NaCl** Na 342.65 mEq/L Cl 342.65 mEq/L	685.30 mOsm/L	**Indications:** Hypertonic NaCl injections are indicated for severe sodium depletion accompanied by abnormal neurologic functioning Used when sodium losses exceed fluid losses	Hypertonic saline solutions must be given with extreme care and should be administered only in critical care areas Strict I & O Assess for fluid overload Monitor renal function
3.0% NacL Na 462 mEq/L Cl 462 mEq/L	924 mOsm/L	Used in crisis associated with Addison's disease Used in diabetic coma	Assess for hypernatremia Contraindicated in CHF, fluid retention, impaired reneal function, and hypernatremia
5.0% NaCl Na 770 mEq/L Cl 770 mEq/L	1,540 mOsm/L	**Incompatibilities:** Amphotericin B Benzquinamide Chlordiazepoxide	Do not administer more than 2 mEq/L/hr The strength and rate of administration of these infusions depends on the patient's age, weight, and clinical condition

Table 13–1 (continued)

Infusion	Osmolarity	Indications and Incompatibilities	Precautions, Comments, Contraindications
pH 5.0 (4.5–7.0) for all strengths		Diazepam Fat emulsions Levarterenol Mannitol Methylprednisolone sodium succinate Phenytoin sodium	
Dextrose in Sodium Chloride Solutions **5% dextrose in 0.45 NaCl** Dextrose 252.52 mOsm/L Na 69.3 mEq/L Cl 69.3 mEq/L	391.12 mOsm/L	**Indications:** Indicated for shock and circulatory insufficiency until plasma volume expander is available Treats severe dehydration Replaces fluid losses from burns	Strict I & O Daily weight Monitor for fluid overload Monitor for electrolytes with prolonged therapy Use with caution in the elderly Use with caution in patients with renal obstruction and patients with renal disease
5% dextrose in 0.9 NaCl Dextrose 252.52 mOsm/L Na 154 mEq/L Cl 154 mEq/L	560.52 mOsm/L	With hypertonic dextrose in saline solutions, the concentrations and rate are determined by the patient's weight, circulatory status, and electrolyte-acid-base balance.	Contraindicated in conditions associated with fluid retention Use with extreme caution in patients with diabetes Contraindicated in diabetic coma
10% dextrose in 0.9 NaCl Dextrose 505.04 mOsm/L Na 154 mEq/L Cl 154 mEq/L pH 4.0 (3.5–6.5) for all strengths	813.04 mOsm/L	**Incompatibilities:** Amphotericin B Ampicillin sodium Amsacrine Diazepam Erythromycin lactobinate Mannitol Phenytoin Warfarin Whole blood	

Table 13–1 (continued)

Infusion	Osmolarity	Indications and Incompatibilities	Precautions, Comments, Contraindications
5% dextrose in Ringer's injection Dextrose 252.52 mOsm/L Na 147.5 mEq/L Cl 156 mEq/L K 4 mEq/L Ca 4.5 mEq/L pH 4.0	564.52 mOsm/L	**Indications:** Provides calories from dextrose and spares protein with electrolyte composition similar to that of plasma Replaces ECF losses and replaces electrolytes **Incompatibilities:** Refer to isotonic Ringer's solution	Contraindicated in renal failure Use with caution in patients with CHF Monitor electrolytes Use with caution in hypernatremic and hypercalcemic patients
5% dextrose and lactated Ringer's injection Dextrose 252.52 mOsm/L Na 130 mEq/L Cl 109 mEq/L K 4 mEq/L Ca 3 mEq/L Lactate 28 mEq/L pH 5.0	526.52 mOsm/L	**Indications:** Treats mild metabolic acidosis Provides 170 kcal from dextrose and 9 kcal from lactate per liter Replaces fluid losses from burns	Dextrose and lactated Ringer's infusions are contraindicated in lactic acidosis Use with caution in metabolic or respiratory alkalosis Use with caution in patients with hepatic insufficiency Monitor for circulatory overload Contraindicated in diabetic ketoacidosis Contraindicated in diabetic ketoacidosis Because of lactate, excess administration could cause metabolic acidosis
10% dextrose and lactated Ringer's injection Dextrose 505.04 mOsm/L remaining constituents same as 5% solution	779.04 mOsm/L	Treats mild metabolic acidosis Provides 340 kcal from dextrose Spares protein Replaces fluid losses from burns **Incompatibilities:** Refer to isotonic lactated Ringer's solution	

Table 13–1 (continued)

Infusion	Osmolarity	Indications and Incompatibilities	Precautions, Comments, Contraindications
Electrolyte Solutions **5% dextrose and Electrolyte # 75 injection** Dextrose 252.52 mOsm/L Na 40 mEq/L Cl 48 mEq/L K 35 mEq/L Lactate 20 mEq/L Phosphate (as HPO$_4^*$)15 mEq/L pH 5.0	410.52 mEq/L	**Indications:** Fluid replacement Fluid and electrolyte maintenance Treats mild metabolic acidosis	With all electrolyte infusions, monitor electrolytes carefully, monitor for fluid overload; and perform hemodynamic monitoring in patients with renal, and cardiovascular impairment
5% dextrose and Plasma-Lyte 56® Dextrose 252.52 mOsm/L Na 40 mEq/L Cl 40 mEq/L K 13 mEq/L Mg 3 mEq/L Acetate 16 mEq/L pH 5.5	364.52 mOsm/L	Fluid replacement Fluid and electrolyte maintenance	
5% dextrose and Plasma-Lyte M® Dextrose 252.52 mEq/L Na 40 mEq/L Cl 40 mEq/L K 16 mEq/L Ca 5 mEq/L Mg 3 mEq/L	380.52 mOsm/L	Fluid replacement Fluid and electrolyte maintenance Treats very mild metabolic acidosis	

Table 13–1 (continued)

Infusion	Osmolarity	Indications and Incompatibilities	Precautions, Comments, Contraindications
Acetate 12 mEq/L Lactate 12 mEq/L pH 5.0			
5% dextrose and Plasma-Lyte 148® Dextrose 252.52 mOsm/L Na 140 mEq/L Cl 98 mEq/L K 5 mEq/L Mg 3 mEq/L Acetate 27 mEq/L Gluconate 23 mEq/l pH 5.0	548.52 mOsm/L	Fluid replacement solutions Electrolyte replacement	With all electrolyte infusions, monitor electrolyte levels, maintain strict I & O, assess for hypernatremia, and monitor for fluid overload
5% dextrose and Plasma-Lyte R® Dextrose 252.52 mEq/L Na 140 mEq/L Cl 103 mEq/L K 10 mEq/L Ca 5 mEq/L Mg 3 mEq/L Acetate 47 mEq/L Lactate 8 mEq/L pH 5.0	568.52 mOsm/L	Fluid replacement solutions Electrolyte replacement	Because of the addition of lactate, contraindicated in patients with liver impairment
Invert Sugar as Fructose and Dextrose Solutions **5% Travert® and Electrolyte #2 injection** Dextrose 252.52 mOsm/L	433.02 mOsm/L	**Indications:** Provide calories in the form of carbohydrates More rapidly metabolized and can be administered more rapidly than dextrose	These infusions are equimolar mixtures of fructose and dextrose Contraindicated for patients with fructose intolerance Strict I & O Use with caution in patients with conditions associated with fluid overload

Table 13–1 (continued)

Infusion	Osmolarity	Indications and Incompatibilities	Precautions, Comments, Contraindications
Na 56 mEq/L Cl 56 mEq/L K 25 mEq/L Mg 6 mEq/L Lactate 25 mEq/L Phosphate (as HPO$_4$) 12.5 mEq/L pH 4.5 **10% Travert® and Electrolyte #2 injection** Dextrose 505.04 mOsm/L Electrolytes are same as 5% solution	685.54 mOsm/L	Use for diabetic patients because insulin is not required for the metabolism of these carbohydrate forms Supply electrolytes at the maintenance level Provide fluid replacement and maintenance **Incompatibilities:** Aminophylline Amobarbital Ampicillin sodium Blood products Diazepam Penicillin G Phenytoin Warfarin Thiopental sodium	Do not use small peripheral veins for administration Do not exceed 1g/kg/hr Monitor for lactic acidosis Contraindicated in patients with gout because hyperuricemia may occur as an adverse reaction to the invert sugar Assess for fluid overload The 10% solution delivers more calories in less fluid (up to 3 L/day is safe and provides 340 kcal/L)
Mannitol 10% mannitol solution 15% mannitol solution 20% mannitol solution	549 mOsm/L 823 mOsm/L 1,098 mOsm/L	**Indications:** Osmotic diuretic Reduces intraocular, intracranial, and intraspinal pressures by raising plasma osmolality and causing fluids in these areas to diffuse back into the plasma and intravascular space Used to measure glomerular filtration rate Promotes excretion of toxic substances Promotes diuresis during oliguric phase of acute renal failure **Incompatibilities:** Refer to isotonic mannitol infusions	Contraindicated in anuria Contraindicated in patients who are severly dehydrated Use with extreme caution in patients with congestive heart failure or pulmonary edema Use filter with 15% and 20% solution Strict I & O with output measurements every 30 to 60 minutes Hemodynamic monitoring Monitor electrolytes and BUN Weigh daily, or more frequently

Table 13–1 (continued)

Infusion	Osmolarity	Indications and Incompatibilities	Precautions, Comments, Contraindications
Amino Acid (Protein) Solutions Aminess® Aminosyn® Branch-amin® FreAmine® HepaAmine® Nephramine® Novamine® ProcalAmine® RenAmine® Travasol® TrophaAmine®	Range from 400 mOsm/L to 1,600 mOsm/L	**Indications:** These are nutritional agents indicated for use when oral routes of nutrition are not possible or are inadequate due to disease, surgery, severe infections, chemotherapy, or severe anorexia Refer to Chapter 13 for complete information on the use of these products **Incompatibilities:** Do not add anything without consultation with a pharmacist	There are numerous precautions and guidelines associated with use of these products: refer to Chapter 13, which covers various hyperalimentation and total parenteral nutrition formulas These hypertonic preparations range in amino acid content from 3.5% to 10%, with or without electrolytes. They also are available in preparations with 5% to 50% dextrose

Alcohol in Dextrose and Water Infusions
5% alcohol and 5% dextrose in water
Alcohol 252.52 mOsm/L
Dextrose 252.52 mOsm/L
pH 4.5
 	
10% alcohol and 5% dextrose in water
Alcohol 505.04 mOsm/L
Dextrose 252.52 mOsm/L
	1,010.08 mOsm/L
	
	757.56 mOsm/L
		Indications:
		Caloric provisions are: dextrose 3.4 kcal/g. alcohol 5.6 kcal/ml
		Fluid replacement
		
		Incompatibilities:
		Check with pharmacist before mixing anything with these infusions
			Contraindicated in
			  alcoholism
			  diabetic coma
			  epilepsy
			  urinary tract infections
			Use with caution in diabetes mellitus
			Monitor for intoxication
			Monitor for hyperglycemia
			Monitor for glycosuria
			Strict I & O
			
			Drug Interactions:
			There are many drug interactions because of the alcohol in these infusions. Many medications are potentiated or have a reduced effect when given concurrently with alcohol infusions. Note the medications the patient is taking and determine untoward interactions.

Table 13–1 (continued)

Infusion	Osmolarity	Indications and Incompatibilities	Precautions, Comments, Contraindications
Alkalinizing Agents		**Indications:**	Contraindicated with
Sodium bicarbonate 5% 595 mEq/L (0.595/mL)	595 mOsm/L	Alkalinizing agent for temporary treatment of severe metabolic acidosis	acidosis (respiratory) alkalosis (metabolic and respiratory)
		Increases plasma bicarbonate and buffers excess hydrogen ion concentration	edema hypertension
Sodium bicarbonate 7.5% 892.50 mEq/L (0.893/mL)	893 mOsm/L	Dosage corresponds to degree of acidosis according to pH (<7.25), PO_2, PCO_2, and electrolytes	hypocalcemia hypochloremia impaired renal function
		Treats hyperkalemia	
Sodium bicarbonate 8.4% 999.60 mEq/L (0.999/mL) pH 7.75 (7.0–8.5)	1,000 mOsm/L	Used as a buffer to raise the pH of intravenous infusates	Use with extreme caution in patients with sodium retention
		Treatment for barbiturate and salicylate intoxication	Use with caution in patients on corticosteroids
		Incompatibilities:	Excessive or rapid administration can result in intracranial hemorrhage
		Numerous; consult pharmacist	Extravasation can result in severe tissue damage
			Flush IV line before and after injection

(Source: *Intravenous Infusion Therapy for Nurses: Principles and Practices,* by D. Josephson, 2004, Clifton Park, NY: Delmar/Cengage Learning.)

Due to the aging process, the older client has the potential for heart and renal insufficiency. If the IV is infused too rapidly, the client's lungs become congested indicating complications of pulmonary edema and congestive heart failure. Since the kidneys cannot effectively rid the body of fluids, IV solutions accumulate in the body causing lung congestion. The heart attempts to compensate for the needs of the body and pumps harder and faster to propel the fluids through the body leading to congestive heart failure.

PEDIATRIC CONSIDERATIONS

Play therapy assists a child in understanding the purpose of IV therapy. Play with the child as she tapes and maintains an IV (without needles) on a doll or teddy bear. Explain the IV in simple terms appropriate for the child's age. Remind the child that this is one of the things nurses do to help sick people get better.

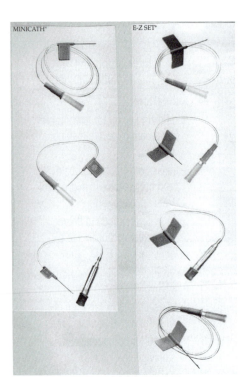

Figure 13–1 Winged Needle Infusion Set. (Source: *Intravenous Infusion Therapy for Nurses: Principles and Practices*, by D. Josephson, 2004, Clifton Park, NY: Delmar/Cengage Learning.)

Intravenous pump alarms cause anxiety and fear in younger and older children. Children may be frightened by the alarm sounds. Remind children that the alarm sound is not an emergency and does not mean that they are in danger or that their condition is worsening.

The winged needle (see Figure 13–1) is very effective in accessing surface veins in an infant or small child's head. When used in a child's head, the winged needle is referred to as a scalp-vein needle. Winged needles or butterfly needles are usually not used with adults other than to deliver a one time medication or to draw blood. Sometimes they are used for short term venous access of 24 hours or less.

PREPARING THE IV BAG AND TUBING

Manufacturers are constantly updating IV administration equipment to stay on the cutting edge of technology. To stay current with new IV equipment and administration techniques, the nurse consistently attends continuing education opportunities. Refer to Box 13–1 to review preparing an IV bag and tubing for administration of IV fluids.

Box 13–1 Preparing the IV Bag And Tubing

1. Prepare the new bag by removing its protective cover. Check the expiration date on the bag and assess for cloudiness or leakage.

2. Open the new infusion set. Unroll tubing and close roller clamp.

3. Spike the bag with the tip of the new tubing and compress the drip chamber to fill halfway.

4. Open the roller clamp, remove the protective cap from the end of the tubing, and slowly flush solution completely through the tubing. (This process is called "priming the tubing.")

5. Close the roller clamp and replace the cap protector.

6. Apply gloves.

7. Remove the old tubing and replace it with new tubing.

8. Discard the old tubing and IV bag.

9. Remove gloves and dispose of them with all used materials.

10. Apply a label to the tubing with date and time of change. Calculate IV drip rates, set the IV pump for administration rate, and begin infusion at the pre-scribed rate.

DETERMINING THE IV FLOW RATE

IV administration of fluids and medications is so routine that nurses frequently overlook po-tential risks. Each health care provider's IV order includes date and time, name of IV solution, administration route, dosage of IV solution, volume to infuse, rate of infusion, length of time for infusion, and health care provider's signature. The nurse is responsible for calculating the correct flow rate and administering the IV fluid at the appropriate rate.

Drip Calculations

The nurse figures drip calculations to determine the correct drops of IV fluid per minute for the correct IV infusion rate. While not necessary for most infusions due to IV pumps control-ling infusion rates, nurses must understand the calculations to determine drip rates in case the IV pumps fail to operate correctly. There are two pieces of information the nurse needs for the calculation: infusion rates per hour in milliliters and drop factor found on the package of the administration set. Each IV tubing manufacturer will provide the number of drops per milliliter (drop factor).

The IV drip rate is calculated by using algebraic equations. Some sources divide the IV rate in milliliters per hour by 60 minutes per hour and then multiply by the drop factor per milliliter to determine the drops/minute.

$$\text{Flow Rate} = \frac{\text{Volume} \times \text{Set Calibration}}{\text{Time}}$$

Alternatively, the nurse can simplify the equation by dividing the drop factor, which could be 10, 15, 20, or 60, by 60 minutes per hour. The resulting fraction is then multiplied by the IV rate per hour to determine the drops per minute for that particular administration set and IV rate.

Example: The doctor orders Normal Saline at 150 mL per hour. The tubing has a drop factor of 15 drops per milliliter. Placing the drop factor over 60 (15/60), the nurse obtains a fraction of ¼. Multiplying the rate, 150 mL / hour by ¼ equals 37.5 and rounded appropriately equals 38 drops per minute (one can not give partial drops). This skill is especially helpful in home health care situations where the IV fluid and medications are sometimes infused per gravity, without an electronic infusion device. In these situations, simple IV drip monitors, such as flow regulators, are available as a safety device. In modern hospitals, even if the power fails to the facility, a back up power source maintains the myriad of life-saving equipment present in the health care facility. Thus, it would be rare for nurses to have to count drops to control IV rates.

Calculating drip rates, while not as essential as in the past, is a skill for which nurses must attain proficiency because of the serious complications of infusing an IV too rapidly. Following are some calculations for review practice.

Setting the IV Flow Rate

- Check calibration and drops per milliliter (gtt/mL) of each infusion set.

$$\text{Flow Rate} = \frac{\text{Volume} \times \text{Set Calibration}}{\text{Time}}$$

Example:
- The order reads 1000 mL D₅W with 20 mEq KCL over 8 hours.
  Drop factor is 15 gtt/mL
  Divide 1000 mL by 8 hours to obtain 125 mL/hour.

$$\frac{125 \text{mL/hour} \times 15 \text{gtts /mL}}{60 \text{ minutes}} = \frac{31.25 \text{gtts}}{\text{minute}} \text{ or } \frac{31 \text{gtts}}{\text{minute}}$$

- Determine the hourly rate by dividing total volume by total hours.

Example 1:
- The order reads 1000 mL D$_5$W with 20 mEq KCL over 8 hours:

$$\frac{1000 \text{ ml}}{8 \text{ hrs}} = 125 \text{ ml/hr}$$

Example 2:
- Three thousand milliliters are ordered for 24 hours:

$$\frac{3000 \text{ mL}}{24 \text{ hrs}} = 125 \text{ mL/hr}$$

- Place a strip of tape on the IV bag that identifies the hourly time periods according to the prescribed rate.
- Calculate the number of drops per minute based on the drop factor of the infusion set so you can quickly identify any malfunctioning of the IV pump.

MAINTAINING AN IV SITE

Determine the client's risk for developing complications from IV therapy, such as being very young, old, or having heart or renal failure. If the nurse is knowledgeable of these risk factors, she uses routine focused assessments to monitor for any potential complications.

Observe the IV site for complications of infection, phlebitis, or infiltration. Signs of these would be redness, swelling, pallor, or temperature changes at the IV site and surrounding tissue, and bleeding or drainage. Teach the client about the purpose of the pump alarm to alleviate concern or anxiety when the alarm sounds.

Check that each client has the prescribed fluid, additives, rate, and volume at the beginning of the shift. Check every two hours that the IV tubing connections are attached tightly.

Complications

The administration of IV fluids has potential risks. Some common side effects of IV fluid administration are cellulitis, phlebitis, infiltration, and extravasation.

Cellulitis

Cellulitis is an inflammation or infection of the skin and subcutaneous tissue. The inflammation or infection spreads through the areas where the IV fluid seeps through the tissues. The area is tender, warm, reddened, and swollen. The appearance of the site is charted and the health care provider notified. Cool and moist warm compresses are alternated and, depending on the severity of the cellulitis, antibiotics, analgesics, and antipyretics are started (Josephson, 2004).

Phlebitis

Phlebitis is the inflammation of a vessel. The symptoms are redness, swelling, warmth, pain, and burning at the IV site and along the IV infusion vessel. The vessel can become hard, red, and cordlike (Josephson, 2004). At the first signs of phlebitis the nurse discontinues the IV and documents the IV site appearance and client statements. The nurse follows the facility protocol. Some facilities culture the site and cannula and notify the infection control nurse (Josephson, 2004).

Infiltration

The most common IV complication is infiltration (Josephson, 2004). An infiltration is the escape of IV fluid from the vein into the surrounding tissue. A few reasons for infiltration are puncture of vessel wall, rapid infusion of fluids into the vessel, improper taping of the IV device, or excessive manipulation of the IV device. To prevent vein irritation, the IV is not hung higher than 36 inches above the IV site. The best way to prevent an infiltration is regular assessment of the IV site and good communication with the client. The nurse teaches the client to notify her if there is any discomfort or swelling and the nurse listens to and acts upon the concerns of the client.

The nurse notifies the health care provider when an infiltration occurs. Some infiltrated sites respond best to warm compresses and some to cold. Elevation of the extremity may cause the client more discomfort. For these reasons, it is best to consult a health care provider and seek advice in handling the infiltration (Josephson, 2004).

Vesicant Extravasation

Another potential concern with IV medication administration is giving medications called **vesicants**. These medications cause tissue necrosis upon infiltration. Some examples include various vasopressors (norepinephrine and dopamine), cancer chemotherapeutic agents (doxorubicin, mitomycin C, and vincristine), and electrolyte solutions (calcium chloride, sodium bicarbonate) (Phillips, 2005). Some of the vesicants have antidotes that can help reduce the damage caused to the tissues upon infiltration, and some do not. A health care provider's order is necessary before administering the antidote. Reducing the amount of infiltration through frequent site assessment is essential to preventing loss of motor and sensory function as well as potential amputation. While not consistently considered a vesicant, Phenergan® (promethazine), can cause severe tissue damage and has resulted in amputations when inadvertently administered into an artery (Keene, Buckley, Small, & Geldzabler, 2006) and extensive treatment and follow-up care when extravasating from a vein (Zapp, 2004). The best treatment for a vesicant extravasation is frequent assessment of the IV site and prevention.

ADMINISTERING MEDICATIONS VIA SECONDARY ADMINISTRATION SETS (PIGGYBACK)

Medication administered via a secondary administration set is the most common method of administering medication intravenously. A primary infusion line is present and a piggyback line is attached to the first injection port.

Intermittent Infusion

Intermittent infusions are often added to a continuous infusion line for short, intermittent periods of time. These fluids are generally antibiotics, although other medications also are given intermittently. Sometimes the intermittent fluids are connected as a secondary or piggyback infusion, or they can be connected directly to the IV cap on the catheter with a saline flush before and after the infusion. The piggyback is hung higher than the primary infusion to infuse along with the primary infusion. Some IV pumps are designed to regulate the primary line and the piggy back in their own separate channel. If this type of pump is used the piggyback does not need to be higher than the primary infusion (see Box 13–2).

Box 13–2 Procedure for Administering Medications Via Secondary Administration Sets (Piggyback)

1. Check the health care provider's order or the medication administration record (MAR) for the medication, dosage, time, and route of administration to ensure accurate administration.

2. Review information regarding the drug, including action, purpose, side effects, normal dose, peak onset, and nursing implications, in order to administer the drug safely.

3. Before adding medication to an IV, determine if the additive in the solution of an existing IV line is compatible with the medication.

4. Assess the placement of the IV catheter in the vein to ensure that the medication will enter the vein and not the surrounding tissue.

5. Check the client's drug allergy history. An allergic reaction could occur rapidly and be fatal.

6. Assess that the client understands the purpose of the medication so you can tailor teaching to her learning needs.

7. Assess the compatibility of the piggyback IV medication with the primary IV solution to avoid an adverse reaction such as the formation of precipitate in the IV tubing.

8. Prepare the medication bag by attaching the tubing and priming the tubing with the medication.

9. Hang the piggyback medication bag above the level of the primary IV bag. One way to do this is to lower the primary bag using an extender; this is often found in the piggy back tubing package.

10. Connect the piggyback tubing to the primary tubing at the first injection port on the primary infusion tubing. For a needleless system, remove the cap on port and connect tubing.

The amount of saline necessary for flushing depends on the type of IV access and on institutional policy. Generally, a peripheral catheter requires a 2–5 mL saline flush before and after medication. See Box 13–3 for a hint in remembering how to flush an IV intermittent line or IV line when administering medication. A central line may require a 5–10 mL flush with a 10 mL syringe. A smaller barrel is not advised due to the resulting increase in pressure or pounds per square inch. The addition of heparin as a final flush is recommended only with central lines. The use of heparinized solutions for peripheral flushes are not commonly used. Medication remaining in the tubing after a secondary bag has completely infused may cause incompatibilities when giving other medication through the tubing.

Box 13–3 Flushing an Intermittent Needle or IV Injection Site

One way to remember the order of flushing when administering medications IV is the acronym: SASH.

S = Saline flush

A = Administer medication

S = Saline flush

H = Heparin flush—usually central lines

Intravenous Push Medications

Another method of administering medications is to "push" the medication through a continuous infusion or separately into an IV catheter as shown in Figure 13–2. As with an intermittent infusion, an IV push medication through a saline lock requires flushing before and after with saline. The nurse can also stop a primary IV infusion to administer the IV medication. Flush the IV line before and after with normal saline if the IV push medication and the infusing solution are not compatible.

Dilution of an IV push medication is not always required, but should be investigated prior to administration. Making the medication more dilute may help reduce phlebitis, increase the injection time, and reduce the risk of speed shock. When the medication is injected too rapidly, speed shock occurs. The symptoms of speed shock are flushing of the head and neck with a pounding headache, apprehension, hypertension, dyspnea, tachycardia with dysrhythmias, loss of consciousness, and cardiac arrest.

The nurse assures that the liquid used to dilute the medication is appropriate for the medication. Most medication is safely diluted with saline. However, some medications are not compatible with saline, and dextrose or other solution is used.

Consulting a knowledgeable resource prior to administration is imperative to maintain client safety. There are resource books devoted entirely to IV drug administration (see Gahart [2009] as listed in suggested resources), and the facility's pharmacy is another excellent source of information.

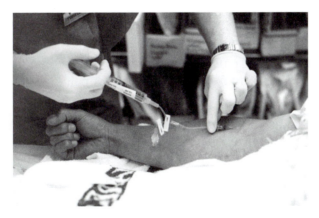

Figure 13–2 IV Push Technique. (Source: *Intravenous Infusion Therapy for Nurses: Principles and Practices*, by D. Josephson, 2004, Clifton Park, NY: Delmar/ Cengage Learning.)

Adding Medications to Infusing IV Bags

Sometimes, the health care provider orders a new additive for a client's IV soon after a new bag of solution is hung. In an effort to reduce medical costs, nurses are sometimes asked to add the new medication or additive to the IV that is currently infusing. While not a common practice, it is one that is recognized as a nursing responsibility. Refer to Box 13–4 for guidelines on adding medication to hanging IV fluids.

Box 13–4 Adding Medication to Hanging IV Fluids

After checking compatibility, concentration requirements, and stability in relation to the fluid and any additive already present in the bag, the nurse proceeds with the addition of the newly ordered medication. The nurse will:

1. Stop the infusion
2. Cleanse the additive port with an antimicrobial cleanser
3. Add the medication through the additive port
4. Gently rock the bag to disperse the medication throughout the solution
5. Restart the infusion according to the health care provider's ordered rate
6. Label the bag with the date, time, nurse's name, drug name and dose, using a ball point pen on the label, not the bag.

THEORY TO PRACTICE

A client has a saline lock for prn use and has an order for morphine sulfate 5 milligrams IV every 3 hours prn. The client requests something for pain.

1. How would the nurse proceed to administer the medication?

The nurse begins flushing the saline lock with normal saline. The client expresses having pain at the IV site and a small area of swelling develops at the insertion site.

2. What action does the nurse take?

3. If the nurse were to give the morphine sulfate through a central line, what changes would he make in the administration technique?

4. Look at an IV medication reference book, such as Gahart, and explain how you would administer the following medications (dilution, dilution solution, rate of administration, incompatibilities, adverse effects, and antidote).

   - famotidine (Pepcid) 20 mg IV push bid
   - ondansetron hydrochloride (Zofran) 4 mg IV push stat
   - hydromorphone hydrochloride (Dilaudid) 2 mg IV push every 4 hours prn pain

DISCONTINUING THE IV AND CHANGING TO A SALINE OR HEPARIN LOCK

Check the health care provider's order for discontinuation of the IV or insertion of a saline lock. If discontinuing an IV and converting it to a saline lock, stop the IV infusion. Open the sterile package containing a needleless adapter saline lock. Loosen IV tubing on the existing IV and remove it. Twist saline lock into the hub of the tubing.

SUMMARY

Administering IV medications and solutions can be complicated and intimidating at times. Obtaining advice from experienced nurses and pharmacists can help assure that the medications are administered properly and the client's safety is maintained. It is important that nurses take time to ask questions, use available resources, and maintain continued education on care of IVs.

CHAPTER REFLECTIONS

1. After reading the chapter on IV administration, what advice do you have for David in the chapter scenario?

2. Compare the State Board of Nursing Standards of the Nurse Practice Act for LPN/VNs and RNs in your state with other states. Share your findings with other peers.

3. What could you do to bring more standardization to the nurse role across the nation? What would you change? What would you leave the same?

Journaling Your Journey

1. Describe your personal experiences with IVs to this point in your career.

2. What is your present comfort level in assessing and maintaining IV sites and equipment and administering IV medications?

3. What intimidates you the most in caring for IVs?

4. What do you still need to learn to increase knowledge and confidence in preparing for your new role in administering IV medications and assessing and maintaining IV lines?

ဢ ဢ ဢ

My Story...

Being an LPN for 9 years before returning to school definitely had its pros and cons! On the positive side, I wasn't afraid or as unsure of myself as others were. I had a solid nursing knowledge base to incorporate additional theories and principles, such as IV therapy skills. Most important, I knew nursing was my niche!

On the other hand, I had acquired a few bad habits I needed to eliminate. Swallowing my pride and admitting to them was not easy! I also had a bit of difficulty stepping out of my LPN role and into my student role.

Patty Emrich, RN

REFERENCES

Adams, M., Holland, L., & Bostwick, P. (2008). *Pharmacology for nurses: A pathophysiologic approach.* Upper Saddle River, N.J.: Pearson Prentice Hall.

Jensen, R. (2008). *Administering intravenous therapy.* Manuscript submitted for publication.

Josephson, D. (2004). Intravenous infusion therapy for nurses: Principles and practice, (2nd ed.). Clifton Park, NY: Thomson Cengage Learning.

Keene, J., Buckley, K., Small, S., & Geldzabler, G. (2006). Accidental intra-arterial injection: A case report, new treatment modalities, and a review of the literature. *Journal of Oral and Maxiloofacial Surgery, 6*(4), 965–968.

Phillips, L. (2005). *Manual of I.V. Therapeutics* (4th ed.). Philadelphia: F. A. Davis.

Zapp, J. (2004). Promethazine hydrochloride: Potential danger of extravasation. *American Journal of Pain Management, 14*(4), 148–150.

SUGGESTED RESOURCES

Altman, G. (2009). Delmar's fundamental and advanced nursing skills (3rd ed.). Clifton Park, NY: Delmar Cengage Learning.

Crawford, M. (2005). Technology and safe medication administration. *American Journal of Nursing, 3,* 37–41.

Curren, A. (2008). Math for meds: Dosages and solutions (10th ed.). Clifton Park, NY: Delmar Cengage Learning.

Gahart, B. & Nazareno, A. (2009). 2010 Intravenous Medications: A Handbook for Nurses and Health Professionals (26th ed.). St. Louis, MO: Mosby.

Hadaway, L. (2007). Infitration and extravasation: Preventing a complication of IV catherterization. *American Journal of Nursing, 107*(8), 64–72.

Huber, C. & Augustine, A. (2009). IV infusion alarms: Don't wait for the beep. *American Journal of Nursing, 109*(4), 32–33.

Pasero, C. (2007). IV opioid range orders for acute pain management. *American Journal of Nursing, 107*(2), 52–59.

Appendix A
Déjà Vu: Nursing Exams Today and the NCLEX-RN Tomorrow

▼ ▼ ▼ ▼ ▼ ▼ ▼

You have successfully taken the National Council Licensure Examination for Practical Nurses (NCLEX-PN). After you graduate from the RN program you will take the National Council Licensure Examination for Registered nurses (NCLEX-RN) to legally practice as a licensed RN. The RN program equips you with knowledge and critical thinking skills for success on the NCLEX. Your role in preparing for the NCLEX-RN is to diligently apply yourself in your educational experience by reading your textbooks, attending class, utilizing learning opportunities in the clinical experiences, improving critical thinking skills, and interacting frequently with the nursing program faculty, clinical nurses, and clients. These preparation steps also equip students for the next step in a nursing career.

The purpose of the NCLEX is to assess the entry-level competence of nursing candidates. The National Council of State Boards of Nursing (NCSBN) routinely updates the NCLEX to keep the testing content current and consistent with new technological advances. For example, in 1994 the NCSBN introduced computerized testing in place of the previous paper-and-pencil exam. On April 1, 2003, the NCSBN (2003) changed the question format on the NCLEX-RN to include alternate item response questions. The current NCLEX exam tests the cognitive ability levels of knowledge, comprehension, application, and analysis as applied in four major categories of client needs (safe, effective care environment, health promotion and maintenance, psychosocial integrity, and physiological integrity). Cognitive ability means the mental process the person uses to determine the correct answer on the exam. Since nursing is the application of skills and knowledge, most exam questions are written at the application or higher level. Four integral components of the nursing practice (nursing process, caring, communication and documentation, and teaching/learning) are integrated and tested throughout the client needs categories.

By adding the alternate item response questions, the exam utilizes opportunities provided by technology to assess candidate clinical expertise and ability other than the standard multiple-choice questions. The NCLEX now incorporates charts, tables, and graphic images into the test questions. Some of the alternate item response questions require the candidate to complete math equations to correctly calculate an answer. These alternate item response questions are added to the standard multiple-choice questions on the NCLEX.

The entire NCLEX exam is computerized. Four different types of questions are used on the NCLEX exams: multiple-choice, multiple-response, fill-in-the-blank, and hot spot. The terminology for these types of questions may be new, but the formatting has probably been seen at some time in one's educational experience. Examples of these types of questions are discussed and a few samples presented. In the question example section, questions covering similar content are given for each type of alternate question in order to see how the responses vary.

The multiple-choice questions pose a question, and the examinee chooses the best answer from four choices. Each of the four choices has a small circle in front of the choice. The examinee chooses the desired choice by left clicking the mouse in one of the circles or selecting the numbered item from the number keypad. See a computerized example of a multiple-choice question in Figure A–1.

The multiple-response questions pose a question with a list of four to seven choices. The question is followed by the phrase "Select all that apply" and the examinee chooses all the choices that correctly answer the question. There may be one or more correct choices. The computerized multiple-response questions have square boxes in front of the choices rather than circles, as in the multiple-choice questions (Figure A–2 A and C). To choose the answer choices, left click the mouse in all the correct squares that answer the question correctly. To deselect the choice, click the square again and the mark disappears. You must choose all of the correct answers for the question to be counted as correct.

Multiple-Choice (one answer):

The nurse listens to the client's apical impulse. The nurse is listening at the cardiac landmark known as (the):

○ 1. aortic area.

○ 2. Erb's point.

○ 3. tricuspid area.

⊙ 4. mitral area.

Select the best response. Click the Next [N] button on the Enter key to confirm answer and proceed.   Item 1
                              Next [N]   Calculator [O]

Figure A–1 NCLEX multiple-choice question example.

Multiple-Response:

The nurse assesses the client's heart sounds by listening to the cardiac landmarks, or sites on the chest where the heart sounds are best heard. What are the names of these sites?

Select all that apply.

☐ 1. Aortic Area

☐ 2. Erb's point

☐ 3. Bachmann's bundle

☐ 4. Costochondral junction

☐ 5. Pulmonic area

☐ 6. Xiphoid process

Select all that apply. Click **Next** to confirm your answer and proceed to the next question.

Item 2

Next   Calculator

A client is admitted with an obstruction in the jejunum. When assessing the client, the nurse will probably not hear active bowel sounds in what areas?

Select all that apply.

☐ 1. Right upper quadrant

☐ 2. Periumbilical region

☐ 3. Epigastric region

☐ 4. Left lower quadrant

☐ 5. Left upper quadrant

Select all that apply. Click **Next** to confirm your answer and proceed to the next question.

Item 3

Next   Calculator

Figure A–2 A and C: NCLEX multiple response question example. (continues)

Remember, when scoring the NCLEX, no partial credit is given for multiple-response questions. All the correct responses must be marked, or no credit is given for the question (see Figure A–2 B and D).

See Figure A–2 for some multiple-response questions for practice. Remember, there is *more than one correct answer* to each of the questions.

The third type of NCLEX question is fill-in-the-blank. The examinee is posed a question and requested to mathematically calculate the answer then type the answer in the space. Only the number with a decimal point is written in the space; no unit of measurement or other characters are permitted. A calculator is available by clicking on the button labeled "Calculator." Any rounding of numbers is only done at the end of the calculation. A sample practice question is in Figure A–3.

Multiple-Response:

The nurse assesses the client's heart sounds by listening to the cardiac landmarks, or sites on the chest where the heart sounds are best heard. What are the names of these sites?

Select all that apply.

☑ 1. Aortic Area

☑ 2. Erb's point

☐ 3. Bachmann's bundle

☐ 4. Costochondral junction

☑ 5. Pulmonic area

☐ 6. Xiphoid process

Select all that apply. Click **Next** to confirm your answer and proceed to the next question.

Item 2

| Next | Calculator |

A client is admitted with an obstruction in the jejunum. When assessing the client, the nurse will probably not hear active bowel sounds in what areas?

Select all that apply.

☑ 1. Right upper quadrant

☐ 2. Periumbilical region

☐ 3. Epigastric region

☑ 4. Left lower quadrant

☑ 5. Left upper quadrant

Select all that apply. Click **Next** to confirm your answer and proceed to the next question.

Item 3

| Next | Calculator |

Figure A–2 B and D: NCLEX multiple response question answer. (continued)

Fill-in-the Blank:

The nurse is to administer 15 milligrams per kilogram of phenytoin sodium (Dilantin) to a pediatric child. The child weighs 20 pounds. How many milligrams does the nurse administer?

Answer: 136   milligrams

Click **Next** to confirm your answer and proceed to the next question.

Item 4

| Next | Calculator |

Figure A–3 NCLEX fill-in-the blank question example.

The fourth type of NCLEX question is the hot-spot question that poses a problem and a figure (See Figure A–4 A and C). The examinee is requested to use the computer mouse to locate and mark an area on the figure. The cursor is placed on the desired area of the figure, the left mouse button is clicked, and an X appears on the figure as the answer to the hot-spot question (See Figure A–4 B and D). To deselect the answer, the examinee places the cursor on the X and left clicks the mouse and the X is removed.

A key to passing the NCLEX-RN is to understand the question format and consistently practice NCLEX-style questions throughout your education experience. To be successful on the NCLEX exam, some tutors recommend completing 100 practice questions a day until consistently scoring 85 percent or higher. Students find that routinely practicing NCLEX questions also helps their course exam performance resulting in an improved grade. The student is more readily able to critically think through questions and thus obtain the correct response. Several NCLEX review books provide the rationale for the answers to the book's review questions. Other NCLEX tutors suggest that time spent reviewing rationales enhances one's ability to critically think through question content. The answer rationale helps students review the background information for each question and assists in logically analyzing each answer option. If rationale for the correct answer is not familiar, thoroughly review the question content in a textbook. Some NCLEX review resources assist a student in developing individualized focused reviews with specific text resources and content to review. Remember that each individual has a different learning style, and not one way of study fits all.

TEST-TAKING STRATEGIES

Nursing faculty at the University of West Georgia conducted a research study and developed a course to improve their school's NCLEX-RN scores and assist students in passing the NCLEX-RN. To parallel their program philosophy, the course attempted to integrate the student's body, mind, and spirit. The purpose of the research study was to "increase self-awareness, promote a positive attitude toward passing the NCLEX-RN, and provide specific strategies for test taking and stress reduction" (Mills, Wilson, & Bar, 2001, p. 360).

The university faculty's literature review showed that most programs designed to assist students in passing the NCLEX included test-taking practice and instruction. Students are encouraged to review a set number of questions on a routine basis and then review content in general or content missed on the exam. The literature (Poorman, Webb, Mastorovich, & Molcan, 1999; Saxton, Nugent, & Pelikan, 1999) also supports reviewing the rationale on questions students miss when taking practice tests.

The faculty then designed a course to assist students in passing the NCLEX-RN that included completing a minimum of 1,200 multiple-choice questions and reviewing the rationales for questions they missed. The course also included "cognitive restructuring, relaxation, visualization, and positive self-affirmations" (Mills et al., 2001, p. 361).

Hot Spot:

Practice Item Type #4: Hot Spot Item

The nurse is assessing the S_2 sound. Identify the area where the nurse places the stethoscope to listen for the closure of the semilunar heart valves.

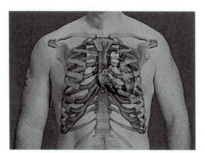

Place the mouse on the correct spot on the figure and click. Then click **Next** to confirm your answer and proceed to the next question.

Click in the figure to indicate your selection. Click the Next [N] button or the Enter key to confirm answer and proceed.   Item 5

Next   Calculator

Hot Spot:

A 50-year-old male is admitted with cholecystitis. The results of the endoscopic retrograde cholangiopancreatography confirm the diagnosis. Identify the area of the body affected by cholecystitis.

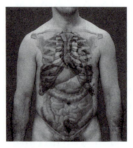

Place the mouse on the correct spot on the figure and click. Then click **Next** to confirm your answer and proceed to the next question.

Click in the figure to indicate your selection. Click the Next [N] button or the Enter key to confirm answer and proceed.   Item 6

Next   Calculator

Figure A–4 A and C: NCLEX hot spot question example. (continues)

Hot Spot:

Practice Item Type #4: Hot Spot Item

The nurse is assessing the S_2 sound. Identify the area where the nurse places the stethoscope to listen for the closure of the semilunar heart valves.

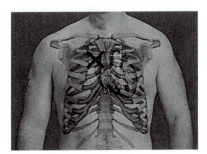

Place the mouse on the correct spot on the figure and click. Then click **Next** to confirm your answer and proceed to the next question.

Click in the figure to indicate your selection. Click the Next [N] button or the Enter key to confirm answer and proceed.   Item 5

Next   Calculator

Hot Spot:

A 50-year-old male is admitted with cholecystitis. The results of the endoscopic retrograde cholangiopancreatography confirm the diagnosis. Identify the area of the body affected by cholecystitis.

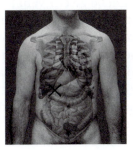

Place the mouse on the correct spot on the figure and click. Then click **Next** to confirm your answer and proceed to the next question.

Click in the figure to indicate your selection. Click the Next [N] button or the Enter key to confirm answer and proceed.   Item 6

Next   Calculator

Figure A–4 B and D: NCLEX hot spot question answer. (continued)

According to Mills et al. (2001), "cognitive restructuring focuses on assisting students to understand that cognition, emotion, and behavior are integrated" (p. 367). In other words, what one thinks, how one feels, and how one acts are all intertwined. For example, if a student feels he does not test well he may feel anxious prior to and when taking an exam and, consequently, receive a lower grade on the exam. If the student's thinking is changed so that he knows he has some strategies to improve his test-taking skills, the knowledge decreases his anxiety and results in improved test scores. Or, perhaps as he is taking the exam he comes to a question that he does not know the content. He may feel his anxiety and negative thoughts returning. If so, he can do self-talk, such as, "I have studied the subject content for this exam. I am not familiar with the content on this question, but that does not mean I will not reason out the correct answer. I will know the content of other test questions." The student then relaxes and concentrates on the rest of the exam. The student needs to learn to recognize prominent, recurring negative thoughts and replaces them with factual, positive, and uplifting thoughts.

The University of West Georgia nursing faculty suggested deep-breathing and shoulder-stretching exercises to assist with relaxation. The students were encouraged to do 30 deep breathing exercises of inhaling for four seconds and then exhaling for eight seconds. They were also encouraged to visualize the testing situation in an effort to desensitize them from the anxiety of the testing situation. Some students included progressive muscle relaxation and music therapy. Progressive muscle relaxation is consciously relaxing a group of muscles and then moving to another set of muscles, until the entire body is relaxed. For example, you can consciously relax tense forehead muscles, then jaw muscles, and so forth. Some students included other relaxation techniques such as lighting candles or taking a warm bath.

Diane Billings (2007) suggests seven steps for successful test taking. The first step is to learn as much as possible about the exam. When is the exam? How much time is allowed for taking the exam? Where will the exam be given? What is the result of the test score? How will the score affect the course grade or nursing licensure? Learning as much as possible about the exam prepares you psychologically to take the test.

The second step is to determine the type of questions on the exam. One prepares differently if all the answers are multiple choice as compared to essay. The previous section explained the type of questions that are on the NCLEX exam so you can be prepared for success.

The third step is to prepare for the exam. The standard guideline is to study two to three hours for each course credit. Be present and actively involved in class discussion and activity. Take notes, then review the notes within 24–48 hours after class to add content and clarify. Comparing class notes with two or three peers helps clarify any remaining questions and fill in any missing content. Study a set period of time each day rather than cramming at the last minute. Content retention is better if one consistently studies throughout the semester rather than a day or two before exams. Start a study group of compatible people who know the rules of the study group and who come prepared to study and contribute to the group. Ask clinical application questions for the clinical setting rather than memorize facts.

The fourth step is to read the test instructions and questions carefully. Quickly scan the entire exam to see the format of the test. Do all the questions count the same number of points?

If a question is difficult to understand, paraphrase the questions in your own words or under-line the key points of the question. Determine what is being asked before choosing an answer. If you do not know the answer, eliminate all the choices you think are incorrect and then determine the correct choice. If you cannot answer the question, do not spend excessive time trying to determine the answer. Move on to the next question and then return after complet-ing the last question. Even though this is an effective way for many to take an exam in the classroom, keep in mind that after answering a question on the NCLEX, you cannot go back to a previous question.

The fifth step is to manage anxiety. Rest before the exam. If the exam is given around a meal time, eat a snack or meal prior to taking the exam. These two suggestions prepare the brain for processing the exam content. Practice the relaxation techniques previously discussed.

The sixth step is to check the exam results and review the exam. Attend a test review ses-sion if offered. Ask questions to comprehend the content rather than attempting to obtain another point. Gain knowledge by learning the reason the question was missed and to apply in the clinical setting when caring for a client. Make an appointment with the instructor to review the exam if a test review is not given. Write down content areas that need further study. Prepare yourself in such a way that if content is repeated, you will have the correct answer not only on the exam but also when providing client care in critical situations.

The NCLEX-RN exam also includes analysis, application, delegation, and prioritization questions. An analysis question includes content that needs to be studied, and the informa-tion to answer the question will need to be mentally broken down and processed in order to obtain the correct answer. Do not agonize over the potential answers, but assimilate the information needed to answer the question and mentally review the information learned from hours of study. Rely on what you have learned and know as fact to deduce the correct answer.

To answer an application question correctly, the student must take information he knows and accurately apply it to a clinical situation. When answering an application question, the student asks himself, What do I need to know, and What would I do in a particular clinical situation? For example, if you were shopping and saw an elderly woman fall headfirst on the concrete floor, what information would you have to know, and how would you apply that information to assist the elderly woman? You would need to know the symptoms of brain hemorrhage and possible cervical fracture and assess for these symptoms. You would also need to know appropriate nursing actions. You would then choose the best option to cor-rectly answer the test question.

Continuing this same scenario with a prioritization question, the student has to decide the best nursing actions to take with the elderly woman. What should the student do first? What should he not do? How should the woman be handled? How should she not be handled? For what symptoms should you assess first, prior to moving her?

The thought process for a delegation question includes these questions: Whom do I need to ask for assistance? Whom do I need to call? To whom can I delegate certain responsibilities? What are the delegatee's abilities?

You will have plenty of opportunity to practice using these thought processes in clinical situations and as you take exams throughout your nursing education experience. By practicing NCLEX review questions, you can sharpen your thought processes and be better equipped to successfully take the NCLEX-RN.

Several techniques for success on the NCLEX-RN have been shared. However, remember that no special techniques can replace knowledge. Practice time management and make reading the textbooks, studying the textbooks' content, and applying your acquired knowledge in the clinical setting a priority in the next few semesters.

The NCLEX-RN is challenging. Your nursing education has provided you with many opportunities to learn the required content to be successful on the NCLEX-RN. With your newly acquired nursing knowledge and knowledge of the alternate questions on the NCLEX-RN, you are preparing yourself for success on the NCLEX-RN exam and a rewarding nursing career.

REFERENCES

Billings, D. (2007). *Seven steps for test-taking success.* American Journal of Nursing (AJN), *107*(4), 72AAA–72CCC.

Ellis, C., & MacLaren, A. (2005). *Rational emotive behavior therapy: A therapist's guide* (2nd ed.). San Luis Obispo, CA: Impact Publishers.

Mills, L., Wilson, C., & Bar, B. (2001). A holistic approach to promoting success on NCLEX-RN. *Journal of Holist Nursing, 19*(4), 360–374.

National Council of State Boards of Nursing (NCSBN). (2003). *Facts about alternate item formats and the NCLEX examinations* [On-line]. Available: www.ncsbn.org

National Council of State Boards of Nursing (NCSBN). (2007). *2007 NCEX-RN® detailed test plan.* Retrieved 5/5/09 at http://ncsbn.org

Poorman, S., Webb, C., Mastorovich, M., & Molcan, K. (1999). *A good thinking approach to the NCLEX and other nursing exams.* Pittsburgh, PA: STAT Nursing Consultants.

Saxton, D., Nugent, P., & Pelikan, P. (2005). *Mosby's comprehensive review of nursing for NCLEX-RN* (18th ed.). St. Louis, MO: Mosby.

Wendt, A. (2004). *Updates on the NCLEX-PN® examination.* The Journal of Practical Nursing, 3, 22–23.

SUGGESTED RESOURCES

Davis, M., Eshelman, E., McKay, M., & Fanning, P. (2008). *The relaxation and stress reduction workbook* (6th ed.). Oakland, CA: New Harbinger Publications.

Jegede, K. (2004). *Milestone: Getting your license: A test of knowledge and nerves.* American Journal of Nursing (AJN), *104*(4), 72CCC–72DDD.

National Council of State Boards of Nursing (NCSBN). (2007). *2007 NCEX-RN® detailed test plan.* Retrieved 5/5/09 at http://ncsbn.org

Poorman, S., Mastorovich, M., Webb, C., & Molcan, K. (2002). *Good thinking: Test taking and study skills for nursing students* (2nd ed.). Pittsburgh, PA: STAT Nursing Consultants.

Wendt, A. (2005). *What's new with the NCLEX.* American Journal of Nursing (AJN), *105*(4), 72AAA–72BBB.

Appendix B
Medication Preparation and Administration Competency for Registered Nurses

▼ ▼ ▼ ▼ ▼ ▼ ▼

Just the word math is enough to frighten some people. Several individuals consider themselves math illiterate and live with a math phobia. However, it is inevitable that nurses will need math skills during their nursing career. All nurses, regardless of their clinical area of practice, administer medications. There are many situations in the nursing profession that require nurses to work with numbers and basic calculations, such as measuring daily intakes and outputs, calorie and carbohydrate counts, weights, and vital signs; reviewing lab results; and administering medication. Every nurse is expected to be competent in basic math skills for the purpose of administering accurate medication dosages and, most importantly, providing safe, quality care to each client.

PREVENTION OF MEDICATION ERRORS

Situations frequently require the nurse to convert one system of measurement to another while administering medications. There are many different ways that a medication prescription is ordered and filled. The nurse receives an order from the physician written in milligrams, but the pharmacist provides the medication in grains. In that case, the nurse converts the ordered dose of medication accurately to verify that the correct dosage is administered. The rate of medication errors that occur and the consequences of those situations are frightening. Approximately 1.3 million medication errors occur in the United States every year (Karch, 2003). Approximately 44,000 to 98,000 deaths occur every year from medication errors in the United States (Strand, 2003). To put this into perspective, 42,000 people die in traffic accidents each year (Strand). These numbers undeniably indicate the tremendous responsibility nurses have for assuring clients' safety during medication administration. "Because nurses are the ones who predominantly administer medications to patients, they are often the last potential barrier between a mediation error (such as the wrong medications given at the wrong time) and serious harm" (Hughes & Edgerton, 2005, p. 79). The clients count on nurses to be responsible and competent caregivers.

As nurses, we take responsibility for our actions. In many cases the errors could have been prevented. Nurses who lack the competency to do dosage calculations in medication preparation and administration present a danger to their clients. Nursing programs offer a variety of methods to review and sharpen math skills, but the student is expected to come in with a strong understanding of basic math. Appendix B serves to reintroduce some basic math skills needed in nursing.

Nursing students make two common errors in dosage calculations (Twiname & Boyd, 2002). The first one is due to errors in basic math skills such as decimals, fractions, and percentages. The second one is misunderstanding the parts of a calculation problem. This might include the extra, or unrelated information, in a scenario to calculate a client's medication dose. According to Hughes and Edgerton (2005), there is a significant decrease in errors if nurses do not have to calculate a dose when administering medications.

We will review basic medication administration rules and guidelines that should be understood even before any calculations take place. Remember, the "seven rights" include: right client, right drug, right dose, right time, and right route, right to refuse, and right documentation. See Figure B–1 for a visual in remembering the drug administration rights. These steps are always paramount in the nurse's mind to prevent medication administration errors. Remember that medications are checked at least three times in the preparation of administering them to the client. Know the acceptable abbreviations for weights, values, and measurement conversions in order to administer medications in a competent fashion. These safeguards protect nurses and clients from medication administration errors. Generally speaking, if a medication error is made, one of these client rights was not followed. The medication administration process is taken seriously and the seven guidelines followed.

These basic math skills are the foundation for all dosage calculations in medication preparation and administration in health care (Pickar, 2004).

Knowledge of basic math (addition, subtraction, multiplication, and division), ratios and percentages, and basic problem-solving skills is essential as one begins the nursing education program.

Seven Rights of Drug Administration	Example
Right Client	*Can you tell me your name?*
Right Drug	*Captropril*
Right Dose	*25 mg*
Right Route	*P.O. tid*
Right Time	*1:00 P.M.*
Right to Deny or Refuse	*I would prefer not to take that until I know more about the medicine.*
Right Documentation	*The nurse properly documents medication administration and uses the acceptable abbreviations for weights, values, and measurement conversions.*

Figure B–1 Seven Rights of Drug Administration.

BASIC MATH PRETEST

It is important to know exactly what areas you understand and what areas require more effort as you decide what to review for dosage-calculation tests. The following 50-question pretest evaluation can indicate where your strengths and areas for improvement lie when dealing with dosage calculations. It will take you approximately an hour and a half to complete this pretest. You will need a piece of scrap paper, a pencil, a calculator, and a quiet place to work.

Mathematics Pretest Evaluation

Instructions: Carry decimals to the third decimal place and round to the second place. Always express fractions in their lowest possible form.

1. $1517 + 0.63 =$ _____

2. Express the value of $0.7 + 0.035 + 20.006$ rounded to two decimal places. _____

3. $9.5 + 17.06 + 32 + 41.11 + 0.99 =$ _____

4. $\$19.69 + \$304.03 =$ _____

5. $93.2 - 47.09 =$ _____

6. $1005 - 250.5 =$ _____

7. Express the value of $17.156 - 0.25$ rounded to two decimal places. _____

8. $509 \times 38.3 =$ _____

9. $\$4.12 \times 42 =$ _____

10. $17.16 \times 23.5 =$ _____

11. $972 \div 27 =$ _____

12. $2.5 \div 0.001 =$ _____

13. Express the value of $\frac{1}{4} \div \frac{3}{8}$ as a fraction reduced to lowest terms. _____

14. Express $\frac{1500}{240}$ as a decimal. _____

15. Express 0.8 as a fraction. _____

16. Express $\frac{2}{5}$ as a percentage. _____

17. Express 0.004 as a percentage. _____

18. Express 5% as a decimal. _____

19. Express $33\frac{1}{3}\%$ as a ratio in lowest terms. _____

20. Express $1:50$ as a decimal. _____

21. $\frac{1}{2} + \frac{3}{4} =$ _____

22. $1\frac{2}{3} + 4\frac{7}{8} =$ _____

23. $1\frac{5}{6} - \frac{2}{9} =$ _____

24. Express the value of $\frac{1}{100} \times 60$ as a fraction. _____

25. Express the value of $4\frac{1}{4} \times 3\frac{1}{2}$ as a mixed number. _____

26. Identify the fraction with the greatest value: $\frac{1}{150}, \frac{1}{200}, \frac{1}{100}$. _____

27. Identify the decimal with the lowest value: $0.009, 0.19, 0.9$. _____

28. $\frac{6.4}{0.02} =$ _____

29. $\frac{.02 + 0.16}{.4 - 0.34} =$ _____

30. Express the value of $\frac{3}{12 + 3} \times 0.25$ as a decimal. _____

31. 8% of 50 = _____

32. $\frac{1}{2}$% of 18 = _____

33. 0.9% of 24 = _____

Find the value of X. Express your answer as a decimal.

34. $\dfrac{1:1000}{1:100} \times 250 - X$ _____

35. $\dfrac{300}{150} \times 2 = X$ _____

36. $\dfrac{2.5}{5} \times 1.5 = X$ _____

37. $\dfrac{1,000,000}{250,000} \times X = 12$ _____

38. $\dfrac{0.51}{1.7} \times X = 150$ _____

39. $X = (82.4 - 52)\dfrac{3}{5}$ _____

40. $\dfrac{\frac{1}{150}}{\frac{1}{300}} \times 1.2 = X$ _____

41. Express $\frac{2}{10}$ as a fraction in the lowest terms. _____

42. Express 2% as a ratio in lowest terms. _____

43. If 5 equal medication containers contain 25 tablets total, how many tablets are in each container? _____

44. A person is receiving 0.5 milligrams of a medication four times a day. What is the total amount of medication in milligrams given each day?_____

45. If 1 kilogram equals 2.2 pounds, how many kilograms does a 66-pound child weigh?_____

46. If 1 kilogram equals 2.2 pounds, how many pounds are in 1.5 kilograms? (Express your answer as a decimal.)_____

47. If 1 centimeter equals $\frac{3}{8}$ inch, how many centimeters are in $2\frac{1}{2}$ inches? (Express your answer as a decimal.)_____

48. If 2.5 centimeters equal 1 inch, how long in centimeters is a 3-inch wound? _____

49. This diagnostic test has a total of 50 problems. If you answer 5 problems incorrectly, what percentage will you have answered correctly?_____

50. For every 5 female student nurses in a nursing class, there is 1 male student nurse. What is the ratio of female to male student nurses?_____

(From Pickar, 2004, pp. 2–4).

After completing the pretest, go to the last page of this appendix to check your answers. If you get 43 questions or more correct, you are ready to begin with medication preparation and administration questions. If you get fewer than 43 questions correct, you need to begin some basic math review. This does not mean that you cannot do dosage calculations or that you will make a bad nurse; it simply means you need more practice and, maybe, some help with this component of your education. The pretest assesses your math skills and competency level. It will give you some idea of what areas you need to review in order to be competent and provide safe medication preparation and administration as you progress through your nursing program and your nursing career.

BASIC MATH FOR REVIEW

A review of fractions and decimals provide you with a good foundation for solving more complicated calculations.

Adding and Subtracting Fractions

A fraction consists of two numbers (a numerator and a denominator) that identify a portion of another whole number or, figuratively, a piece of the pie. Always write a fraction in its lowest possible form, or terms.

Example:

$$\frac{8}{12} = \frac{2}{3} \text{ or } \frac{25}{50} = \frac{1}{2}$$

To add or subtract fractions, first change the two denominators to the lowest common denominator.

Example:

$$\frac{2}{8} + \frac{1}{2} \text{ becomes } \frac{2}{8} + \frac{4}{8}$$

In the example, 1/2 was changed to 4/8 by multiplying both the numerator and the denominator by 4. Now both fractions share the denominator 8, and now can be added. Last, always reduce the fraction to its lowest possible form.

Example:

$$\frac{2}{8} + \frac{4}{8} = \frac{6}{8} \text{ can be reduced to } \frac{3}{4}$$

Multiplying Fractions

When multiplying fractions, begin first with reducing the fractions where ever possible, then multiply the numerators together, and then multiply the denominators together. Reduce the answer (the product) to its lowest form.

Example:

$$\frac{125}{250} \times \frac{2}{3} =$$

First, reduce the fractions when possible: $\frac{125}{250} = \frac{1}{2}; \frac{2}{3}$ is already in its lowest form. At this point, multiply across the numerators and then multiply across the denominators.

Example:

$$\frac{1 \times 2}{2 \times 3} = \frac{2}{6} \text{ (reduced to its lowest form) } \frac{1}{3}$$

To divide fractions, invert the second fraction, or the divisor, and then change *divide* to *multiply*. Cancel or reduce all terms as much as possible. Then, multiply numerators and denominators across. Reduce the answer to its lowest form.

Example:

$$\frac{2}{6} \div \frac{3}{9} =$$

$$\frac{2}{\overset{\cancel{6}}{2}} \times \frac{\overset{3}{\cancel{9}}}{3} = \frac{6}{6} = 1$$

PRACTICE WITH FRACTIONS

1. Circle all of the fractions that are equal when reduced to their lowest form:

$$\frac{1}{5} = \frac{20}{200} \quad \frac{2}{6} = \frac{1}{3} \quad \frac{2}{4} = \frac{1}{2} \quad \frac{3}{4} = \frac{6}{8} \quad \frac{33}{66} = \frac{1}{2} \quad \frac{125}{250} = \frac{2}{3} \quad \frac{1}{4} = \frac{250}{1000}$$

2. Change the following fractions to whole or mixed numbers (always reduce to the lowest terms).

$$\frac{36}{12} = \underline{\hspace{1cm}} \quad \frac{11}{11} = \underline{\hspace{1cm}} \quad \frac{66}{33} = \underline{\hspace{1cm}} \quad \frac{125}{25} = \underline{\hspace{1cm}}$$

$$\frac{15}{2} = \underline{\hspace{1cm}} \quad \frac{50}{3} = \underline{\hspace{1cm}}$$

3. Write the following fractions using the specified denominators.

$$\frac{2}{4} \text{ converted to eighths} = \underline{\hspace{1cm}}$$

$$\frac{1}{5} \text{ converted to fifteenths} = \underline{\hspace{1cm}}$$

$$\frac{2}{3} \text{ converted to twelfths} = \underline{\hspace{1cm}}$$

4. A nursing student gets 40 questions correct on a 50-question exam. Write the student's score in a fraction format. Reduce the fraction to its lowest form to show the portion of the exam the student got correct._____

5. In a nursing class there are 5 men and 45 women. What fraction of the students are women? Reduce the fraction to the lowest terms._____

6. Add or subtract the following fractions. Reduce to the lowest form.

$$\frac{2}{4} + \frac{1}{3} = \underline{\hspace{1cm}}$$ $$\frac{2}{4} - \frac{1}{4} = \underline{\hspace{1cm}}$$

$$\frac{1}{5} + \frac{2}{7} = \underline{\hspace{1cm}}$$ $$\frac{6}{8} - \frac{2}{4} = \underline{\hspace{1cm}}$$

$$\frac{3}{9} + \frac{6}{12} = \underline{\hspace{1cm}}$$ $$\frac{3}{6} - \frac{2}{9} = \underline{\hspace{1cm}}$$

7. Multiply or divide the following fractions. Reduce to the lowest form.

$$\frac{3}{8} \times \frac{2}{6} = \underline{\hspace{1cm}}$$ $$\frac{25}{75} \div \frac{2}{5} = \underline{\hspace{1cm}}$$

$$\frac{7}{21} \times \frac{1}{7} = \underline{\hspace{1cm}}$$ $$\frac{11}{33} \div \frac{2}{3} = \underline{\hspace{1cm}}$$

$$\frac{25}{75} \times 6 = \underline{\hspace{1cm}}$$ $$\frac{1}{30} \div \frac{2}{3} = \underline{\hspace{1cm}}$$

Decimals

Some key decimal notes are:
Adding zeros after the last digit of a decimal fraction *does not* change its value.

Example:

$$0.50 \text{ is the same as } 0.5$$

Always add a zero to the left of the decimal point to avoid errors and possibly missing the decimal point.

Adding a zero between the decimal point and the first digit of a decimal fraction *does* change its value.

Example:

$$0.05 \text{ is different from } 0.5$$

To convert a fraction to a decimal, divide the numerator by the denominator.

Example:

$$\frac{76}{100} = 76 \div 100 = 0.76$$

To change a decimal to a fraction, write the decimal number as a whole number in the position of the numerator (on top), then write the denominator as the number 1 with as many zeros after it as there were places behind the decimal point. Reduce to the lowest form.

Example:

$$0.125 = \frac{125}{1000} = \frac{1}{8}$$

To add or subtract decimal fractions, line up the decimal points and add zeros to make them even.

Example:

$$
\begin{array}{r}
7.250 \\
+32.500 \\
\hline
39.750
\end{array}
$$

When multiplying numbers with decimals, first multiply the numbers and then add the decimal from right to left, one space for each decimal in the original numbers.

Example:

$$7.50 \times 12 = 90.00 \text{ or } 8.25 \times 2.75 = 22.6875$$

(Source: *Dosage Caclulations*, 7th Ed., G. Pickar, 2004, pp. 26–29, Clifton Park, NY: Delmar/ Cengage Learning.)

PRACTICE WITH DECIMALS

Convert the following numbers to their opposite form in the space provided.

Fraction: $\frac{2}{3}$ _____ $\frac{25}{250}$ _____ $5\frac{1}{3}$ _____

Decimal: 0.95 _____   0.33 _____   1.25 _____

Table B–1 Important conversions

Household measurements	Apothecary system	Metric system
1 tsp	1 dram (60 minims)	4–5 mL
2 tbsp	1 oz (8 drams)	30 mL
1 glass/measuring cup	8 oz	240 mL
1 quart	32 ounces	1,000 mL (1 liter)
15–16 drops	15–16 minims	1 mL
	1 gr	60–65 mg
	15 gr	1 g (1,000 mg)
	1/60 gr	1 mg
1 oz	8 drams	30 grams
1 gtt	1 m	0.06–0.07 mL
2.2 lb		1 kg (1,000 grams)
1 in		2.5 cm

DOSAGE CALCULATION

Once you have completed the necessary review, you are ready to move on to practicing dosage calculation.

Medication Weight, Values, and Measurements

In order to understand and be able to administer the correct dosages of medication, it is important to know the different weights, values, and measurements used for medications (see Table B–1). Know each system and how to convert between systems.

Dosage Calculations

If you have established a method or formula for dosage calculations that you understand and know consistently produces the correct answers, then continue to use that method. If you do not have a current method that leads to success and are one of the many who find math challenging or fear dosage calculations, then take this opportunity to grow and develop math skills for safe, competent medication preparations and administration.

Many people are familiar with the *ratio and proportion* formulas. The formula typically used for this method is:

$$\frac{D \,(\text{desired})}{H \,(\text{have})} \times Q \,(\text{quantity}) = X$$

Another method used for calculations is called *dimensional analysis,* or the *factor method.* This is a method that is used safely with all dosage calculations. In order to use this formula, review the following steps:

1. SETUP: Dimensional analysis problems are set up like fractions. First, decide what it is you need to know. Then set up the fractions so that the unwanted units of measurement can be canceled out. Continue to write these fractions until all the units present in the question and the ones that you need to find are in the fractions.

2. Next, cross out the units in each fraction that cancel each other out, leaving nothing but the wanted quantity.

3. Finally, do the basic math. Solve the problem by using basic math—no algebra required! Multiply the numbers across the top and then across bottom. Divide the top number by the bottom number. It is as simple as that!

4. When you are done, make sure your answer makes sense. Think about whether the dose should be larger or smaller than what is available. The answer should always seem realistic. If it does not, recalculate the problem.

Example: The client is to receive 40 mg of Lasix every morning. The dose on hand is 20 mg tablets. How many tablets will the nurse administer?

$$\frac{\text{Tabs}}{\text{Dose}} = \frac{1\,\text{tab}}{20\,\text{mg}} \times \frac{40\,\text{mg}}{\text{dose}} = \frac{40\,\text{tabs}}{20\,\text{mg dose}} = \frac{2\,\text{tabs}}{\text{dose}}$$

Example: The client is to receive 500 mg of X drug q 4h. The label reads "1gram/5mL." How many mL will the nurse administer per dose?

$$\frac{\text{mL}}{\text{Dose}} = \frac{5\,\text{mL}}{1\,\text{mg}} \times \frac{1\,\text{gm}}{1{,}000\,\text{mg}} \times \frac{500\,\text{mg}}{\text{dose}} = \frac{5}{2} = \frac{2.5\,\text{mL}}{\text{dose}}$$

Example: The physician orders 125 mL/hour of 5% dextrose in water with 40 mEq of kcl. The drop factor for the IV administration tubing is 15 gtt/mL. The nurse will correctly set the drip rate to run at how many drops per minute?

$$\frac{\text{gtt}}{\text{min}} = \frac{15\,\text{gtt}}{1\,\text{mL}} \times \frac{125\,\text{mL}}{1\,\text{hr}} \times \frac{1\,\text{hr}}{60\,\text{min}} = 31.25, \text{ which rounds to } 31\,\frac{\text{gtt}}{\text{min}}$$

PRACTICE WITH DOSAGE CALCULATIONS

1. The physician has ordered 0.25 mg digoxin (Lanoxin). You have available 0.125 mg tablets. How many tablets will you give? _____

2. Warfarin (Coumadin) 10 mg is prescribed. You have available 2.5 mg tablets. How many tablets will you give? _____

3. Phenytoin (Dilantin) 300 mg is prescribed. You have available Dilantin suspension 125 mg/5 cc. How many mL will you give? _____

4. Ibuprofen (Motrin) 0.8 g is prescribed. Motrin 400 mg tablets are available. How many tablets will you give? _____

5. Acetaminophen (Tylenol) gr X is prescribed. You have available Tylenol Elixer labeled 160 mg/teaspoon. How many mL will you give? _____

6. Nitroglycerin grains 1/150 is prescribed. Nitroglycerin 0.4 mg tablets are available. How many tablets will you give? _____

7. Glyburide (Diabeta) 5 mg is ordered. You have available 1.25 mg tablets. How many tablets will you give? _____

8. Morphine sulfate 7 mg IV was ordered for pain. Morphine sulfate is available in 10 mg per mL. How many mL would you administer? _____

9. Midazolam (Versed) 3 mg IM was ordered pre-op. You have available Versed 2 mg/mL. How many mL will you administer IM? _____

10. The nurse practitioner ordered 125 mg of methylprednisone (Solu-Medrol) IM for severe inflammation. Powder in a 0.5 gram vial is available. You would reconstitute it according to the vial directions so that each 8 mL will contain 0.5 grams of Solu-Medrol. How many mL will you give in order to give 125 mg? _____

11. The physician prescribed 25 mg of chlondiazepoxide (Librium) IM. You will need to add 2 cc diluent to make it 100 mg/2 mL. How many mL will you give? _____

12. The physician prescribed imipenem and cilastatin sodium (Primaxin IM) Primaxin 600 mg IM every 12 hours. The drug available is 750 mg/mL. How many mL will you give? _____

13. The physician prescribes Rocephin 125 mg I.M. Rocephin is supplied in a 250 mg vial. The label states to reconstitute Rocephin in a 250-mg vial with 2.4 mL of diluent to yield 100 mg/mL. How many mL will you give? _____

SUMMARY

The general rule of thumb is to practice, practice, and practice. When students and nurses stop using these math skills, they begin to lose their confidence, competency skills, and comprehension of the dosage calculation process. Brown (2002) believes that an emphasis on math in real-life situations improves medication administration competency skills. In the nursing clinicals, take every opportunity to practice dosage calculation problems, even when the calculations have already been completed by the pharmacy. Use your time with mentors to discuss your problem areas and do problem solving together. As your understanding of dosage calculations grows, so too will your confidence, competence, and the safety of clients. Always remember, safety first! But remember too that mistakes can and do happen. Everyone is human and can err in this process. Placing blame is easy, but accepting the consequences and responsibility for errors and moving forward to find solutions to prevent them from reoccurring takes accountability and dedication to your clients and to the nursing profession (Swihart, 2004).

BASIC MATHEMATICS PRETEST EVALUATION ANSWER KEY

1. 1517.63
2. 20.74
3. 100.66
4. $323.72
5. 46.11
6. 754.5
7. 16.91
8. 19,494.7
9. $173.04
10. 403.26
11. 36
12. 2500
13. $\frac{2}{3}$
14. 6.25
15. $\frac{4}{5}$
16. 40%
17. 0.4%
18. 0.05
19. 1:3
20. 0.02
21. $1\frac{1}{4}$
22. 6 13/24
23. $1\frac{11}{18}$
24. 3/5
25. $14\frac{7}{8}$

26. $\frac{1}{100}$
27. 0.009
28. 320
29. 3
30. 0.05
31. 4
32. 0.09
33. 0.22
34. 25
35. 4
36. 0.75
37. 3
38. 500
39. 18.24
40. 2.4
41. $\frac{1}{5}$
42. 1:50
43. 5 tablets
44. 2 milligrams
45. 30 kilograms
46. 3.3 pounds
47. $6\frac{2}{3} = 6.67$ centimeters
48. 7.5 centimeters
49. 90%
50. 5:1

PRACTICE WITH FRACTIONS ANSWER KEY

1. Circled are $\dfrac{2}{6} = \dfrac{1}{3}, \dfrac{2}{4} = \dfrac{1}{2}, \dfrac{3}{4} = \dfrac{6}{8}, \dfrac{33}{66} = \dfrac{1}{2}$, and $\dfrac{1}{4} = \dfrac{250}{1000}$

2. $3, 1, 2, 5, 7\dfrac{1}{2}$, and $16\dfrac{2}{3}$

3. $\dfrac{4}{8}, \dfrac{3}{15}$, and $\dfrac{8}{12}$

4. $\dfrac{4}{5}$

5. $\dfrac{9}{10}$

6. Addition column is $\dfrac{5}{6}, \dfrac{17}{35}$, and $\dfrac{5}{6}$; subtraction column is $\dfrac{1}{4}, \dfrac{1}{4}$, and $\dfrac{5}{18}$

7. Multiplication column is $\dfrac{1}{8}, \dfrac{1}{21}$, and 3; division column is $\dfrac{5}{6}, \dfrac{1}{2}$, and $\dfrac{1}{20}$

PRACTICE WITH DECIMALS ANSWER KEY

Fraction row: $\dfrac{95}{100}, \dfrac{33}{100}$, and $\dfrac{125}{100}$

Decimal row: 0.66, 0.1, and 5.33

PRACTICE WITH DOSAGE CALCULATIONS ANSWER KEY

1. 2 tablets
2. 4 tablets
3. 12 mL
4. 2 tablets
5. 18.75 mL
6. 1 tablet
7. 4 tablets
8. 0.7 mL

9. 1.5 mL

10. 2 mL

11. 1.4 mL

12. 0.8 mL

REFERENCES

Brown, D. (2002). Does 1+1 still equal 2? A study of the mathematic competencies of associate degree nursing students. *Nurse Educator, 27*(3), 132–135.

Hughes, R. & Edgerton, E. (2005). First, do no harm. *AJN, 105*(5), 79–84.

Karch, A. (2003). *Lippincott's guide to preventing medication errors.* Philadelphia: Lippincott Williams & Wilkins.

Pickar, G. (2004). *Dosage calculations* (7th ed.). Clifton Park, NY: Thomson Delmar Learning.

Strand, R. D. (2006). *Death by prescription.* Nashville, TN: Thomas Nelson Publishers.

Swihart, D. (2004). First do no harm: Preventing medical errors. *Advance Online.* Retrieved December 21, 2003, from www.advancefornurses.com/common/editorial/editorial

Twiname, B., & Boyd, S. (2002). *Student nurse handbook: Difficult concepts made easy* (2nd ed.). Upper Saddle River, NJ: Prentice Hall.

Woods, A. (2003). Patient safety: Not a question of competencies. *Nursing Management, 34*(9), 6.

SUGGESTED RESOURCES

Curren, A. (2009). Dimensional analysis for meds (4th ed.). Clifton Park, NY: Delmar Cengage Learning.

Curren, A. (2008). Math for meds: Dosages and solutions (10th ed.). Clifton Park, NY: Delmar Cengage Learning.

Drug calculations for health professionals, www.testandcalc.com

Drug calculations quiz club, www.testandcalc.com

Math Magic for Meds, www.edgt.com

Appendix C
American Nurses Association
Code of Ethics

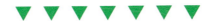

APPROVED AS OF JUNE 30, 2001

The ANA House of Delegates approved these nine provisions of the new *Code of Ethics for Nurses* at its June 30, 2001, meeting in Washington, D.C. In July 2001, the Congress of Nursing Practice and Economics voted to accept the new language of the interpretive statements resulting in a fully approved revised *Code of Ethics for Nurses with Interpretive Statements*.

1. The nurse, in all professional relationships, practices with compassion and respect for the inherent dignity, worth, and uniqueness of every individual, unrestricted by considerations of social or economic status, personal attributes, or the nature of health problems.

2. The nurse's primary commitment is to the patient, whether an individual, family, group, or community.

3. The nurse promotes, advocates for, and strives to protect the health, safety, and rights of the patient.

4. The nurse is responsible and accountable for individual nursing practice and determines the appropriate delegation of tasks consistent with the nurse's obligation to provide optimum patient care.

5. The nurse owes the same duties to self as to others, including the responsibility to preserve integrity and safety, to maintain competence, and to continue personal and professional growth.

6. The nurse participates in establishing, maintaining, and improving health care environments and conditions of employment conducive to the provision of quality health care and consistent with the values of the profession through individual and collective action.

7. The nurse participates in the advancement of the profession through contributions to practice, education, administration, and knowledge development.

8. The nurse collaborates with other health professionals and the public in promoting community, nation, and international efforts to meet health needs.

9. The profession of nursing, as represented by associations and their members, is responsible for articulating nursing values, for maintaining the integrity of the profession and its practice, and for shaping social policy.

Appendix D
The International Council
of Nurses Code of Ethics

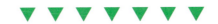

THE ICN CODE OF ETHICS FOR NURSES

An international code of ethics for nurses was first adopted by the International Council of Nurses (ICN) in 1953. It has been revised and reaffirmed at various times since, most recently with this review and revision completed in 2005.

PREAMBLE

Nurses have four fundamental responsibilities: to promote health, to prevent illness, to restore health and to alleviate suffering. The need for nursing is universal.

Inherent in nursing is respect for human rights, including cultural rights, the right to life and choice, to dignity and to be treated with respect. Nursing care is respectful of and unrestricted by considerations of age, colour, creed, culture, disability or illness, gender, sexual orientation, nationality, politics, race or social status.

Nurses render health services to the individual, the family and the community and coordinate their services with those of related groups.

THE ICN CODE

The *ICN Code of Ethics for Nurses* has four principal elements that outline the standards of ethical conduct.

Elements of the Code

1. Nurses and people

The nurse's primary professional responsibility is to people requiring nursing care.

In providing care, the nurse promotes an environment in which the human rights, values, customs and spiritual beliefs of the individual, family and community are respected.

The nurse ensures that the individual receives sufficient information on which to base consent for care and related treatment.

The nurse holds in confidence personal information and uses judgement in sharing this information.

The nurse shares with society the responsibility for initiating and supporting action to meet the health and social needs of the public, in particular those of vulnerable populations.

The nurse also shares responsibility to sustain and protect the natural environment from depletion, pollution, degradation, and destruction.

2. Nurses and Practice

The nurse carries personal responsibility and accountability for nursing practice, and for maintaining competence by continual learning.

The nurse maintains a standard of personal health such that the ability to provide care is not compromised.

The nurse uses judgement regarding individual competence when accepting and delegating responsibility.

The nurse at all times maintains standards of personal conduct which reflect well on the profession and enhance public confidence.

The nurse, in providing care, ensures that use of technology and scientific advances are compatible with the safety, dignity and rights of people.

3. Nurses and the Profession

The nurse assumes the major role in determining and implementing acceptable standards of clinical nursing practice, management, research and education.

The nurse is active in developing a core of research-based professional knowledge.

The nurse, acting through the professional organisation, participates in creating and maintaining safe, equitable social and economic working conditions in nursing.

4. Nurses and Co-workers

The nurse sustains a co-operative relationship with co-workers in nursing and other fields.

The nurse takes appropriate action to safeguard individuals, families and communities when their health is endangered by a co-worker or any other person.

Suggestions for Use of the *ICN Code of Ethics for Nurses*

The *ICN Code of Ethics for Nurses* is a guide for action based on social values and needs. It will have meaning only as a living document if applied to the realities of nursing and health care in a changing society.

To achieve its purpose the *Code* must be understood, internalised and used by nurses in all aspects of their work. It must be available to students and nurses throughout their study and work lives.

Applying the Elements of the *ICN Code of Ethics for Nurses*

The four elements of the *ICN Code of Ethics for Nurses*: nurses and people, nurses and practice, nurses and the profession, and nurses and co-workers, give a framework for the standards of conduct. The following chart will assist nurses to translate the standards into action. Nurses and nursing students can therefore:

- Study the standards under each element of the *Code.*
- Reflect on what each standard means to you. Think about how you can apply ethics in your nursing domain: practice, education, research, or management.
- Discuss the *Code* with co-workers and others.
- Use a specific example from experience to identify ethical dilemmas and standards of conduct as outlined in the *Code*. Identify how you would resolve the dilemmas.
- Work in groups to clarify ethical decision making and reach a consensus on standards of ethical conduct.
- Collaborate with your national nurses' association, co-workers, and others in the continuous application of ethical standards in nursing practice, education, management, and research.

Element of the Code #1: Nurses and People

Practitioners and Managers	Educators and Researchers	National Nurses' Associations
Provide care that respects human rights and is sensitive to the values, customs and beliefs of all people.	In curriculum include references to human rights, equity, justice, solidarity as the basis for access to care.	Develop position statements and guidelines that support human rights and ethical standards.
Provide continuing education in ethical issues.	Provide teaching and learning opportunities for ethical issues and decision making.	Lobby for involvement of nurses in ethics review committees.
Provide sufficient information to permit informed consent and the right to choose or refuse treatment.	Provide teaching/learning opportunities related to informed consent.	Provide guidelines, position statements and continuing education related to informed consent.
Use recording and information management systems that ensure confidentiality.	Introduce into curriculum concepts of privacy and confidentiality.	Incorporate issues of confidentiality and privacy into a national code of ethics for nurses.
Develop and monitor environmental safety in the workplace.	Sensitise students to the importance of social action in current concerns.	Advocate for safe and healthy environment.

Element of the Code #2: Nurses and Practice

Practitioners and Managers	Educators and Researchers	National Nurses' Associations
Establish standards of care and a work setting that promotes safety and quality care.	Provide teaching/learning opportunities that foster life long learning and competence for practice.	Provide access to continuing education, through journals, conferences, distance education, etc.
Establish systems for professional appraisal, continuing education and systematic renewal of licensure to practice.	Conduct and disseminate research that shows links between continual learning and competence to practice.	Lobby to ensure continuing education opportunities and quality care standards.
Monitor and promote the personal health of nursing staff in relation to their competence for practice.	Promote the importance of personal health and illustrate its relation to other values.	Promote healthy lifestyles for nursing professionals. Lobby for healthy work places and services for nurses.

Element of the Code #3: Nurses and the Profession

Practitioners and Managers	Educators and Researchers	National Nurses' Associations
Set standards for nursing practice, research, education and management.	Provide teaching/learning opportunities in setting standards for nursing practice, research, education and management.	Collaborate with others to set standards for nursing education, practice, research and management.
Foster workplace support of the conduct, dissemination and utilisation of research related to nursing and health.	Conduct, disseminate and utilise research to advance the nursing profession.	Develop position statements, guidelines and standards related to nursing research.
Promote participation in national nurses' associations so as to create favourable socio-economic conditions for nurses.	Sensitise learners to the importance of professional nursing associations.	Lobby for fair social and economic working conditions in nursing. Develop position statements and guidelines in workplace issues.

Element of the Code #4: Nurses and Co-workers

Practitioners and Managers	Educators and Researchers	National Nurses' Associations
Create awareness of specific and overlapping functions and the potential for interdisciplinary tensions.	Develop understanding of the roles of other workers.	Stimulate co-operation with other related disciplines.
Develop workplace systems that support common professional ethical values and behaviour.	Communicate nursing ethics to other professions.	Develop awareness of ethical issues of other professions.
Develop mechanisms to safeguard the individual, family or community when their care is endangered by health care personnel.	Instill in learners the need to safeguard the individual, family or community when care is endangered by health care personnel.	Provide guidelines, position statements and discussion fora (forum) related to safeguarding people when their care is endangered by health care personnel.

Dissemination of the *ICN Code of Ethics for nurses*

To be effective the *ICN Code of Ethics for Nurses* must be familiar to nurses. We encourage you to help with its dissemination to schools of nursing, practising nurses, the nursing press and other mass media. The Code should also be disseminated to other health professions, the general public, consumer and policy-making groups, human rights organisations and employers of nurses.

Glossary of Terms Used in the *ICN Code of Ethics for nurses*

Co-worker   Other nurses and other health and non-health related workers and professionals.

Co-operative relationship   A professional relationship based on collegial and reciprocal actions, and behaviour that aim to achieve certain goals.

Family   A social unit composed of members connected through blood, kinship, emotional or legal relationships.

Nurse shares with society   A nurse, as a health professional and a citizen, initiates and supports appropriate action to meet the health and social needs of the public.

Personal health   Mental, physical, social, and spiritual wellbeing of the nurse.

Personal information   Information obtained during professional contact that is private to an individual or family, and which, when disclosed, may violate the right to privacy, cause inconvenience, embarrassment, or harm to the individual or family.

Related groups   Other nurses, health care workers or other professionals providing service to an individual, family or community and working toward desired goals.

Appendix E
National Student Nurses' Association, Inc.
Code of Professional Conduct

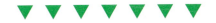

As a member of the National Student Nurses' Association, I pledge myself to:

- Maintain the highest standard of personal and professional conduct.
- Actively promote and encourage the highest level of ethics within nursing education, the profession of nursing, and the student nurses' association.
- Uphold all Bylaws and regulations relating to the student nurses' association at the chapter, state and national levels, reserving the right to criticize rules and laws constructively, but respecting the rules and laws as long as they prevail.
- Strive for excellence in all aspects of decision making and management at all levels of the student nurses' association.
- Use only legal and ethical principles in all association decisions and activities.
- Ensure the proper use of all association funds.
- Serve all members of the student nurses' association impartially, provide no special privilege to any individual member, and accept no personal compensation from another member or non-member.
- Maintain the confidentiality of privileged information entrusted or known to me by virtue of an elected or appointed position in the association.
- Refuse to engage in, or condone, discrimination on the basis of race, gender, age, citizenship, religion, national origin, sexual orientation, or disability.
- Refrain from any form of cheating or dishonesty, and take action to report dishonorable practices to proper authorities using established channels.
- Always communicate internal and external association statements in a truthful and accurate manner by ensuring that there is integrity in the data and information used by the student nurses' association.
- Cooperate in every reasonable and proper way with association volunteers and staff, and work with them in the advocacy of student rights and responsibilities and the advancement of the profession of nursing.

- Use every opportunity to improve faculty understanding of the role of the student nurses association.
- Use every opportunity to raise awareness of the student nurses' association's mission, purpose, and goals at the school chapter level.
- Promote and encourage entering nursing students to join and become active in NSNA.
- Promote and encourage graduating seniors to continue their involvement by joining professional nurses' associations upon licensure as Registered Nurses.

Reprinted with permission, National Student Nurses' Association, Inc. 45 Main St, Suite 606, Brooklyn, NY, 11201, www.nsna.org. Adopted by the 1999 National Student Nurses' Association House of Delegates, Pittsburgh, PA at the 47th Annual NSNA Convention.

REFERENCES

American Society of Association Executives and the National Society for Fund Raising Executives.

Appendix F
National Student Nurses' Association, Inc.
Code of Academic and Clinical Conduct

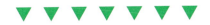

PREAMBLE

Students of nursing have a responsibility to society in learning the academic theory and clinical skills needed to provide nursing care. The clinical setting presents unique challenges and responsibilities while caring for human beings in a variety of health care environments.

The Code of Academic and Clinical Conduct is based on an understanding that to practice nursing as a student is an agreement to uphold the trust with which society has placed in us. The statements of the Code provide guidance for the nursing student in the personal development of an ethical foundation and need not be limited strictly to the academic or clinical environment but can assist in the holistic development of the person.

A CODE FOR NURSING STUDENTS

As students are involved in the clinical and academic environments we believe that ethical principles are a necessary guide to professional development. Therefore within these environments we:

Advocate for the rights of all clients.

Maintain client confidentiality.

Take appropriate action to ensure the safety of clients, self, and others.

Provide care for the client in a timely, compassionate and professional manner.

Communicate client care in a truthful, timely and accurate manner.

Actively promote the highest level of moral and ethical principles and accept responsibility for our actions.

Promote excellence in nursing by encouraging lifelong learning and professional development.

Treat others with respect and promote an environment that respects human rights, values, and choice of cultural and spiritual beliefs.

Collaborate in every reasonable manner with the academic faculty and clinical staff to ensure the highest quality of client care.

Use every opportunity to improve faculty and clinical staff understanding of the learning needs of nursing students.

Encourage faculty, clinical staff, and peers to mentor nursing students.

Refrain from performing any technique or procedure for which the student has not been adequately trained.

Refrain from any deliberate action or omission of care in the academic or clinical setting that creates unnecessary risk of injury to the client, self, or others.

Assist the staff nurse or preceptor in ensuring that there is full disclosure and that proper authorizations are obtained from clients regarding any form of treatment or research.

Abstain from the use of alcoholic beverages or any substances in the academic and clinical setting that impair judgment.

Strive to achieve and maintain an optimal level of personal health.

Support access to treatment and rehabilitation for students who are experiencing impairments related to substance abuse and mental or physical health issues.

Uphold school policies and regulations related to academic and clinical performance, reserving the right to challenge and critique rules and regulations as per school grievance policy.

Reprinted with permission, National Student Nurses' Association, Inc. 45 Main St, Suite 606, Brooklyn, NY, 11201, www.nsna.org. Adopted by the 1999 National Student Nurses' Association House of Delegates, Nashville, TN on April 6, 2001.

Index

▼ ▼ ▼ ▼ ▼ ▼ ▼